Food Allergy

Guest Editor

ANNA NOWAK-WĘGRZYN, MD

IMMUNOLOGY AND ALLERGY CLINICS OF NORTH AMERICA

www.immunology.theclinics.com

Consulting Editor
RAFEUL ALAM, MD, PhD

February 2012 • Volume 32 • Number 1

SAUNDERS an imprint of ELSEVIER, Inc.

W.B. SAUNDERS COMPANY

A Division of Elsevier Inc.

1600 John F. Kennedy Blvd., • Suite 1800 • Philadelphia, PA 19103-2899.

http://www.theclinics.com

IMMUNOLOGY AND ALLERGY CLINICS OF NORTH AMERICA Volume 32, Number 1

February 2012 ISSN 0889–8561, ISBN-13: 978-1-4557-3877-9

Editor: Rachel Glover
Developmental Editor: Teia Stone

Immunology and Allergy Clinics of North America (ISSN 0889–8561) is published quarterly by Elsevier Inc., 360 Park Avenue South, New York, NY 10010-1710. Months of issue are February, May, August, and November. Periodicals postage paid at New York, NY and additional mailing offices. Subscription prices are $294.00 per year for US individuals, $417.00 per year for US institutions, $139.00 per year for US students and residents, $361.00 per year for Canadian individuals, $202.00 per year for Canadian students, $518.00 per year for Canadian institutions, $409.00 per year for international individuals, $518.00 per year for international institutions, $202.00 per year for international students. To receive student/resident rate, orders must be accompanied by name of affiliated institution, date of term, and the *signature* of program/residency coordinator on institution letterhead. Orders will be billed at individual rate until proof of status is received. Foreign air speed delivery is included in all *Clinics* subscription prices. All prices are subject to change without notice. **POSTMASTER:** Send address changes to *Immunology and Allergy Clinics of North America,* Elsevier Health Sciences Division, Subscription Customer Service, 3251 Riverport Lane, Maryland Heights, MO 63043. **Customer Service: 1-800-654-2452 (U.S. and Canada); 314-447-8871 (outside U.S. and Canada). Fax: 314-447-8029. E-mail: journalscustomerservice-usa@elsevier.com (for print support); journalsonlinesupport-usa@elsevier.com (for online support).**

Reprints. For copies of 100 or more, of articles in this publication, please contact the Commercial Reprints Department, Elsevier Inc., 360 Park Avenue South, New York, New York 10010-1710. Tel. (212) 633-3812, Fax: (212) 462-1935, E-mail: reprints@elsevier.com.

Immunology and Allergy Clinics of North America is covered in MEDLINE/PubMed (Index Medicus), Current Contents/Life Sciences, Science Citation Index, ISI/BIOMED, Chemical Abstracts, and EMBASE/Excerpta Medica.

Printed and bound by CPI Group (UK) Ltd, Croydon, CR0 4YY
Transferred to Digital Print 2012

Contributors

ANTONELLA CIANFERONI, MD, PhD
Assistant Professor of Pediatrics, Allergy and Immunology Division, The Children's
Hospital of Philadelphia, University of Pennsylvania, Philadelphia, Pennsylvania

SCOTT COMMINS, MD, PhD
The Asthma and Allergic Diseases Center, University of Virginia Health System,
Charlottesville, Virginia

A.L. COX, MD
Assistant Professor, Division of Pediatric Allergy and Immunology, Mount Sinai Medical
Center, New York, New York

ROSEMARIE H. DEKRUYFF, PhD
Associate Professor, Harvard Medical School; Division of Immunology, Children's
Hospital, Boston, Massachusetts

DAVID M. FLEISCHER, MD
Division of Pediatric Allergy and Immunology, National Jewish Health, Denver, Colorado

SHUBA IYENGAR, MD
Division of Pulmonary Medicine, Massachusetts General Hospital, Boston,
Massachusetts

KIRSI M. JÄRVINEN, MD, PhD
Division of Allergy and Immunology and Center for Immunology and Microbial Diseases,
Albany Medical College, Albany, New York

JENNIFER S. KIM, MD
Division of Allergy and Immunology, Department of Pediatrics, Jaffe Food Allergy
Institute, Mount Sinai School of Medicine, New York, New York

ARUNIMA KOHLI, BS
Division of Immunology and Allergy, Department of Pediatrics, Stanford University,
Stanford, California

GEORGE N. KONSTANTINOU, MD, PhD, MSc
Division of Allergy and Immunology, Department of Pediatrics, Jaffe Food Allergy
Institute, Mount Sinai School of Medicine, New York, New York; Department of
Allergy, 424 General Military Training Hospital, Thessaloniki, Greece

JENNIFER J. KOPLIN, PhD
Murdoch Childrens Research Institute, The Royal Children's Hospital, Melbourne,
Victoria, Australia

XIU-MIN LI, MD, MS
Department of Pediatrics, Jaffe Food Allergy Institute, Mount Sinai Hospital, New York,
New York

JAY A. LIEBERMAN, MD
Fellow, Division of Allergy and Immunology, Department of Pediatrics, Mount Sinai School
of Medicine, New York, New York

MADHAN MASILAMANI, PhD
Division of Allergy and Immunology, Department of Pediatrics, Jaffe Food Allergy
Institute; Immunology Institute, Mount Sinai School of Medicine, New York, New York

C. MULLARKEY, BS
Division of Behavioral and Developmental Health, Department of Pediatrics, Mount Sinai Medical Center, New York, New York

ANTONELLA MURARO, MD, PhD
Chief, Food Allergy Referral Center, Department of Pediatrics, Padua General University Hospital, Padua, Italy

KARI C. NADEAU, MD, PhD
Director, Stanford Food Allergy Program, Division of Immunology and Allergy, Stanford University, Stanford, California

N.L. RAVID, BA
Mount Sinai School of Medicine, New York, New York

HUGH A. SAMPSON, MD
Professor of Pediatrics, Director, Jaffe Food Allergy Institute Division of Allergy and Immunology, Department of Pediatrics, Mount Sinai School of Medicine, New York, New York

E. SHEMESH, MD
Associate Professor, Division of Behavioral and Developmental Health, Department of Pediatrics, Mount Sinai Medical Center, New York, New York

WAYNE SHREFFLER, MD, PhD
Pediatric Allergy and Immunology, Center for Immunology and Inflammatory Disorders, Massachusetts General Hospital, Boston, Massachusetts

S.H. SICHERER, MD
Professor, Division of Pediatric Allergy and Immunology, Mount Sinai Medical Center, New York, New York

DALE T. UMETSU, MD, PhD
The Prince Turki al Saud Professor, Harvard Medical School; Director, Children's Hospital Asthma Center, Division of Immunology, Children's Hospital, Boston, Massachusetts

JULIA ANN WISNIEWSKI, MD
Department of Pediatrics, Division of Allergy and Immunology, University of Virginia, Charlottesville, Virginia

Contents

The default response of the mucosal immune system to antigens derived from food is one of active immune tolerance carried out by regulatory T cells and induced by dendritic cells residing in the intestinal mucosa. This tolerance response must be inhibited or bypassed to generate allergic sensitization in experimental food allergy and this has been achieved by 3 main approaches: genetic modifications, experimental adjuvants, and bypassing oral tolerance by administering the antigen through alternative routes. This article discusses the implications of these approaches for understanding the mechanisms of sensitization to food allergens in human disease.

Food allergy is an emerging epidemic in the United States and the Western world. The determination of factors that make certain foods allergenic is still not clearly understood. Only a tiny fraction of thousands of proteins and other molecules is responsible for inducing food allergy. In this review, the authors present 3 examples of food allergies with disparate clinical presentations: peanut, soy, and mammalian meat. The potential relationships between allergen structure and function, emphasizing the importance of cross-reactive determinants, immunoglobulin E antibodies to the oligosaccharides, and the immune responses induced in humans are discussed.

The rise in food allergy prevalence in developed countries is evident from anecdotal reports but has been difficult to document and until recently good quality prevalence data were lacking. Although most emerging risk factors seem related to the "modern lifestyle" the reasons for the rise in food allergy prevalence remain poorly understood. The incidence of food allergy–related anaphylaxis is rising particularly in children younger than 5 years of age. Emerging studies are better designed to assess the true prevalence of IgE-mediated food allergy using formal population sampling

particularly important because a misdiagnosis could lead to life-threatening reactions or to unnecessary restrictive diets. However, allergy tests currently used in clinical practice have limited accuracy, and an oral food challenge, considered as the gold standard, is often required to confirm or exclude a food allergy. This article reviews several promising novel approaches for the diagnosis of food allergy, such as new molecular diagnostic technologies and functional assays, along with their potential clinical applications.

Food-induced anaphylaxis (FIA) is a serious allergic reaction that may cause death rapidly in otherwise healthy individuals. There is no universal agreement on its definition or criteria for diagnosis. Hospital admissions for FIA have more than doubled in the last decade. Food is one of the most common causes of anaphylaxis, with most surveys indicating that food-induced reactions account for 30% to 50% of cases. The most commonly implicated foods are peanut, tree nuts, milk, eggs, sesame seeds, fish, and shellfish. The only life-saving treatment for anaphylaxis is allergen avoidance, and epinephrine injection if an anaphylactic event occurs.

THE CLINICS ARE NOW AVAILABLE ONLINE!

Access your subscription at:
www.theclinics.com

FORTHCOMING ISSUES

May 2012
Angioedema
Bruce L. Zuraw, MD,
Guest Editor

August 2012
Obesity
Anurag Agrawal, MD,
Guest Editor

RECENT ISSUES

February 2011
Occupational Asthma
David I. Bernstein, MD,
Guest Editor

August 2011
Rhinitis
Michael A. Kaliner, MD,
Guest Editor

May 2011
Immunodeficiencies
Mark Ballow, MD, Guest Editor

Foreword

Is Food Allergy Giving Me a Headache?

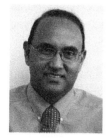

Rafeul Alam, MD, PhD
Consulting Editor

There are some who do not bear cheese well, their constitutions are different, they differ in this respect, that what in their body is incompatible with cheese, is roused and put in commotion by such a thing; and those in whose bodies such a humor happens to prevail in greater quantity and intensity, are likely to suffer the more from it.

—*Hippocrates, ca. 460 BC–ca. 370 BC*

Food is essential for our survival, yet more than 2000 years ago Hippocrates recognized that certain foods can be bad for some of us. One interesting aspect of food allergy is that it is suspected not only in genuine allergic diseases but also in many other health conditions including migraine headache, epilepsy, mania, autism, gout, dyspepsia, irritable bowel syndrome, hypertension, and others. Some of these conclusions were made based on the results from an elimination diet. The problem with this approach is that these elimination diets usually eliminate most of the foods leading to caloric restriction. The latter is known to induce cellular regeneration through deceleration of mTOR function and induction of autophagy.[1,2] As a consequence, caloric restriction extends lifespan in animals.

Immunologically, food represents one of the first foreign antigens for a newborn. Food ingestion triggers a vigorous educational program for the immune system in the gut mucosa. There has been tremendous progress in our understanding of the gut mucosal immunity, and its response to gut microbiome and food. Along with this progress, we observed paradigm-shifting discoveries in food allergy. These discoveries changed our understanding of the development of food allergy and are beginning

Supported by NIH grants R56AI077535, PPG HL 36577, and N01 HHSN272200700048C.

Immunol Allergy Clin N Am 32 (2012) xiii–xiv
doi:10.1016/j.iac.2011.12.002
0889-8561/12/$ – see front matter © 2012 Elsevier Inc. All rights reserved.

to change our management approach. To update us on these exciting discoveries, Dr Anna Nowak-Węgrzyn, a leader in the field, has invited an outstanding group of experts. This is an exciting time for food allergy research.

Rafeul Alam, MD, PhD
Division of Allergy and Immunology
National Jewish Health and
University of Colorado Denver Health Sciences Center
1400 Jackson Street
Denver, CO 80206, USA

E-mail address:
AlamR@NJHealth.org

REFERENCES

1. Madeo F, Tavernarakis N, Kroemer G. Can autophagy promote longevity? Nat Cell Biol 2010;12:842–6.
2. Blagosklonny MV. Calorie restriction: decelerating mTOR-driven aging from cells to organisms (including humans). Cell Cycle 2010;9:683–8.

Preface

Food Allergy Guidelines and Beyond

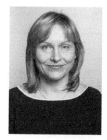

Anna Nowak-Węgrzyn, MD
Guest Editor

Allergic reactions to milk were first described by Hippocrates more than two thousand years ago; however, it is only in the past two decades that food allergy has emerged as an important public health problem affecting people of all ages in societies with a western lifestyle, such as US, Canada, UK, Australia, and Western Europe.[1,2] The overall prevalence of food allergy increased by 18% from 1997 to 2007 in US children. In particular, peanut allergy tripled over the similar period in the US, Canada, UK, and Australia. Eosinophilic esophagitis (EoE) epidemics have been recognized in children and adults in the past decade; diagnosis of food allergy in EoE is especially challenging due to the lack of a noninvasive diagnostic test.[3] Food allergy is the most common cause of the anaphylaxis in the outpatient setting for all ages and may lead to fatalities.[4–6] The diagnosis of food allergy requires labor-intense, medically supervised oral food challenges that carry a risk for anaphylaxis and are not readily available to all patients.[7] Finally, there is no cure for food allergy; management relies on food avoidance and timely treatment of acute reactions. Food avoidance is difficult to adhere to; it affects the quality of life and may result in nutritional deficiencies. The growing recognition of the burden of food allergies and challenges in diagnosis and management are driving multifaceted research approaches. This special issue of the *Immunology and Allergy Clinics of North America* gives an overview of the relevant recent advances in food allergy.

Diagnosis and management of food allergy can vary between clinical practice settings. To promote the best clinical practices, the National Institute of Allergy and Infectious Diseases (NIAID) sponsored clinical guidelines for the diagnosis and management of food allergy in the United States.[8] An expert panel and coordinating committee representing 34 professional organizations, federal agencies, and patient advocacy groups developed the guidelines during a 2-year period. The 43 guidelines were based on an independent literature review and expert clinical opinion. The guidelines provide concise recommendations on how to diagnose and manage food allergy and treat acute food allergy reactions. They also identify gaps in the current scientific knowledge and

Immunol Allergy Clin N Am 32 (2012) xv–xix
doi:10.1016/j.iac.2011.12.001
0889-8561/12/$ – see front matter © 2012 Elsevier Inc. All rights reserved.

immunology.theclinics.com

Table 1
Guidelines for the diagnosis and management of food allergy in the United States: Report of the NIAID-sponsored expert panel[8]: The key points[a]

Definitions	Food allergy (FA) is an adverse health effect arising from a specific immune response. FA results in IgE-mediated, immediate reactions (anaphylaxis) as well as a variety of chronic diseases (eg, eosinophilic esophagitis, food protein-induced enterocolitis syndrome) in which IgE may not play an important role.

Epidemiology and Natural History

Children	FA is more common in children than adults. Among the most common food allergies in children, milk, egg, wheat and soy allergies often resolve in childhood; peanut, tree nut, fish, and shellfish allergies can resolve, but are more likely to persist. Peanut allergy prevalence has increased during recent decades and now affects 1%–2% of young children.
Adults	Adult FA can reflect persistence of childhood allergies or de novo sensitization to food allergens encountered after childhood. FA that starts in adult life tends to persist. In adults, shellfish allergy (2.5%), fish allergy (0.5%), peanut (0.6%), and tree nut (0.5%) allergy are the most common. Adults and some children also experience "cross-reactivity" between certain aeroallergens and certain foods (oral allergy/pollen food allergy syndrome) detailed in the guidelines. Milk, egg, wheat, and soy allergies often resolve in childhood; peanut, tree nut, fish, and shellfish allergies can resolve, but more likely persist.
Comorbidities	FA may coexist with asthma, atopic dermatitis, eosinophilic esophagitis (EoE), and exercise-induced anaphylaxis. FA is associated with severe asthma, increased risk of severe exacerbations, and hospitalization. FA disrupts quality of life. FA is not a common trigger of eczema in adults. EoE is a chronic remitting/relapsing condition that is commonly associated with sensitization to foods. EoE involves localized eosinophilic inflammation of the esophagus. In some patients, avoidance of specific foods will result in normalization of histopathology. In children, EoE presents with feeding disorders, vomiting, reflux symptoms, and abdominal pain. In adolescents and adults, EoE most often presents with dysphagia and esophageal food impactions. One third of patients with *exercise-induced anaphylaxis* report reactions triggered by foods; exercise-induced anaphylaxis has a natural history marked by frequent recurrence of episodes.
Risk Factors for Severe Anaphylaxis	Fatal food allergic reactions are usually caused by *peanut, tree nuts, and seafood*, but have also occurred from milk, egg, seeds, and other foods. Fatalities have been associated with: age (teenagers and young adults), delayed treatment with epinephrine, and comorbid asthma. Severity of future allergic reactions is not accurately predicted by past history. There are no laboratory tests to predict severity of future reactions. Food taken on an empty stomach, exercise, alcohol, NSAIDs, and anti-acid agents may increase severity of an allergic reaction. Therapy with beta-blockers may decrease effectiveness of epinephrine in anaphylaxis.

(continued on next page)

Table 1 *(continued)*	
Diagnosis	FA is suspected when typical symptoms (eg, urticaria, edema, wheezing, mouth itch, cough, nausea/vomiting, anaphylaxis, etc) occur within minutes to hours of food ingestion. A detailed history of the reaction to each incriminated food is essential for proper diagnosis.
	Children less than 5 years old with moderate to severe atopic dermatitis should be considered for FA evaluation for milk, egg, peanut, wheat, and soy, if one or more of the following conditions are present:
	Persistent AD despite optimized management and topical therapy, **or**
	Reliable history of an immediate reaction after ingestion of a specific food.
	A medically supervised food challenge is considered the most specific test for food allergy.
	Tests for food-specific IgE assist in diagnosis, but should not be relied on as a sole means to diagnose food allergy. The medical history and exam are recommended to aid in diagnosis. Limitations of food-specific IgE testing:
	Positive tests are not intrinsically diagnostic and reactions sometimes occur with negative tests.
	Testing "food panels" without considering history is often misleading.
	Several tests *are not recommended*, including food-IgG/IgG₄, total IgE, applied kinesiology, and electrodermal testing.
Prevention	The recommendations follow the 2008 AAP Clinical Report.[10] Breastfeeding is encouraged for all infants; hydrolyzed infant formulas are suggested for infants "at risk,"[b] and complementary foods, including potential allergens, are not restricted after 4–6 months of age (not applicable for infants experiencing allergic reactions). Maternal diet during pregnancy should be healthy and balanced; avoidance of potential food allergens is not recommended.
Management	
Avoidance	Education about food avoidance is critical to prevent reactions.
Immunizations	Patients with egg allergy can be immunized with influenza vaccines containing a low dose of egg protein.
	Yellow fever and rabies vaccines are contraindicated in persons with a history of urticaria, angioedema, asthma, or anaphylaxis to egg proteins. Allergy evaluation and testing can provide insight into the potential for risk to an individual.
Anaphylaxis	Management of anaphylaxis relies on prompt administration of epinephrine, observation for 4–6 hours or longer following treatment, education on avoidance, early recognition, treatment, medical identification jewelry, and follow-up with a primary health care provider and consideration for consultation with an allergist-immunologist.
	Prescription for epinephrine autoinjectors and patient education advice includes having two doses available, switching from 0.15 to 0.3 mg fixed-dose autoinjectors at approximately 25 kg (55 lbs) in context of patient-specific circumstances, having a written emergency plan, and providing supporting educational material.[11,12]

[a] The summary of the Food Allergy Guidelines has been discussed with the members of the Adverse Reactions to Foods Committee, American Academy of Allergy, Asthma & Immunology.
[b] Infants at risk are defined as having one or more immediate family member (parent, sibling) with atopic disorder.

identify and provide guidance on points of current controversy in patient management (**Table 1**). Internationally, the World Allergy Organization (WAO) Special Committee on Food Allergy published WAO Diagnosis and Rationale for Action against Cow's Milk Allergy in 2008.[9] Clinical practice guidelines on food allergy in children and young people were developed by the National Institute for Health and Clinical Excellence.

Table 2	
Web-based resources for medical professionals and patients	
Guidelines	
Guidelines for the diagnosis and management of food allergy in the United States a. Complete report b. Summary c. Summary for the patients, families and caregivers	www.niaid.nih.gov/topics/foodAllergy/
National Institute for Health and Clinical Excellence (NICE), published Feb 2011: Evidence-based clinical guideline on Diagnosis and assessment of food allergy in children and young people in primary care and community settings	http://guidance.nice.org.uk/CG116
World Allergy Organization (WAO): Diagnosis and Rationale for Action against Cow's Milk Allergy (DRACMA), 2008	http://www.worldallergy.org/publications/ WAO_DRACMA_guidelines.pdf
Education Materials	
Food Allergy Education Program on the Consortium for Food Allergy Research (CoFAR) website	https://web.emmes.com/study/cofar/ EducationProgram.htm
Patient Organizations	
Food Allergy and Anaphylaxis Network (FAAN)	http://www.foodallergy.org/
Food Allergy Initiative (FAI)	http://www.faiusa.org/
Kids With Food Allergies (KFA)	www.kidswithfoodallergies.org/

These guidelines are intended for use predominantly in primary care within the National Health Service and community settings in England, Wales, and Northern Ireland. The European Academy of Allergy and Clinical Immunology has created a task force that is currently developing guidelines for the diagnosis and management of food allergy that will be complementary with the NIAID US Food Allergy Guidelines. The NIAID Food Allergy Guidelines are available online (http://www.niaid.nih.gov/topics/foodallergy/) in a full format, as an executive summary, and a lay-language summary for patients, families, and caregivers. Additional web-based resources are listed in **Table 2**.

The articles in this issue of *Clinics* address many important problem areas identified by the Food Allergy Guidelines and show new horizons in food allergy research. Food allergy is a rapidly developing field of allergy and immunology that is approaching a critical mass necessary for the major breakthrough: finding the cure.

Anna Nowak-Węgrzyn, MD
Department of Pediatrics
Division of Allergy and Immunology
Jaffe Food Allergy Institute
Mount Sinai School of Medicine
Box 11988, One Gustave Levy Place
New York, NY 10029, USA

E-mail address:
anna.nowak-wegrzyn@mssm.edu

REFERENCES

1. Sicherer SH, Sampson HA. Food allergy: recent advances in pathophysiology and treatment. Annu Rev Med 2009;60:261–77.
2. Branum AM, Lukacs SL. Food allergy among children in the United States. Pediatrics 2009;124(6):1549–55.
3. Liacouras CA, Furuta GT, Hirano I, et al. Eosinophilic esophagitis: Updated consensus recommendations for children and adults. J Allergy Clin Immunol 2011.
4. Sicherer SH. Epidemiology of food allergy. J Allergy Clin Immunol 2011;127(3): 594–602.
5. Decker WW, Campbell RL, Manivannan V, et al. The etiology and incidence of anaphylaxis in Rochester, Minnesota: a report from the Rochester Epidemiology Project. J Allergy Clin Immunol 2008;122(6):1161–5.
6. Bock SA, Munoz-Furlong A, Sampson HA. Fatalities due to anaphylactic reactions to foods. J Allergy Clin Immunol 2001;107(1):191–3.
7. Nowak-Wegrzyn A, Assa'ad AH, Bahna SL, et al. Work group report: oral food challenge testing. J Allergy Clin Immunol 2009;123(Suppl 6):S365–83.
8. Boyce J, Assa'ad AH, Burks AW, et al. Guidelines for the diagnosis and management of food allergy in the United States: Summary of the NIAID sponsored expert panel report. J Allergy Clin Immunol 2010;126(Suppl 6):S1–58.
9. Fiocchi A, Schunemann HJ, Brozek J, et al. Diagnosis and Rationale for Action Against Cow's Milk Allergy (DRACMA): a summary report. J Allergy Clin Immunol 2010;126(6):1119–28.
10. Greer FR, Sicherer SH, Burks AW. Effects of early nutritional interventions on the development of atopic disease in infants and children: the role of maternal dietary restriction, breastfeeding, timing of introduction of complementary foods, and hydrolyzed formulas. Pediatrics 2008;121(1):183–91.
11. Sampson HA, Munoz-Furlong A, Campbell RL, et al. Second symposium on the definition and management of anaphylaxis: summary report–second National Institute of Allergy and Infectious Disease/Food Allergy and Anaphylaxis Network symposium. Ann Emerg Med 2006;47(4):373–80.
12. Simons FE, Ardusso LR, Bilo MB, et al. World Allergy Organization anaphylaxis guidelines: summary. J Allergy Clin Immunol 2011;127(3):587–93.

Mechanisms of Allergic Sensitization to Foods: Bypassing Immune Tolerance Pathways

M. Cecilia Berin, PhD

KEYWORDS

- Oral tolerance • Dendritic cell • Adjuvant • Epicutaneous
- Innate immunity • iT_{reg}

The mucosal immune system is constantly exposed to antigens derived from food ingestion and the endogenous flora. Although the intestine is densely packed with memory T cells, there is little evidence of T-cell activation in response to dietary antigens or commensal flora. As can be observed after infection with an enteropathogen, the mucosal immune system is capable of mounting a vigorous immune response when appropriate. The homeostatic balance of tolerance and immunity is modulated by many factors in the intestine and when perturbed can result in the breach of tolerance and development of inappropriate allergic sensitization to food proteins. This article outlines factors identified using in vivo experimental approaches that break or bypass immune tolerance and promote the development of food allergy.

ORAL TOLERANCE

The phenomenon of oral tolerance was described by Wells and Osborne in 1911. The investigators showed that guinea pigs could not be made anaphylactic to proteins that were present in the diet.[1,2] Their experiments showed that prior feeding could suppress humoral responses, and subsequent studies by Chase[3] showed that prior feeding could suppress a cell-mediated delayed-type hypersensitivity response. Feeding of antigen was shown to elicit suppressor T cells in the Peyer patches and spleens of mice.[4,5] Transfer of CD4$^+$ or CD8$^+$ T cells could confer tolerance to naive recipients,[6–8] demonstrating that tolerance is an active immunologic process. Mice can be made systemically nonresponsive to antigens after a single high-dose feed of antigen (50–100 mg) or 5 daily feeds of low-dose antigen (0.5–1 mg daily). High

Pediatric Allergy and Immunology, Mount Sinai School of Medicine, Box 1198, One Gustave L. Levy Place, New York, NY 10029, USA
E-mail address: Cecilia.Berin@mssm.edu

Immunol Allergy Clin N Am 32 (2012) 1–10
doi:10.1016/j.iac.2011.10.001
0889-8561/12/$ – see front matter © 2012 Elsevier Inc. All rights reserved.

doses favor deletion of antigen-specific T cells, whereas low doses favor the development of regulatory T (T_{reg}) cells.[9] The phenomenon of oral tolerance has also been demonstrated in humans using neoantigens.[10,11]

Many different phenotypes of T cells have been shown to have regulatory activity using both in vitro and in vivo assays. Adoptive transfer experiments indicate that both CD4+ and CD8+ T cells have the capacity to transfer tolerance to naive mice. Oral feeding of mice or humans induces a CD4+ T-cell subset termed helper T-cell (T_H) subtype 3, characterized by expression of transforming growth factor β (TGF-β), interleukin (IL) 4, and IL-10 and that is regulatory through a TGF-β–dependent mechanism in mice.[7,12] Although thymus-derived natural T_{reg} cells expressing Foxp3 have been shown to be dispensable for tolerance,[13] feeding of antigen can induce antigen-specific CD4+ CD25+ Foxp3+ T cells (induced T_{reg} [iT_{reg}] cells) that mediate suppression through TGF-β.[14] Transfer studies have shown that several subsets are capable of transferring tolerance, but deletion studies have indicated that iT_{reg} cells are critical for oral tolerance. Hadis and colleagues[15] recently demonstrated that ablation of Foxp3+ T cells with diphtheria toxin after antigen feeding (using DEREG mice that express the diphtheria toxin receptor selectively on Foxp3+ cells) resulted in reversal of tolerance.

The induction of regulatory T cells by fed antigen is mediated by intestinal dendritic cells (DCs). Early studies showed that expansion of DCs with Flt3L could decrease the threshold of antigen needed to induce oral tolerance.[16] Under baseline conditions, there are 2 developmentally distinct subsets of DCs in the intestine that can be discriminated based on the expression of CD103 and CX3CR1.[17,18] The latter population extends dendrites across the intestinal epithelium and can directly sample luminal contents.[19] Of these 2 populations, only the CD103+ DCs have been shown to migrate from the lamina propria to the draining lymph node.[17,18] Therefore, only the CD103+ subset has access to naive T cells to initiate an immune response. Worbs and colleagues[20] showed that the CD103+ DC subset initiated oral tolerance in the draining mesenteric lymph node in a CCR7-dependent manner. Although this migrating DC subset was necessary for the induction of tolerance, CX3CR1+ resident DCs also have a role in tolerance induction, presumably by expanding the Foxp3+ T_{reg} cells in the lamina propria that are initially induced in the mesenteric lymph node.[15]

Oral administration of antigens is particularly effective for the induction of immunologic tolerance. This finding prompted the question of what was unique about the phenotype of gastrointestinal DCs that could promote the development of T_{reg} cells from naive T cells. Mesenteric lymph node DCs expressing CD103 promote the development of Foxp3+ CD4+ T cells with gut-homing potential, and this is mediated through TGF-β and retinoic acid.[21,22] CD103+ DCs in the draining mesenteric lymph node also express the enzyme indolamine 2,3-dioxygenase. Inhibition of this enzyme inhibits the development of iT_{reg} cells in vitro, and suppression of the enzyme in vivo prevents the development of oral tolerance.[23]

The data summarized above demonstrate that tolerance is an active immunologic antigen-specific process that is initiated in response to antigens delivered by the oral route. It is thought that food allergy results from a failure of tolerance. Sensitization is also an active immunologic process, and it has not been definitively determined if food allergy is the result of defective tolerance pathways or overactive mechanisms promoting sensitization. For example, blockade of the regulatory costimulatory molecule cytotoxic T-lymphocyte antigen 4 (CTLA-4) in mice does not convert tolerance to sensitization when antigen is provided without an adjuvant but does enhance sensitization when antigen is given in the context of an adjuvant.[24] The balance of these 2 distinct pathways is likely to be important. Food allergy has been described in a subset of patients with IPEX (immune dysregulation, polyendocrinopathy, enteropathy, X-linked) syndrome lacking Foxp3$^+$ T$_{reg}$ cells,[25] although clinical manifestations include severe enteropathy that is distinct from IgE-mediated food allergy in otherwise immunologically competent individuals.

ANIMAL MODELS OF FOOD ALLERGY

Advances in food allergy research have been hampered by limitations of available experimental models. Injection of food antigens into mice or rats has been useful to assess the relative allergenicity of the antigens but does not provide insight into the mechanism by which oral ingestion of a food protein can induce allergic sensitization rather than tolerance.[26] An ideal model has been proposed to be one in which oral exposure in the absence of an adjuvant leads to the generation of allergen-specific IgE and oral reexposure leads to symptoms of systemic anaphylaxis. This has not yet been described in mice. Spontaneous food allergy has been shown to occur in dogs, but the symptoms are primarily cutaneous.[27,28] The lack of ability to orally sensitize mice in the absence of an adjuvant might suggest that environmental factors that function as adjuvants must be present for sensitization to occur. Alternatively, sensitization may occur via nonoral routes. A third explanation is that genetic predisposition is present in human subjects with food allergy but not in laboratory mice. Two models of transgenic mice have been found to develop sensitization to oral antigens in the absence of an adjuvant. IL-9-transgenic mice that have an intestinal mastocytosis develop sensitization to ovalbumin given orally in the absence of systemic priming or adjuvant.[29] Mice expressing a modified IL-4 receptor (lacking a functional inhibitory immunoreceptor tyrosine-based motif [ITIM]) also develop sensitization to ovalbumin given orally without adjuvant.[30] Genetic studies of human subjects with food allergies are needed to identify potential susceptibility loci.

MECHANISM OF ACTION OF ADJUVANTS

Feeding mice clinically relevant food allergens such as peanut, milk, or egg proteins in the absence of an adjuvant does not generally result in allergic sensitization or clinical reactivity to the food; however, sensitization in response to a single high-dose feed of peanut has been reported.[31] IgE production is a side effect of the mucosal adjuvant cholera toxin (CT), and Snider and colleagues[32] first demonstrated that mice fed with antigen plus CT developed antigen-specific IgE antibodies and underwent systemic anaphylaxis when rechallenged with the antigen in vivo. CT has subsequently been used to sensitize mice to several foods, including peanut, milk, egg, lupin, and shrimp to name a few.[33–37]

CT is an effective mucosal adjuvant that induces protective immune responses such as IgG antibodies and cytotoxic T-cell responses as well as allergic sensitization, but it is also a useful tool for examining immune mechanisms of sensitization versus tolerance. Feeding of CT leads to a significant upregulation of IL-1β and IL-6 locally within the intestine, and administration of IL-1β at the same time as antigen administration abrogated oral tolerance.[38] The role that IL-1β and IL-6 may play in the sensitization response to CT has not been established, nor is the source of these proinflammatory cytokines known. Feeding of CT alters the migration of DCs from the lamina propria to the mesenteric lymph node and enhances the maturation of the migrating DCs,[39] resulting in enhanced T-cell priming. The CD103$^+$ DC subset that is normally tolerogenic was shown to be the main target of CT in vivo.[40] Upregulation of OX40L on this DC subset was responsible for the enhanced production of IL-4 and IL-13, but not interferon-γ or IL-17, from responder T cells. Therefore, OX40L on this DC subset seemed to be selectively responsible for the allergic sensitization component of the adjuvant activity of CT.[40] Within the lamina propria it has been found that allergic sensitization is associated with an expansion of CD11b[+] DCs and a relative reduction of CD103[+] DCs.[41] These data indicate that the phenotype of the gastrointestinal DC determines the outcome of sensitization versus tolerance to foods.

The mucosal adjuvant CT is an experimental tool that is highly effective at sensitizing mice to food antigens, but it is unlikely to play a role in human food allergic disease. Staphylococcal enterotoxin B (SEB) is a toxin produced by some strains of *Staphylococcus aureus*. SEB can be found as a contaminant in the food supply and is frequently found to be produced by *S aureus* strains colonizing the lesional skin of patients with atopic dermatitis.[42] Ganeshan and colleagues[43] described the use of oral SEB as an adjuvant promoting allergic sensitization to ovalbumin and peanut in mice. This finding was associated with an increase in T_H2 cytokine expression and a decrease in TGF-β and Foxp3 expression in splenocytes restimulated in vitro with antigen. Yang and colleagues[44] have shown that SEB acts directly on DCs, upregulates TIM-4 expression, and thereby drives T_H2 cytokine expression in responder T cells.

Studies using experimental adjuvants illuminate mucosal immune pathways that when modulated can shift the immune response from tolerance to allergic sensitization. This is illustrated in **Fig. 1**. The contribution of the mucosal immune pathways to human disease remain to be confirmed, but screening environmental factors for their ability to modulate molecules such as OX40L or TIM-4 on gastrointestinal DCs may identify factors potentially responsible for the steep increase in the incidence of food allergy in recent years.

SENSITIZATION THROUGH NONORAL ROUTES

The incidence of peanut allergy has increased sharply at the same time as infant feeding guidelines were implemented to suggest delaying introduction of peanut

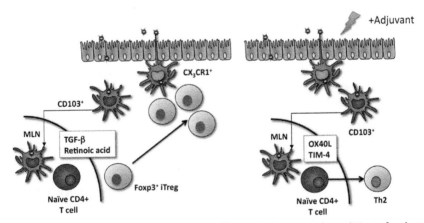

Fig. 1. Role of mucosal DCs in tolerance and allergy. Under normal conditions, food antigens are acquired by CD103[+] DCs that migrate to the draining mesenteric lymph node (MLN) and present antigens to naive T cells. The induction of Foxp3[+] iT$_{reg}$ cells is promoted by retinoic acid and TGF-β from the CD103[+] DCs. These T$_{reg}$ cells home to the lamina propria, where they are expanded by resident CX3CR1 DC/macrophages. In the presence of an adjuvant, CD103[+] DCs change their phenotype and upregulate markers including OX40L that promote the induction of T_H2-skewed CD4[+] T cells. TIM-4 has also been shown to be upregulated on DCs after adjuvant exposure and promotes T_H2 skewing.

into the diet. Although this may be coincidental, it has also been noted that sensitization rates to peanut are substantially different in 2 genetically similar populations that differ in the time of introduction of peanut in the diet, with early introduction being associated with lower rates of sensitization to peanut.[45] Household peanut exposure has been shown to be a risk factor for peanut sensitization in children, independent of maternal peanut consumption.[46] This finding has led to the hypothesis that oral exposure is tolerance generating by default, but exposure via other routes may be preferentially sensitizing. One such route of interest has been the skin, in part because of the interesting finding that children with a positive peanut challenge test result were significantly more likely to have used creams containing peanut oil than atopic or normal controls.[47]

There are conflicting data from mouse models about whether the skin is an inherently proallergenic tissue. Supporting the idea that the skin is inherently proallergenic are findings of adjuvant-independent sensitization to clinically relevant food allergens including hazelnut, cashew nut, and milk whey proteins.[48–50] Other investigators have reported that effective sensitization through the skin is dependent on tape stripping of the skin, which leads to upregulation of cytokines, including IL-21 and TSLP.[51,52] The latter data suggest that the skin is not inherently sensitizing but show that other physiologic processes such as mechanical injury and inflammation can take the place of adjuvants. Furthermore, desensitization has been demonstrated in response to antigens delivered through the skin of sensitized mice.[53]

In experiments using the milk allergen α-lactalbumin, it has been observed that an adjuvant is necessary to induce sensitization in the absence of mechanical injury.[54] An adjuvant is necessary to drive antigen-bearing dermal DCs to the draining lymph node. It is speculated that several physiologic factors may take the place of an adjuvant in human disease, including mechanical injury such as that induced by scratching of the skin or by intrinsic adjuvant activity of strong allergens such as peanuts or tree nuts as described in the next section.

DIRECT EFFECTS OF FOOD ALLERGENS ON THE INNATE IMMUNE SYSTEM

In addition to identifying factors that increase susceptibility to allergic sensitization, there is a great deal of interest in determining what makes certain foods such potent allergens. Shreffler and colleagues[55] found that peanut extract could lead to activation of human DCs and enhance the T_H2 skewing potential of the DCs. The investigators identified glycan structures on Ara h 1 as critical for this function, and the receptor on the DC was found to be DC-SIGN. A similar ability to induce T_H2 skewing through modulation of the DC phenotype was shown for Ber e 1 (from Brazil nut) using mouse DCs and T cells.[56] Binding of allergens to DC-SIGN on human DCs was found to be common to glycan structures of several relevant allergens, and the interaction between allergen and DC-SIGN resulted in activation of signaling pathways in the DC.[57] Thus, common allergens may have self-adjuvant activity by binding to pattern recognition receptors on antigen-presenting cells. Food processing can also enhance the innate activity of food allergens. Extensive heating results in the formation of advanced glycation end products through the Maillard reaction. Processing of the model allergen ovalbumin in this manner results in enhanced uptake and presentation by DCs that is mediated through macrophage scavenger receptors I and II.[58,59] Peanut and other nut extracts have been found to have anaphylactoid effects in mice through complement-mediated activation of macrophages.[60] This was speculated to have the effect of amplifying IgE-triggered reactions, but this innate activity may also contribute to sensitization. Complement has been shown to enhance the

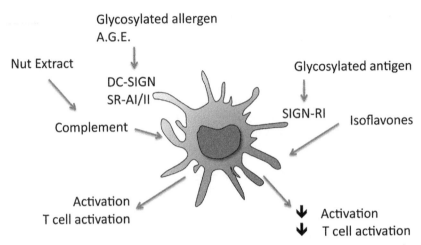

Fig. 2. Innate activity of food allergens. Food allergens may alter their own presentation by altering the phenotype of antigen-presenting cells including DCs and macrophages. Binding of glycosylated allergens or those bearing advanced glycation end products (A.G.E.) to DC-SIGN or scavenger receptor I or II (SR-AI/II) results in activation of DCs and enhanced activation of effector T cells. Nut extracts induce complement that activates macrophages, which may enhance effector T-cell activation. Binding of glycosylated antigens to SIGN-R1 facilitates tolerance, whereas isoflavones found in soy directly inhibit DC presentation to and activation of T cells.

activation of effector $CD4^+$ T cells.[61] Antigen-presenting cells are not the only targets of food allergens. Milk sphingolipids were recently found to activate invariant natural killer T cells and induce the release of IL-4 and IL-13.[62] This innate source of T_H2 cytokines could facilitate the development of an antigen-specific T_H2-skewed $CD4^+$ T-cell response that would promote class switching of antigen-specific B cells to IgE production.

In addition to having innate effects that promote sensitization, some foods have been found to have immunomodulatory effects that suppress sensitization. Isoflavones present in soy have been shown to suppress allergic sensitization by inhibiting the activation of mouse and human DCs.[63] Zhou and colleagues[64] demonstrated that a heavily glycosylated modified antigen that bound to the innate receptor SIGN-R1 could promote tolerance through selective presentation by regulatory DCs in the intestinal lamina propria. These modulatory effects of food antigens on cells of the innate immune system may contribute to their relative potency as food allergens (**Fig. 2**).

SUMMARY

The default response of the mucosal immune system to food antigens is one of tolerance. This tolerance can be broken by experimental adjuvants such as SEB and CT, and finding physiologic triggers that can modulate the same immune pathways may provide insight into environmental factors that promote allergic sensitization. There is currently controversy over whether exposure through routes such as the skin would promote sensitization over tolerance. The immune outcome of exposure through the skin or other routes may be dependent on the innate immune modulatory activity of food allergens.

REFERENCES

1. Wells HG, Osborne TB. The biological reactions of the vegetable proteins. I. Anaphylaxis. J Infect Dis 1911;8:66–124.
2. Wells HG. Studies on the chemistry of anaphylaxis (III). Experiments with isolated proteins, especially those of the hen's egg. J Infect Dis 1911;9(2):147–71.
3. Chase MW. Inhibition of experimental drug allergy by prior feeding of the sensitizing agent. Proc Soc Exp Biol Med 1946;61:257–9.
4. Ngan J, Kind LS. Suppressor T cells for IgE and IgG in Peyer's patches of mice made tolerant by the oral administration of ovalbumin. J Immunol 1978;120(3):861–5.
5. Mattingly JA, Kaplan JM, Janeway CA Jr. Two distinct antigen-specific suppressor factors induced by the oral administration of antigen. J Exp Med 1980;152(3):545–54.
6. Chen Y, Inobe J, Weiner HL. Induction of oral tolerance to myelin basic protein in CD8–depleted mice: both CD4+ and CD8+ cells mediate active suppression. J Immunol 1995;155(2):910–6.
7. Chen Y, Kuchroo VK, Inobe J, et al. Regulatory T cell clones induced by oral tolerance: suppression of autoimmune encephalomyelitis. Science 1994;265(5176):1237–40.
8. Miller A, Lider O, Roberts AB, et al. Suppressor T cells generated by oral tolerization to myelin basic protein suppress both in vitro and in vivo immune responses by the release of transforming growth factor beta after antigen-specific triggering. Proc Natl Acad Sci U S A 1992;89(1):421–5.
9. Chen Y, Inobe J, Marks R, et al. Peripheral deletion of antigen-reactive T cells in oral tolerance. Nature 1995;376(6536):177–80.
10. Husby S, Mestecky J, Moldoveanu Z, et al. Oral tolerance in humans. T cell but not B cell tolerance after antigen feeding. J Immunol 1994;152(9):4663–70.
11. Kraus TA, Toy L, Chan L, et al. Failure to induce oral tolerance to a soluble protein in patients with inflammatory bowel disease. Gastroenterology 2004;126(7):1771–8.
12. Fukaura H, Kent SC, Pietrusewicz MJ, et al. Induction of circulating myelin basic protein and proteolipid protein-specific transforming growth factor-beta1-secreting Th3 T cells by oral administration of myelin in multiple sclerosis patients. J Clin Invest 1996;98(1):70–7.
13. Mucida D, Kutchukhidze N, Erazo A, et al. Oral tolerance in the absence of naturally occurring Tregs. J Clin Invest 2005;115(7):1923–33.
14. Curotto de Lafaille MA, Kutchukhidze N, Shen S, et al. Adaptive Foxp3+ regulatory T cell-dependent and -independent control of allergic inflammation. Immunity 2008;29(1):114–26.
15. Hadis U, Wahl B, Schulz O, et al. Intestinal tolerance requires gut homing and expansion of FoxP3+ regulatory T cells in the lamina propria. Immunity 2011;34(2):237–46.
16. Viney JL, Mowat AM, O'Malley JM, et al. Expanding dendritic cells in vivo enhances the induction of oral tolerance. J Immunol 1998;160(12):5815–25.
17. Bogunovic M, Ginhoux F, Helft J, et al. Origin of the lamina propria dendritic cell network. Immunity 2009;31(3):513–25.
18. Schulz O, Jaensson E, Persson EK, et al. Intestinal CD103+, but not CX3CR1+, antigen sampling cells migrate in lymph and serve classical dendritic cell functions. J Exp Med 2009;206(13):3101–14.
19. Niess JH, Brand S, Gu X, et al. CX3CR1-mediated dendritic cell access to the intestinal lumen and bacterial clearance. Science 2005;307(5707):254–8.

20. Worbs T, Bode U, Yan S, et al. Oral tolerance originates in the intestinal immune system and relies on antigen carriage by dendritic cells. J Exp Med 2006;203(3): 519–27.
21. Coombes JL, Siddiqui KR, Arancibia-Carcamo CV, et al. A functionally specialized population of mucosal CD103+ DCs induces Foxp3+ regulatory T cells via a TGF-beta and retinoic acid-dependent mechanism. J Exp Med 2007; 204(8):1757–64.
22. Jaensson E, Uronen-Hansson H, Pabst O, et al. Small intestinal CD103+ dendritic cells display unique functional properties that are conserved between mice and humans. J Exp Med 2008;205(9):2139–49.
23. Matteoli G, Mazzini E, Iliev ID, et al. Gut CD103+ dendritic cells express indoleamine 2,3-dioxygenase which influences T regulatory/T effector cell balance and oral tolerance induction. Gut 2010;59(5):595–604.
24. van Wijk F, Hoeks S, Nierkens S, et al. CTLA-4 signaling regulates the intensity of hypersensitivity responses to food antigens, but is not decisive in the induction of sensitization. J Immunol 2005;174(1):174–9.
25. Torgerson TR, Linane A, Moes N, et al. Severe food allergy as a variant of IPEX syndrome caused by a deletion in a noncoding region of the FOXP3 gene. Gastroenterology 2007;132(5):1705–17.
26. Ladics GS, Knippels LM, Penninks AH, et al. Review of animal models designed to predict the potential allergenicity of novel proteins in genetically modified crops. Regul Toxicol Pharmacol 2010;56(2):212–24.
27. Jackson HA, Jackson MW, Coblentz L, et al. Evaluation of the clinical and allergen specific serum immunoglobulin E responses to oral challenge with cornstarch, corn, soy and a soy hydrolysate diet in dogs with spontaneous food allergy. Vet Dermatol 2003;14(4):181–7.
28. Jackson HA, Hammerberg B. Evaluation of a spontaneous canine model of immunoglobulin E-mediated food hypersensitivity: dynamic changes in serum and fecal allergen-specific immunoglobulin E values relative to dietary change. Comp Med 2002;52(4):316–21.
29. Forbes EE, Groschwitz K, Abonia JP, et al. IL-9- and mast cell-mediated intestinal permeability predisposes to oral antigen hypersensitivity. J Exp Med 2008; 205(4):897–913.
30. Mathias CB, Hobson SA, Garcia-Lloret M, et al. IgE-mediated systemic anaphylaxis and impaired tolerance to food antigens in mice with enhanced IL-4 receptor signaling. J Allergy Clin Immunol 2011;127(3):795–805.e1–6.
31. Proust B, Astier C, Jacquenet S, et al. A single oral sensitization to peanut without adjuvant leads to anaphylaxis in mice. Int Arch Allergy Immunol 2008;146(3): 212–8.
32. Snider DP, Marshall JS, Perdue MH, et al. Production of IgE antibody and allergic sensitization of intestinal and peripheral tissues after oral immunization with protein Ag and cholera toxin. J Immunol 1994;153(2):647–57.
33. Li XM, Serebrisky D, Lee SY, et al. A murine model of peanut anaphylaxis: T- and B-cell responses to a major peanut allergen mimic human responses. J Allergy Clin Immunol 2000;106(1 Pt 1):150–8.
34. Roth-Walter F, Berin MC, Arnaboldi P, et al. Pasteurization of milk proteins promotes allergic sensitization by enhancing uptake through Peyer's patches. Allergy 2008;63(7):882–90.
35. Martos G, Lopez-Exposito I, Bencharitiwong R, et al. Mechanisms underlying differential food allergy response to heated egg. J Allergy Clin Immunol 2011; 127(4):990–7.e1–2.

36. Foss N, Duranti M, Magni C, et al. Assessment of lupin allergenicity in the cholera toxin model: induction of IgE response depends on the intrinsic properties of the conglutins and matrix effects. Int Arch Allergy Immunol 2006;141(2):141–50.

37. Capobianco F, Butteroni C, Barletta B, et al. Oral sensitization with shrimp tropomyosin induces in mice allergen-specific IgE, T cell response and systemic anaphylactic reactions. Int Immunol 2008;20(8):1077–86.

38. Williamson E, Westrich GM, Viney JL. Modulating dendritic cells to optimize mucosal immunization protocols. J Immunol 1999;163(7):3668–75.

39. Anjuere F, Luci C, Lebens M, et al. In vivo adjuvant-induced mobilization and maturation of gut dendritic cells after oral administration of cholera toxin. J Immunol 2004;173(8):5103–11.

40. Blazquez AB, Berin MC. Gastrointestinal dendritic cells promote Th2 skewing via OX40L. J Immunol 2008;180(7):4441–50.

41. Smit JJ, Bol-Schoenmakers M, Hassing I, et al. The role of intestinal dendritic cells subsets in the establishment of food allergy. Clin Exp Allergy 2011;41(6):890–8.

42. Cardona ID, Cho SH, Leung DY. Role of bacterial superantigens in atopic dermatitis: implications for future therapeutic strategies. Am J Clin Dermatol 2006;7(5): 273–9.

43. Ganeshan K, Neilsen CV, Hadsaitong A, et al. Impairing oral tolerance promotes allergy and anaphylaxis: a new murine food allergy model. J Allergy Clin Immunol 2009;123(1):231–8.e4.

44. Yang PC, Xing Z, Berin CM, et al. TIM-4 expressed by mucosal dendritic cells plays a critical role in food antigen-specific Th2 differentiation and intestinal allergy. Gastroenterology 2007;133(5):1522–33.

45. Du Toit G, Katz Y, Sasieni P, et al. Early consumption of peanuts in infancy is associated with a low prevalence of peanut allergy. J Allergy Clin Immunol 2008; 122(5):984–91.

46. Fox AT, Sasieni P, du Toit G, et al. Household peanut consumption as a risk factor for the development of peanut allergy. J Allergy Clin Immunol 2009;123(2): 417–23.

47. Lack G, Fox D, Northstone K, et al. Factors associated with the development of peanut allergy in childhood. N Engl J Med 2003;348(11):977–85.

48. Birmingham NP, Parvataneni S, Hassan HM, et al. An adjuvant-free mouse model of tree nut allergy using hazelnut as a model tree nut. Int Arch Allergy Immunol 2007;144(3):203–10.

49. Gonipeta B, Parvataneni S, Tempelman RJ, et al. An adjuvant-free mouse model to evaluate the allergenicity of milk whey protein. J Dairy Sci 2009;92(10): 4738–44.

50. Parvataneni S, Gonipeta B, Tempelman RJ, et al. Development of an adjuvant-free cashew nut allergy mouse model. Int Arch Allergy Immunol 2009;149(4): 299–304.

51. Jin H, Oyoshi MK, Le Y, et al. IL-21R is essential for epicutaneous sensitization and allergic skin inflammation in humans and mice. J Clin Invest 2009;119(1): 47–60.

52. Oyoshi MK, Larson RP, Ziegler SF, et al. Mechanical injury polarizes skin dendritic cells to elicit a T(H)2 response by inducing cutaneous thymic stromal lymphopoietin expression. J Allergy Clin Immunol 2010;126(5):976–84, 984.e1–5.

53. Dioszeghy V, Mondoulet L, Dhelft V, et al. Epicutaneous immunotherapy results in rapid allergen uptake by dendritic cells through intact skin and downregulates the allergen-specific response in sensitized mice. J Immunol 2011;186(10): 5629–37.

54. Dunkin D, Berin MC, Mayer L. Allergic sensitization can be induced via multiple physiologic routes in an adjuvant-dependent manner. J Allergy Clin Immunol 2011. [Epub ahead of print].

55. Shreffler WG, Castro RR, Kucuk ZY, et al. The major glycoprotein allergen from Arachis hypogaea, Ara h 1, is a ligand of dendritic cell-specific ICAM-grabbing nonintegrin and acts as a Th2 adjuvant in vitro. J Immunol 2006;177(6):3677–85.

56. Kean DE, Goodridge HS, McGuinness S, et al. Differential polarization of immune responses by plant 2S seed albumins, Ber e 1, and SFA8. J Immunol 2006; 177(3):1561–6.

57. Hsu SC, Chen CH, Tsai SH, et al. Functional interaction of common allergens and a C-type lectin receptor, dendritic cell-specific ICAM3-grabbing non-integrin (DC-SIGN), on human dendritic cells. J Biol Chem 2010;285(11):7903–10.

58. Hilmenyuk T, Bellinghausen I, Heydenreich B, et al. Effects of glycation of the model food allergen ovalbumin on antigen uptake and presentation by human dendritic cells. Immunology 2010;129(3):437–45.

59. Ilchmann A, Burgdorf S, Scheurer S, et al. Glycation of a food allergen by the Maillard reaction enhances its T-cell immunogenicity: role of macrophage scavenger receptor class A type I and II. J Allergy Clin Immunol 2010;125(1): 175–83.e1–11.

60. Khodoun M, Strait R, Orekov T, et al. Peanuts can contribute to anaphylactic shock by activating complement. J Allergy Clin Immunol 2009;123(2):342–51.

61. Strainic MG, Liu J, Huang D, et al. Locally produced complement fragments C5a and C3a provide both costimulatory and survival signals to naive CD4+ T cells. Immunity 2008;28(3):425–35.

62. Jyonouchi S, Abraham V, Orange JS, et al. Invariant natural killer T cells from children with versus without food allergy exhibit differential responsiveness to milk-derived sphingomyelin. J Allergy Clin Immunol 2011;128(1):102–9.e13.

63. Masilamani M, Wei J, Bhatt S, et al. Soybean isoflavones regulate dendritic cell function and suppress allergic sensitization to peanut. J Allergy Clin Immunol 2011. [Epub ahead of print].

64. Zhou Y, Kawasaki H, Hsu SC, et al. Oral tolerance to food-induced systemic anaphylaxis mediated by the C-type lectin SIGNR1. Nat Med 2010;16(10): 1128–33.

Determinants of Food Allergy

Madhan Masilamani, PhD[a,b], Scott Commins, MD, PhD[c],
Wayne Shreffler, MD, PhD[d],*

KEYWORDS

- Food allergy • Allergen • Plant food allergens
- Animal food allergens • Peanut • Soy
- Cross-reactive carbohydrate determinants • Alpha-gal

As of September 2011, there were 12,273 recognized protein families in the Pfam database, yet only 255 (2.1%) of those families are represented among allergens. Among food allergens, only 71 (0.6%) families are represented (from ~400 described allergens); and among the top 20 families, a mere 0.16% of protein families, account for 80% of all described food allergens (**Table 1**).[1] At the same time, it is not the case that simple elements (ie, primary or secondary structure) are constrained among allergens. For instance, examples of all common polypeptide folds are found without apparent strong overrepresentation of some.[2,3] These observations suggest that there are determinants of food allergy, that is, structural or functional properties of certain proteins that play a significant role in determining what makes them allergens. In this review, the authors briefly review the categorization of food allergens and then draw on 3 examples of food allergies with disparate clinical presentations to discuss the potential relationships between allergen structure and function and the immune responses induced in humans.

WHAT IS A FOOD ALLERGEN?

The simplest definition of an allergen is a substance that causes an allergic reaction, broadly speaking, a hypersensitivity immune response, but usually refers to a type I– or

Funding sources: The Jaffe Food Allergy Institute (M.M.), NIH (S.C., W.S.).
Conflict of interest: The authors have no conflict of interest.
[a] Division of Allergy and Immunology, Department of Pediatrics, The Jaffe Food Allergy Institute, Mount Sinai School of Medicine, Anbg 17-40, One Gustave L Levy Place, New York, NY 10029, USA
[b] Immunology Institute, Mount Sinai School of Medicine, One Gustave L Levy Place, New York, NY 10029, USA
[c] The Asthma and Allergic Diseases Center, University of Virginia Health System, PO Box 801355, Charlottesville, VA 22908, USA
[d] Pediatric Allergy and Immunology, Center for Immunology and Inflammatory Disorders, Massachusetts General Hospital, 55 Fruit Street, CPZS 557, Boston, MA 02114, USA
* Corresponding author.
E-mail address: wshreffler@partners.org

Immunol Allergy Clin N Am 32 (2012) 11–33
doi:10.1016/j.iac.2011.12.003
0889-8561/12/$ – see front matter © 2012 Elsevier Inc. All rights reserved.

Table 1
Common food allergy protein families ranked by number of identified allergens in each family

Family	Source	Rank by Number of Identified Family Members Associated with Food Allergy	Rank by Number of Identified Family Members Associated with Aero/Contact Allergy	Additional Notes
Prolamin superfamily	Plant	1	4	Includes cereal storage (gliadins), 2S albumin (eg, Ara h 2/6), LTPs
Tropomyosin	Animal	2	5	Dominant crustacean allergen
Cupin superfamily	Plant	3	Rare; 1 described inhalant, 1 described contact	Dominant family of legume and nut allergens
Profilin	Plant	4	1	Highly cross-reactive
EF-hand domain	Plant, animal	5	2	For ingestion, exclusively associated with fish, shellfish
PR-10	Plant	6	18	Bet v 1 related
Alpha/beta-caseins	Animal, mammal	7	Not described	Milk allergens
Heveinlike domain	Plant	8	Latex allergy only	Includes some chitinases; latex, banana, avocado
Class I chitinases	Plant	9	Latex allergy only	Latex, banana, avocado (also chestnut, grape, corn)

Oleosins	Plant	10	Not described	?Major sesame, minor peanut, hazelnut allergens
Lipocalin	Animal: arthropod and mammalian	11	6	Beta-lactoglobulin from milk in this family
Beta-1,3-glucanase	Plant	12	Latex (Hev b 2) olive tree pollen	Described in tomato, potato, banana, bell pepper
Papainlike cysteine protease	Plant	13	Der p 1, Der f 1	Kiwi, pineapple, papaya (fairly rare)
Thaumatinlike protein	Plant	14	Cedar/cypress pollen	Apple, cherry, grape, kiwi, pepper
Expansin, C-term	Plant: all grasses	Not described	3	Major allergens of grass pollen
Trypsinlike serine proteases	Animal: arthropod and mammalian	Not described	9	Bee and bumblebee sting, mite and roach inhalant
Enolase	Fungi and plants	Not described	10	—
Expansin, N-term	Plant: all grasses except 1	Very low; 1 food allergen described from kiwi	8	—
Subtillsinlike serine protease	Fungi (1 identified from bacteria)	Very low; 1 food allergen described from musk melon	7	—

Data from Radauer C, Bublin M, Wagner S, et al. Allergens are distributed into few protein families and possess a restricted number of biochemical functions. J Allergy Clin Immunol 2008;121(4):847–52.

immunoglobulin E (IgE)–mediated hypersensitivity response. This definition is vague, allowing for both principal and proximate causes. In practical terms, allergens are defined by being recognized by IgE from patients. Some allergens included by this definition are not very potent inducers of primary allergic immune responses, in other words, they are weak allergenic immunogens; but if IgE capable of binding them is present (perhaps because of cross-reactivity with a strong immunogen), they can trigger effector responses. Other structures (eg, some glycans discussed later) are inducers of IgE and are recognized by IgE in binding assays but may be impotent triggers of allergic responses. A molecule with the capacity to induce sensitization and trigger reactions has been termed a *complete allergen*[3]; Ara h 2 from peanut seems to meet this definition. Mal d 1, by contrast, is an incomplete allergen because it can trigger reactions by being cross-reactive with the dominant aeroallergen from birch pollen, Bet v 1, but is not an important immunogen. It is important to recognize that defining allergens purely by the IgE response may overlook the importance of molecules that predominantly stimulate T cells or other immune cells and the potential importance of that for the pathogenesis of both IgE- and perhaps non–IgE-mediated food allergy.

Food allergens, for this review, include molecules, mostly proteins, that are recognized by IgE and found in the diet, whether or not they are complete allergens. We recognize that defining what is a food allergen is greatly influenced by culture and circumstance. Many proteins that may not be important at all as food allergens in a particular culture may be significant in another population, and proteins that are rarely or never described as food allergens in patients may be capable of being an allergen under contrived conditions or experimental models, particularly when combined with strong T helper (Th)-2 adjuvants. That said, by recognizing that there is significant homology across many plant and animal taxa that are sources of food, one can be impressed by the observation that some protein families are significantly overrepresented (eg, prolamins) and that some species of plant or animal are also overrepresented as strongly polarizing allergen sources in many cultures (eg, crustaceans, peanut).

STRUCTURAL FEATURES

It seems intuitive that structural features, including stability during food processing and digestion, are important factors in determining allergenic potency of ingested molecules. The food-pollen syndromes, best represented by PR-10 sensitization, exemplify this concept as the structural instability of those proteins correlates with the observation that cooking destroys allergenicity and that ingestion of any form is rarely if ever associated with systemic reactions. Digestibility, on the other hand, as a predictor of food allergenicity has been tested empirically with mixed results.[4–7] There are multiple potential explanations for the weak correlation between digestibility and food allergenicity, including limitations of in vitro systems used to mimic digestion, food matrix effects that are lost when assessing purified proteins, alteration of protein structure during protein preparation, relative abundance of proteins in whole food, and others. However, whatever the explanation, we know that IgE-mediated activation of effector cells requires cross-linking and, therefore, interaction with multivalent ligands that must, therefore, possess a complex structure. Food allergens, thus, must either survive or bypass digestion in sufficient amounts to provoke immune responses.

Protein glycosylation has been shown to contribute to protein stability,[8,9] although it is also likely to enhance immunogenicity in other ways. That glycosylation can enhance the allergic immunogenicity of proteins has been demonstrated by creating neoconjugates of specific glycans to non-glycosylated carrier proteins.[10] The immunogenicity of nonmammalian glycans had already been suggested by the demonstration of ubiquitous glycan-specific antibodies in humans from a variety of clinical contexts as well as in murine models.[11,12] These structures are antigenic structures that are distinct from endogenous glycans. Much like the glycans that underlie ABO blood group incompatibility, responses to them are simply not edited out during immune development and can therefore induce immune responses. Some glycans are recognized by specific innate immune pattern receptors within the C-type lectin receptor (CLR) family, and this seems to enhance or modulate their immunogenicity, as discussed later.

Lipid binding is a common feature of both food and respiratory allergens.[13] Many prolamins (the largest food allergen group, including nonspecific lipid transfer proteins, 2S albumins, prolamin storage proteins, and α-amylase/trypsin inhibitors), lipocalins, and some cupins interact with lipids; and this may protect them from degradation and enhance their absorption from the gastrointestinal (GI) tract.[14] The lipocalin milk allergen, β-lactoglobulin, for example, is more stable when lipid bound.[15]

Macromolecular aspects of protein structure are also known to be relevant in the context of food allergen immune responses and mucosal immunity more broadly. Particulate antigens are predominantly processed and presented in Peyer patches via specialized microfold cell uptake, and this can be a route of strong humoral immune induction. In contrast, soluble antigens can be efficiently absorbed across the intestinal epithelium and tend to be less immunogenic. Mammalian milk is a complex colloidal fluid in which caseins (α, β, κ) are largely contained in large micelles that are in suspension and are predominantly presented to the immune system via Peyer patches, whereas whey proteins (eg, β-lactoglobulin and α-lactalbumin) are highly soluble and rapidly transported across the intestinal epithelium. One functional consequence of this in an animal model of milk allergy is that caseins are more potent inducers of antibodies, including IgE; but for animals sensitized to both casein and whey proteins, it is the whey proteins that induce stronger systemic allergic reactions on exposure, possibly because they are so rapidly absorbed.[16] Many food allergens have a tendency to aggregate because of the presence of repetitive sequences, rheomorphic structures, or the ability to oligomerize.[17] This tendency may favor their capacity to induce sensitization in the gut by being preferentially presented in Peyer patches.

FUNCTIONAL FEATURES

In addition to passive aspects of structure, part of what may make an allergen potent may be what immunostimulatory capacity it has intrinsically or by intimate association with other molecules. Some of the same features that enhance immunogenicity by increasing stability or aggregation (eg, glycosylation, lipid binding) might also stimulate innate immune responses.

Examples of pathways that are directly stimulated by allergens are growing in literature. For example, glycans in house dust mite extract induce Th2 differentiation via binding to the C-type lectin Dectin-2 on dendritic cells (DC) and the subsequent production of cysteinyl leukotrienes.[18] The mannose receptor (MR), another CLR, binds to and mediates the internalization of a variety of allergens, such as Der p1 and p2 (house dust mite) and Ara h1 (peanut). MR also mediated Der p1–induced Th2 skewing by human monocyte derived DCs (MoDC) through the upregulation of indoleamine 2,3-dioxygenase (IDO) activity.[19]

IDO has also been associated with immune tolerance, particularly, although not exclusively, in models of Th1 inflammation. In fact, many pathways or mediators (eg, CLRs, thymic stromal lymphopoietin (TSLP), OX40 ligand (OX40L), retinoic acid) that under some conditions have been associated with Th2 induction have also been implicated in tolerance. In both the induction of Treg and Th2, the suppression of interleukin (IL)-12 and other features of alternative DC activation may be shared. As an example, the activation of the CLR SIGNR1 (the murine paralogue of DC-SIGN) on lamina propria DC (LPDC) had a tolerogenic rather than a Th2-skewing effect: bovine serum albumin (BSA) coupled with mannoside (Man-BSA) selectively targeted SIGNR1-expressing LPDC and induced the production of IL-10, which promoted the generation of CD4+ type 1 regulatory T cells. In mice sensitized with BSA, treatment with Man-BSA substantially reduced the BSA-induced anaphylactic response.[20]

Additional examples of functional allergen properties include the cystein protease allergens, including both respiratory and food allergens from plants (see below), signaling via protease activated receptors (PARs),[21] and the functional mimicry of MD-2 by the dust mite allergen, Der p 2, possibly modulating TLR4 sensitivity to natural ligands.[22]

PLANT FOOD ALLERGENS

About 65% of the plant food allergens belongs to one of the following classes of structurally related protein superfamilies: (1) the prolamin superfamily; (2) the cupin superfamily; and (3) the pathogenesis-related proteins (PR-10) family, of which Bet v 1 is the best known.[23,24]

The prolamin superfamily includes seed storage proteins of cereals, lipid transfer proteins (LTPs), alpha-amylase/protein inhibitors and 2S albumins. Their 3-dimensional (3D) structure consists of a compact tertiary structure with 4 alpha-helices stabilized by disulfide bridges and a central cavity for lipid binding. There are 8 conserved cysteine residues with cys-cys and cys-X-cys motifs. Despite their homologous structures, the sequence similarity is low between members of the prolamin superfamily. The seed storage proteins/prolamins of wheat are known to cause baker's asthma and celiac diseases. The alpha-amylase/trypsin inhibitors from several cereals, such as wheat, barley, and rice, are shown to be involved in allergy. Some of the clinically relevant allergenic proteins that belong to this protein superfamily are the following: Ara h 2, Ara h 6, Sin a 1, Ber e 1, Ses i 2, Jug v 1, and so forth. The nonspecific LTPs are known to be major food allergens in fruits from the Rosacea family. The presence of specific IgE to LTP is considered to be a significant risk factor for allergy and may even serve as a diagnostic marker.[25]

The prominent allergens of the cupin superfamily of proteins are the 7S (vicilins) and 11S globulins. The 7S globulins include Ara h 1, Jug r 2, and Ses i 3. Some examples of 11S globulins are Ara h 3, soybean glycinins, Ber e 2, Cor a 9, and Fag e 1.[14] The 3D structure of proteins that belong to the cupin family consists of a series of antiparallel β-sheets associated with α-helix and forms a cavity (cuplike structure, hence the name cupin; *cupa* in Latin means "barrel").[26] This structure is also found in several proteins of the lipocalin family involved in the transport of hydrophobic ligands, including β-lactoglobulin of milk. Profilins are highly conserved, small, actin-binding proteins that are ubiquitously expressed in all eukaryotic cells.[27]

Plant profilins share about 70% of the amino acid sequence homology among themselves. Profilins consist of a compact globular structure with central 7 stranded antiparallel beta sheets enclosed by alpha helices.[28] Because of its conserved amino acid sequences, about 20% to 30% of all patients with tree pollen allergies react to profilin.[29,30] Moreover, sensitization to profilin is considered a risk factor for developing multiple pollen-associated food allergies.[25]

Bet v 1–related proteins are ubiquitously distributed and comprised of 8 superfamilies that include PR-10, major latex proteins, and proteins involved in alkaloid biosynthesis. The 3D conformation of the Bet v 1–related proteins provides a large, Y-shaped hydrophobic pocket that binds to plant steroids.[31]

ANIMAL FOOD ALLERGENS

Although in theory all proteins have the potential to become allergens, this is not usually the case. In fact, before an epitope can result in an allergenic response, it requires that the human immune system has first discriminated self from nonself. This requirement is likely to be particularly true when related to animal food allergens. For instance, any antibody response in humans to vertebrate tropomyosins might be expected to cause autoimmune disease.[24] Others have alluded to the notion that allergy to mammalian proteins likely approaches the limit of the human immune system to discriminate self from foreign antigens.[32] Thus, unlike most plant allergens, almost all the animal food allergen families have an equivalent or counterpart in the human protein repertoire that may influence the human immune system response. Recent work has classified animal food allergens into 3 main families: tropomyosins, EF-hand proteins, and caseins.[24] In each of these 3 main animal food allergen families, the ability to act as an allergen seems to be related to the relative identity to human homologs such that proteins closely related to human homologs are significantly less likely to be allergenic. In the 3 families of allergens analyzed, proteins with a sequence identity of roughly 54% to human homologs were all allergenic, whereas those with a sequence identity greater than 63% to human homologs were rarely allergenic.[24] In keeping with this finding, others have suggested that a low degree of similarity to a host's proteome is required for immunogenicity.[33]

Of the tropomyosin family, the animal food allergenic varieties are reportedly confined to invertebrate groups, namely mollusks and arthropods.[24] Although there are 4 types of mammalian muscle tropomyosins, none of these have been reported to be sources of an IgE response in humans.[34] Likewise, no human IgE response has been identified to tropomyosins from birds or fish. The absence of such a response might be expected because these sequences are greater than or equal to 90% identical to at least 1 human tropomyosin.[24]

EF-hand proteins compose the second largest animal food allergen family, and this is largely made up of parvalbumins.[24] Parvalbumins themselves are divided into α- and β-parvalbumins. The α-parvalbumins, generally considered to be nonallergenic, are found primarily in the muscle of fish and amphibians.[24] On the contrary, β-parvalbumins are found in a variety of fish species; retain allergenic potential; and, interestingly, are absent from human muscle.[35]

Of the caseins that have been shown to elicit an IgE response in humans, the general principle is that, again, the closer the sequence in homology to the human equivalent the less likely an IgE response will occur. One exception worth mentioning in the setting of animal food allergy is that of BSA. Sensitization to BSA is the main predictive marker of the cross-reactivity to cow's milk that is present in 73% to 93% of patients with beef allergies, despite the fact that BSA shares 76% identity to its human homolog.[24,36] Cross-reactivity to BSA is frequently outgrown in children, and this may be caused by the high homology to human serum albumin, whereby BSA may elicit a less-effective immune response than other cow's milk proteins (ie, caseins).[37,38]

In sum, it may be that both the source of the food allergen and the route of sensitization are important in determining which protein families predominate, with different families represented in plant versus animal food allergen families.

WHAT CAN WE LEARN FROM 3 DISPARATE EXAMPLES OF FOOD ALLERGY?
Peanut Allergy

In the United States, approximately 1% of the population is peanut allergic, and this prevalence seems to have risen.[39] In several studies, peanut allergen is also disproportionately implicated as a trigger of severe reactions among those who are affected. The humoral immune response to peanut allergens in susceptible individuals is more strongly IgE biased, in comparison, for example, with the immune response to milk allergens, against which atopic individuals tend to make both IgE and IgG. Although atopy is clearly a risk factor for peanut allergy, isolated peanut allergy is common[40] in part because peanut allergy is more persistent than other common food allergies. Contrast that with soy allergy, discussed later, which is rarely an isolated allergy.

There are 12 peanut allergens recognized in Allergome, although several of these include isomers and some distinctly named proteins (eg, Ara h 2 and Ara h 6), are paralogs related as tandem gene duplicates. The major plant allergen families are all represented. For example, Ara h 1, 2, and 6 are prolamins, whereas Ara h 3 is a cupin, Ara h 8 is a PR-10 protein, and Ara h 9 is a profilin. Additional identified allergens include the lectin, peanut agglutinin, and an 18kD oleosin. The most immunodominant allergens, at least in populations with primary peanut allergy, are Ara h 2, Ara h 6 and Ara h 1. Geographic variation in sensitization to specific peanut allergens has been recognized, but it is reactivity to Ara h 2 and Ara h 6 that has increasingly emerged as the major risk factor for significant clinical reactivity.[41]

The major peanut allergen and glycoprotein Ara h 1 induces activation of human DC and enhances the induction of Th2 differentiation by these DC in naïve T cells. Ara h 1 was further shown to bind to the CLR, DC-SIGN. De-glycosylated Ara h 1 lacked this Th2-skewing effect, indicating that allergen-bound carbohydrate structures may act as a Th2-skewing adjuvant.[42] Correspondingly, other studies have reported that glycation of proteins enhances their uptake by DC and their T-cell immunogenicity,[43] as well as their ability to induce Th2 differentiation.[44,45] Incubation of DC with Lewis-x trisaccharides suppressed the production of IL-12,[45] which suggests one mechanism for the enhanced Th2 skewing induced by these glycans.

Peanut extract has also been shown to activate complement in murine and human serum, resulting in the formation of C3a. In susceptible mice, peanut extract induced anaphylactic shock, which was dependent on C3a as well as on platelet-activating factor and histamine. No involvement of DC was shown in this response[46]; however, complement split products can activate DC and regulate adaptive immunity.[47,48]Both C3- and C3a-deficient mice are resistant to asthma in an Aspergillus-induced model.[49]

Soy Allergy

Soy allergy usually manifests in childhood. The prevalence of soy allergy in adults is still poorly described[40] but estimated to be around 0.3% to 0.4%.[50,51] Soy allergy is spontaneously resolved in about 50% of children with soy allergies by 7 years of age.[52] Allergic symptoms to soy may include atopic dermatitis, enterocolitis, and other IgE-mediated multisystem reactions.[53,54] Even though soy is recognized as one of the big 8 food allergens, it is rather uncommon to see allergic reactions exclusive to soy.[55] Soy allergy is often present in individuals who are allergic to multiple foods and birch pollen.[56] About 6% of atopic children[57] and 10% to 14% of infants with a cow milk allergy also suffer from concomitant soy allergy.[58–60] Moreover, anaphylaxis caused by soy is very rare.[57,61] Isolated soy allergy seems to be rare; for example, 88% of children with soy allergies also have peanut allergies.[52]

Soybean Allergens and Their Cross-Reactivity with Other Allergenic Proteins

Soybeans contain allergens that belong to all the categories of the protein superfamilies previously discussed. So far, about 28 potential allergens have been identified based on IgE binding from patients with a soy allergy.[62,63] Among them, 16 proteins are characterized as allergens by the Allergome database. However, the reactivity of these allergens is highly variable among individual patients with no correlation with severity of symptoms. Only a few of them are recognized as major allergens by the International Union of Immunologic Societies of Allergen Nomenclature Subcommittee: Gly m 1, Gly m 2, Gly m 3, and Gly m 4. Other dominant allergens in soy are the soybean Kunitz trypsin inhibitor, the thiol-protease Gly m Bd 30k, the alpha subunit of β-conglycinin (BC, Gly m 5), the acidic chain of the major storage protein glycinin (G, Gly m 6) G1 subunit, the basic chain of the G2 subunit,[64] and 2S albumin. For a full list of allergenic proteins in soy, refer to article by L'Hocine and colleagues.[65]

Gly m1 and Gly m2 are soybean hull proteins and have been shown to be aeroallergens. These proteins, in addition to the Kunitz trypsin inhibitor, have been implicated in the development of allergic asthma.[66] Gly m 1 (also known as Gly m Bd30K/P34 or P34) is a soybean vacuolar protein.[67,68] Gly m Bd30K shares a high sequence similarity to thiol proteinases of the papain family. Another notable member of this group is Der p 1, which is the major allergen in the dust mite. Birch pollen–related allergens, Gly m 3 and Gly m 4, belong to the profilin family of proteins. Gly m 3 is highly homologous with Bet v 2, with an amino acid sequence identity of 73%. The IgE-binding epitopes of Gly m 3 are highly conformational because fragments of Gly m 3 fail to bind IgE.[69] Gly m 4, also called as PR-10 protein, and starvation-associated message 22, is a stress-related protein with a 50% homology with Bet v 1. Gly m 4 is a major cross-reactive allergen in patients with a birch pollen allergy.[70] Serum IgE from 85% of patients with birch pollen allergies reacts to Gly m 4.[71] About 10% of Central European patients sensitized to birch pollen are reported to have concomitant soy allergy, mainly caused by cross-reactivity to Gly m 4.[56]

Major seed storage proteins Gly m 5 (β-conglycinin, 7 S) and Gly m 6 (glycinin, 11 S) were found to be major allergens in a cohort of 30 patients with Double-blind, placebo-controlled food challenge (DBPCFC)-confirmed soy allergy, which suggests that these molecules are good diagnostic markers of component-resolved in vitro testing.[64] However, another study by Vissers[72] found high IgE binding to Gly m 4 but not Gly m 5 and Gly m 6. Patients who are allergic to peanuts but clinically non–soy allergic tested positive for Gly m 5 and 6.

Glycinin (11S) and β-conglycinin (7S) belong to storage proteins that belong to the cupin family.[73] Burks and colleagues,[74,75] Ogawa and colleagues,[76] and Beardslee and colleagues[77] all have identified IgE binding to different subunits of β-conglycinin. Changes in the ionic strength and pH alter the conformation structure of glycinin and have significant effect on the immunogenicity in terms of IgG1 binding.[78]

Because soy proteins are considered to be less immunogenic than cow milk protein,[79] soy-based formula is usually used as an alternative in infants with a cow milk allergy. However, it is common to see coexisting soy allergy in patients with a cow milk allergy. Osterballe and colleagues[80] have shown that about 17% of patients with a cow milk allergy are also sensitized to soy. In a study with 10 patients with a cow milk allergy but never exposed to soy, their serum reacted to components in soy extract by competitive inhibition enzyme-linked immunosorbent assay. The authors have identified the cross-reactive protein to be a 30 KD fraction of 11S globulin in soy.[81]

Similarity of Soybean and Peanut Allergens: Why Soy is Less Allergenic than Peanut

Several soy allergens share high sequence homology to their counterparts in peanut (**Table 2**). Soybean β-conglycinin Gly m 5 is the closest homolog of Ara h 1, with 51% amino acid sequence identity and a similar 3D structure. In addition, Ara h 3 and soybean glycinin Gly m 6 share similar 3D structure to that of Ara h 1 despite less sequence homology.[82] However, the incidence of soy allergy is much less than that of peanut.[83] Although fatal events after consumption of soy have been

Table 2
Amino acid homology between peanut and soy allergens

		Soy				
% Similarity *% Identity*		Gly m Conglycinin 7S Globulin	Gly m Glycinin G1 11S Globulin	Gly m Glycinin G2 11S Globulin	2S Albumin 1	2S Albumin 3
Peanut						
Ara h 1	7S globulin	**52.2** *40.0*	23.0 *14.2*	24.0 *13.9*	7.1 *3.8*	6.4 *3.0*
Ara h 2	2S albumin	6.6 *3.4*	7.1 *5.1*	7.4 *4.7*	**44.2** *35.6*	**41.5** *34.8*
Ara h 3	11S globulin	24.9 *15.5*	**65.3** *57.3*	**65.6** *57.2*	7.4 *4.3*	6.7 *4.1*

Homology between peanut and soy allergens as determined by Vector-NTI software.
Numbers in bold represent comparisons of proteins that fall in similar categories.
The percentage of amino acids that are similar or identical are shown as straight and italicized text, respectively.

reported,[84,85] those patients also had severe peanut allergies. In a double-blind, placebo-controlled food challenge study in 30 European patients, 67% of patients with a soy allergy reported concomitant peanut allergy.[86] Because of the high amino acid homology between peanut and soy, soy protein has been tried as an immunotherapeutic agent for peanut allergy in mouse models.[87] In this study, peanut-allergic mice were able to get desensitized with crude soy extract. Intraperitoneal injection of peanut-sensitized mice with soy extract resulted in suppressed immune response to peanut and markedly reduced clinical symptoms on peanut challenge.[87]

Soy protein is potentially allergenic. However, the reaction threshold (ie, safe for 90% of allergic patients) to soy is as high as 400 mg compared with 0.1 mg for peanut.[88,89] In a retrospective study of DBPCFC, Sicherer and colleagues[90] reported that about 28% of children with a soy allergy reacted to an initial dose of 500 mg of soy (200 mg soy protein). Ballmer-Weber and colleagues[86] reported a range of 454 mg to 50 g of soy required to achieve objective allergic symptoms, is at least one order of magnitude higher than observed in peanut allergy. It is not clear why soy protein showed a low reaction threshold and diminished immunoreactivity.

Soy has been a part of staple food in Asia for centuries. Anecdotal evidences suggest that high consumption of traditional soy food, particularly fermented soy food in Far Eastern countries, could account for the lower incidence of several chronic health conditions. Comparatively, much of the soy-food in the Western world is in the form of processed protein isolates and subtle food additives. Investigation of why the incidence and severity of soy allergy is low compared with peanut and other foods would be informative in designing a therapy for other food allergies. It is possible that the intrinsic allergenicity of soy could be different in terms of glycosylation[91,92] and IgE binding.[93] Kroghsbo and colleagues[93] have compared immune response with 7S globulins of peanut, hazelnut, soy, and pea in Brown Norway rats. Peanut 7S globulins induced IgE of higher avidity than other related proteins. Soy induced IgE of least avidity. Susceptibility to heat[74,94] and hydrolysis[95,96] have been shown to result in the reduced allergenicity of soy.

Emerging evidence suggests that the presence of anti-inflammatory phytochemicals in soy could be one of the reasons for their reduced allergenicity. Several phytochemicals are present in soybean: isoflavones, saponins, phytates, sterols, lignans, and so forth. Most of them present as glycosides in soybean. The microbiota in the gut converts glycosides to active aglycones, which have antiinflammatory and immunomodulatory properties. The levels of bioactive phytochemicals are increased in fermented soy food as a result of the hydrolysis of isoflavone glycosides. These immunomodulatory phytochemicals are well known to have beneficial properties in various disorders, including food allergy.[97-99]

MAMMALIAN MEAT ALLERGY
Carbohydrates Induce and Bind IgE

Although the most frequent allergens involved in anaphylactic reactions are proteins found in peanuts, tree nuts, fish, shellfish, bee and wasp venoms, and haptens in drugs and latex,[100-103] carbohydrate moieties are also present in many foods and can induce antiglycan IgE responses.[11] Because carbohydrate moieties can share significant structural homologies beyond that of proteins, they are prone to extensive cross-reactivity. These cross-reactive epitopes are called cross-reactive carbohydrate determinants (CCDs); however, the clinical significance of IgE antibodies directed against them is unclear.[104-106]

The study of carbohydrates as food antigens began in the 1970s when a Japanese group reported the structure of a protease from pineapple stems.[107] It was subsequently shown that this protease, bromelain, contained an oligosaccharide with 2 structural features that had not been found in mammalian glycoproteins: core α1,3-fucose and xylose (**Fig. 1**).[108] In fact, xylose and core-3-linked fucose may be the most common carbohydrate epitopes recognized by human IgE antibodies.[109]

CCDs in Allergy: A Review of the Controversy

The link between plant-based glycans and allergy was made by Aalberse and colleagues[104] in 1981. They showed that IgE from patients' sera cross-reacted with extracts from several foods and insect venoms. This work laid the foundation for later studies, which indicated that asparagine-linked (N-glycans) were involved in IgE binding to honeybee venom phospholipase A$_2$ (PLA$_2$; Api m 1).[110] Ultimately, the structural basis for the cross-reactivity of IgE with insect and plant glycoproteins was shown to be core α1,3-fucose.[111] The binding to Api m 1 from sera of patients with a bee allergy was inhibited by glycopeptides from pineapple stem bromelain.[111]

Current estimates are that 15% to 30% of allergic patients generate specific antigly-can IgE.[105,106,112,113] This frequent occurrence of sensitization to CCDs contrasts with their apparent inability to produce clinical symptoms. Evidence against a significant clinical impact of carbohydrate-directed IgE comes from several aforementioned studies and was recently reviewed.[106,113,114] A clinically benign role for CCDs is now being questioned because several studies have shown the ability of anti-CCD IgE to trigger mediator release from basophils.[115–118] Although preliminary studies in the authors' laboratory using basophils isolated from patients with IgE to alpha-gal showed evidence of activation in response to a carbohydrate antigen, the ability of this IgE antibody to trigger a mediator release in vivo remains an area of active investigation. In the aforementioned study by Mari[113] that examined bromelain sensitization, skin testing to bromelain revealed few positives. This finding may be expected, though, given that degranulation requires cross-linking on the surface of the mast cell and that bromelain contains only one oligosaccharide chain.[119] It has also been suggested that antibodies to uncharged carbohydrate epitopes would have low affinity,[120] rendering skin testing less reliable. However, the evidence that IgE antibodies to CCDs are of low affinity is poor, and recent work has indicated that these antibodies have affinities comparable with IgG antibodies.[121]

Adding to this growing literature, recent work from the authors' group has shown that IgE antibodies specific for the carbohydrate alpha-gal are capable of eliciting serious, even fatal, reactions.[122] The authors subsequently extended that observation by confirming that IgE antibodies to alpha-gal are associated with an unusual form of delayed anaphylaxis, which follows 3 to 6 hours after eating meat that carries

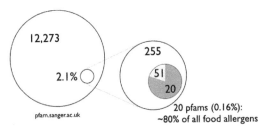

Fig. 1. Protein families present among allergens (255) and food allergens (71) relative to the total number of described family members in the Pfam database. (*Data from* Radauer C, Bublin M, Wagner S, et al. Allergens are distributed into few protein families and possess a restricted number of biochemical functions. J Allergy Clin Immunol 2008;121(4):847–52.)

alpha-gal (eg, beef, pork, or lamb).[123] In contrast to previously described CCD motifs of xylose and core-3-linked fucose, which populate plants and insects, the alpha-gal epitope is abundantly expressed on cells and tissues of nonprimate mammals.[124,125] This expression pattern makes alpha-gal potentially clinically relevant either as a food allergen (eg, beef, pork, lamb) or as an inhaled allergen (eg, cat, dog).[123,126]

Galactose-α-1,3-Galactose (Alpha-Gal): Epitope Characteristics and Clinical Relevance

Although alpha-gal has not had a long history within the allergy literature, the alpha-gal epitope and its naturally occurring IgG antibody have been the subject of much important and thoughtful work from other scientific perspectives. Karl Landsteiner speculated about the existence of a blood-group-B–like substance on mammalian cells in the 1930s, and this was likely to be alpha-gal. One can reason this because blood group B antigen and the alpha-gal epitope differ only in that blood group B antigen has a fucose-linked α-1,2 to the penultimate galactose (**Fig. 2**). Likewise, medical and surgical transplant communities are familiar with alpha-gal: the naturally occurring antibody to alpha-gal in humans, apes, and Old World monkeys is responsible for the hyperacute rejection of pig xenografts by binding alpha-gal epitopes on the porcine cells.

Bromelain

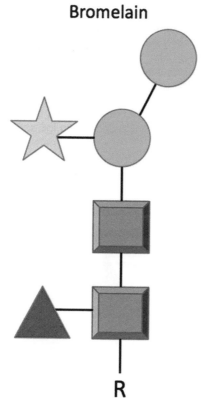

R

Fig. 2. Bromelain showing the core α1,3-fucose (*red triangle*) and xylose (*orange star*) as referenced in the text. NB The oligosaccharide structures are shown in the symbols suggested by the Consortium of Functional Glycomics, such that the blue squares represent N-acetylglucosamine, green circles represent mannose, yellow symbolizes galactose, whereas orange star and red triangle are xylose and fucose, respectively. R, an organic molecule.

The alpha-gal epitope induces the production of a highly specific antigal IgG antibody through continuous antigenic stimulation by carbohydrate antigens on GI bacteria of the normal flora,[127] much akin to the production of antibodies to blood group A or B antigens (**Fig. 3**).[128] Inactivation of the α1,3GT gene is thought to have occurred roughly 28 million years ago,[129] such that humans, apes, and Old World monkeys possess a pseudogene found on chromosome 9. The exon that codes for the main catalytic domain contains 2 point mutations (deletions) that produce a frameshift and a premature stop codon.[130] The result is that although all lower mammals make alpha-gal as a glycosylation product, humans do not and instead produce antigal antibodies.

Recently Identified IgE to Alpha-Gal

While investigating IgE antibodies in the serum of patients who experienced a hypersensitivity reaction to the chimeric monoclonal antibody cetuximab, Chung and colleagues[122] identified control patients without cancer who also had serum IgE antibodies that bound to cetuximab. These IgE antibodies were shown to be specific for an alpha-gal moiety found on the asparagine at position 88 in the murine heavy chain portion of cetuximab. The authors have recently broadened this work and described a cohort of patients with IgE antibodies to alpha-gal who experience delayed symptoms of anaphylaxis, angioedema, or urticaria after eating mammalian meat.[123] This report was the first to identify food allergy related to IgE antibodies to the alpha-gal carbohydrate epitope. Whether IgE to alpha-gal is specific for this moiety only or, as with CCDs, has the ability to bind other epitopes is currently unknown (ie, whether this is actually IgE directed against alpha-gal or IgE that binds alpha-gal and other closely related epitopes). The authors' experience is that patients with IgE to alpha-gal describe no oral allergy syndrome-type symptoms; report generalized urticaria or frank anaphylaxis starting 3 to 6 hours after eating beef, pork, or lamb; and have a consistent pattern of both skin testing and serum IgE antibody results.[114,123]

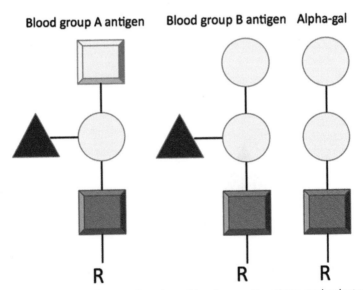

Fig. 3. Comparison of blood group A antigen, blood group B antigen, and galactose-α-1,3-galactose (alpha-gal). Note that the lack of a core fucose residue separates the structure of blood group B antigen from alpha-gal.

The elucidation of IgE to alpha-gal has reversed the conclusion of prior work showing that binding of cat IgA and IgM was caused by an IgE-independent cross-linking with the patients' anti-glycan IgM.[131] In fact, this antiglycan IgM has now been shown to be IgE to alpha-gal.[132] Recent work by Wong and colleagues[133] hinted at the existence of another CCD in mammalian tissue. The authors' description of IgE to alpha-gal in a cohort of patients who report delayed symptoms after eating mammalian meat fits the notion of Wong and colleagues, and alpha-gal may well be a clinically relevant CCD that is specifically found in mammalian tissue.

Evidence for the Role of Tick Bites

Since establishing the assay for IgE antibodies to alpha-gal, large numbers of sera have been screened. The results showed that these IgE antibodies were regionally distributed and that they were also associated with a novel form of anaphylaxis.[122,123] As mentioned, these patients reported delayed symptoms after eating mammalian meat, but they had had no trouble with chicken, turkey, or fish.[114,123] Thus, their symptoms matched the specificity of IgE antibodies present in their serum, which accurately reflected the known distribution of alpha-gal in mammals.[120,123] In most cases, these patients were adults who had consumed red meat for many years before they developed the delayed reactions. The implication was that some new exposure had triggered the production of IgE antibodies to alpha-gal.

Not only did the known distribution of the immediate reactions to cetuximab match to the area of the highest prevalence of Rocky Mountain spotted fever, the authors also heard histories from patients that their reactions to red meat started after receiving multiple tick bites.[134] The authors have reported the evidence that tick bites in the United States can induce IgE antibodies to alpha-gal, and the evidence included, following the response prospectively in 3 cases, a strong correlation with histories of tick bites, epidemiologic evidence that these antibodies are not found in regions where tick bites are rare, and the correlation with IgE antibodies specific for tick proteins.[134] In addition, there is epidemiologic evidence that these IgE antibodies are found in areas where tick bites are common, that the responses correlate with prolonged pruritic reactions to tick bites, and that IgE antibodies to alpha-gal correlate with the presence of IgE antibodies to tick proteins.[134] Furthermore, the currently known distribution of delayed anaphylactic reactions to red meat fits the known distribution of the lone star tick, *Amblyomma americanum*.[134] As the deer population expands, it will be interesting to follow whether there is an increase in the incidence of diagnosed mammalian meat allergy.

Summary of Allergy to Glycans

The discovery of IgE antibodies to the oligosaccharide galactose alpha -1, 3-galactose has made it possible to investigate several novel aspects of allergic disease. The obvious thing is that the glycosylation of therapeutic recombinant molecules, particularly monoclonal antibodies, can create a risk for severe hypersensitivity reactions. In addition, because these IgE antibodies also bind to a wide range of mammalian proteins, the authors recognized the syndrome of delayed anaphylaxis to mammalian meat.[123] However, the most interesting feature of their reactions may be that first symptoms (ie, itching or urticaria) occur 3 to 6 hours after eating meat and would normally be regarded as spontaneous or idiopathic anaphylaxis. Understanding the factors that control the delay may provide real insight into the factors that control anaphylaxis. Moreover, understanding how ticks induce this form of response will be important as we explore the control of IgE antibody responses in general.

SUMMARY

Much has been learned by identifying the molecules that can be recognized by IgE from patients with allergies. Increasingly, by correlating patterns of sensitization with clinical features, it has become possible to distinguish molecules responsible for primary sensitization (complete allergens) from those that are more likely cross-reactive targets. In the case of animal allergens, evolutionary distance seems to be an important factor in determining allergenicity. However, until more is understood regarding the mechanistic details of primary sensitization, including the participation of molecules that stimulate innate immune responses and the repertoire of T-cell antigens, molecules that may or may not themselves be important B-cell antigens, we will not be able to explain fundamental questions, such as why peanut allergy is more severe than soy allergy or why tick exposure is associated with clinically relevant sensitization to a carbohydrate epitope.

ACKNOWLEDGMENTS

The authors would like to thank Youngshin Han, PhD and Galina Grishina, MS for providing the sequence analysis data.

REFERENCES

1. Radauer C, Bublin M, Wagner S, et al. Allergens are distributed into few protein families and possess a restricted number of biochemical functions. J Allergy Clin Immunol 2008;121(4):847–52.e7.
2. Aalberse RC, Stadler BM. In silico predictability of allergenicity: from amino acid sequence via 3-D structure to allergenicity. Mol Nutr Food Res 2006;50(7): 625–7.
3. Aalberse RC. Structural biology of allergens. J Allergy Clin Immunol 2000; 106(2):228–38.
4. Astwood JD, Leach JN, Fuchs RL. Stability of food allergens to digestion in vitro. Nat Biotechnol 1996;14(10):1269–73.
5. Bannon GA. What makes a food protein an allergen? Curr Allergy Asthma Rep 2004;4(1):43–6.
6. Fu T, Abbott UR, Hatzos C. Digestibility of food allergens and nonallergenic proteins in simulated gastric fluid and simulated intestinal fluid-a comparative study. J Agric Food Chem 2002;50(24):7154–60.
7. Herman RA, Woolhiser MM, Ladics GS, et al. Stability of a set of allergens and non-allergens in simulated gastric fluid. Int J Food Sci Nutr 2007;58(2):125–41.
8. Pedrosa C, Felice FG, Trisciuzzi C, et al. Selective neoglycosylation increases the structural stability of vicilin, the 7S storage globulin from pea seeds. Arch Biochem Biophys 2000;382(2):203–10.
9. Wormald MR, Dwek RA. Glycoproteins: glycan presentation and protein-fold stability. Structure 1999;7(7):R155–60.
10. Bencúrová M, Hemmer W, Focke-Tejkl M, et al. Specificity of IgG and IgE antibodies against plant and insect glycoprotein glycans determined with artificial glycoforms of human transferrin. Glycobiology 2004;14(5):457–66.
11. Altmann F. The role of protein glycosylation in allergy. Int Arch Allergy Immunol 2007;142(2):99–115.
12. Faveeuw C, Mallevaey T, Paschinger K, et al. Schistosome N-glycans containing core α3-fucose and core β2-xylose epitopes are strong inducers of Th2 responses in mice. Eur J Immunol 2003;33(5):1271–81.

13. Wilson IB, Zeleny R, Kolarich D, et al. Analysis of Asn-linked glycans from vegetable foodstuffs: widespread occurrence of Lewis a, core alpha1,3-linked fucose and xylose substitutions. Glycobiology 2001;11(4):261–74.
14. Mills EN, Jenkins JA, Alcocer MJC, et al. Structural, biological, and evolutionary relationships of plant food allergens sensitizing via the gastrointestinal tract. Crit Rev Food Sci Nutr 2004;44(5):379–407.
15. Considine T, Patel HA, Singh H, et al. Influence of binding of sodium dodecyl sulfate, all-trans-retinol, palmitate, and 8-anilino-1-naphthalenesulfonate on the heat-induced unfolding and aggregation of beta-lactoglobulin B. J Agric Food Chem 2005;53(8):3197–205.
16. Roth-Walter F, Berin MC, Arnaboldi P, et al. Pasteurization of milk proteins promotes allergic sensitization by enhancing uptake through Peyer's patches. Allergy 2008;63(7):882–90.
17. Breiteneder H, Mills EN. Molecular properties of food allergens. J Allergy Clin Immunol 2005;115(1):14–23 [quiz: 24].
18. Barrett NA, Rahman OM, Fernandez JM, et al. Dectin-2 mediates Th2 immunity through the generation of cysteinyl leukotrienes. J Exp Med 2011;208(3): 593–604.
19. Royer P, Emara M, Yang C, et al. The mannose receptor mediates the uptake of diverse native allergens by dendritic cells and determines allergen-induced T cell polarization through modulation of IDO activity. J Immunol 2010;185(3): 1522–31.
20. Zhou Y, Kawasaki H, Hsu S, et al. Oral tolerance to food-induced systemic anaphylaxis mediated by the C-type lectin SIGNR1. Nat Med 2010;16(10): 1128–33.
21. Reed CE, Kita H. The role of protease activation of inflammation in allergic respiratory diseases. J Allergy Clin Immunol 2004;114(5):997–1008 [quiz: 1009].
22. Trompette A, Divanovic S, Visintin A, et al. Allergenicity resulting from functional mimicry of a Toll-like receptor complex protein. Nature 2009;457(7229):585–8.
23. Mills E, Madsen C, Shewry P. Food allergens of plant origin–their molecular and evolutionary relationships. Trends in Food Science and Technology 2003;(14): 145–56.
24. Jenkins JA, Breiteneder H, Mills EN. Evolutionary distance from human homologs reflects allergenicity of animal food proteins. J Allergy Clin Immunol 2007;120(6): 1399–405.
25. Hoffmann-Sommergruber K, Mills EN. Food allergen protein families and their structural characteristics and application in component-resolved diagnosis: new data from the EuroPrevall project. Anal Bioanal Chem 2009;395(1):25–35.
26. Dunwell JM, Purvis A, Khuri S. Cupins: the most functionally diverse protein superfamily? Phytochemistry 2004;65(1):7–17.
27. Witke W. The role of profilin complexes in cell motility and other cellular processes. Trends Cell Biol 2004;14(8):461–9.
28. Radauer C, Willerroider M, Fuchs H, et al. Cross-reactive and species-specific immunoglobulin E epitopes of plant profilins: an experimental and structure-based analysis. Clin Exp Allergy 2006;36(7):920–9.
29. Ballmer-Weber BK, Wangorsch A, Bohle B, et al. Component-resolved in vitro diagnosis in carrot allergy: does the use of recombinant carrot allergens improve the reliability of the diagnostic procedure? Clin Exp Allergy 2005;35(7):970–8.
30. Lüttkopf D, Ballmer-Weber BK, Wüthrich B, et al. Celery allergens in patients with positive double-blind placebo-controlled food challenge. J Allergy Clin Immunol 2000;106(2):390–9.

31. Marković-Housley Z, Degano M, Lamba D, et al. Crystal structure of a hypoallergenic isoform of the major birch pollen allergen Bet v. 1 and its likely biological function as a plant steroid carrier. J Mol Biol 2003;325(1):123–33.

32. Spitzauer S. Allergy to mammalian proteins: at the borderline between foreign and self? Int Arch Allergy Immunol 1999;120(4):259–69.

33. Kanduc D, Lucchese A, Mittelman A. Individuation of monoclonal anti-HPV16 E7 antibody linear peptide epitope by computational biology. Peptides 2001;22(12): 1981–5.

34. Ayuso R, Lehrer SB, Tanaka L, et al. IgE antibody response to vertebrate meat proteins including tropomyosin. Ann Allergy Asthma Immunol 1999;83(5): 399–405.

35. Wild LG, Lehrer SB. Fish and shellfish allergy. Curr Allergy Asthma Rep 2005;5(1): 74–9.

36. Restani P, Beretta B, Fiocchi A, et al. Cross-reactivity between mammalian proteins. Ann Allergy Asthma Immunol 2002;89(6 Suppl 1):11–5.

37. Fiocchi A, Restani P, Riva E, et al. Meat allergy: I–Specific IgE to BSA and OSA in atopic, beef sensitive children. J Am Coll Nutr 1995;14(3):239–44.

38. Werfel SJ, Cooke SK, Sampson HA. Clinical reactivity to beef in children allergic to cow's milk. J Allergy Clin Immunol 1997;99(3):293–300.

39. Liu AH, Jaramillo R, Sicherer SH, et al. National prevalence and risk factors for food allergy and relationship to asthma: results from the National Health and Nutrition Examination Survey 2005-2006. J Allergy Clin Immunol 2010;126(4): 798–806.e13.

40. Sicherer SH. Epidemiology of food allergy. J Allergy Clin Immunol 2011;127(3): 594–602.

41. Nicolaou N, Poorafshar M, Murray C, et al. Allergy or tolerance in children sensitized to peanut: prevalence and differentiation using component-resolved diagnostics. J Allergy Clin Immunol 2010;125(1):191–7.e1–13.

42. Shreffler WG, Castro RR, Kucuk ZY, et al. The major glycoprotein allergen from Arachis hypogaea, Ara h 1, is a ligand of dendritic cell-specific ICAM-grabbing nonintegrin and acts as a Th2 adjuvant in vitro. J Immunol 2006;177(6): 3677–85.

43. Ilchmann A, Burgdorf S, Scheurer S, et al. Glycation of a food allergen by the Maillard reaction enhances its T-cell immunogenicity: role of macrophage scavenger receptor class A type I and II. J Allergy Clin Immunol 2010;125(1): 175–83.e1–11.

44. Hilmenyuk T, Bellinghausen I, Heydenreich B, et al. Effects of glycation of the model food allergen ovalbumin on antigen uptake and presentation by human dendritic cells. Immunology 2010;129(3):437–45.

45. Hsu S, Tsai T, Kawasaki H, et al. Antigen coupled with Lewis-x trisaccharides elicits potent immune responses in mice. J Allergy Clin Immunol 2007;119(6): 1522–8.

46. Khodoun M, Strait R, Orekov T, et al. Peanuts can contribute to anaphylactic shock by activating complement. J Allergy Clin Immunol 2009;123(2):342–51.

47. Carroll MC. The complement system in regulation of adaptive immunity. Nat Immunol 2004;5(10):981–6.

48. Hawlisch H, Belkaid Y, Baelder R, et al. C5a negatively regulates toll-like receptor 4-induced immune responses. Immunity 2005;22(4):415–26.

49. Drouin SM, Corry DB, Hollman TJ, et al. Absence of the complement anaphylatoxin C3a receptor suppresses Th2 effector functions in a murine model of pulmonary allergy. J Immunol 2002;169(10):5926–33.

50. Becker W, Brasseur D. Opinion of the Scientific Panel on Dietetic Products, Nutrition and Allergies on a request from the Commission relating to the evaluation of allergenic foods for labeling purposes. The EFSA Journal 2004;32:1–197.
51. Zuidmeer L, Goldhahn K, Rona RJ, et al. The prevalence of plant food allergies: a systematic review. J Allergy Clin Immunol 2008;121(5):1210–8.e4.
52. Savage JH, Kaeding AJ, Matsui EC, et al. The natural history of soy allergy. J Allergy Clin Immunol 2010;125(3):683–6.
53. Kattan JD, Cocco RR, Järvinen KM. Milk and soy allergy. Pediatr Clin North Am 2011;58(2):407–26, x.
54. Sicherer SH, Sampson HA. Food allergy: recent advances in pathophysiology and treatment. Annu Rev Med 2009;60:261–77.
55. Bruno G, Giampietro PG, Guercio MJD, et al. Soy allergy is not common in atopic children: a multicenter study. Pediatr Allergy Immunol 1997;8(4):190–3.
56. Mittag D, Vieths S, Vogel L, et al. Soybean allergy in patients allergic to birch pollen: clinical investigation and molecular characterization of allergens. J Allergy Clin Immunol 2004;113(1):148–54.
57. Magnolfi CF, Zani G, Lacava L, et al. Soy allergy in atopic children. Ann Allergy Asthma Immunol 1996;77(3):197–201.
58. Bhatia J, Greer F, American Academy of Pediatrics Committee on Nutrition. Use of soy protein-based formulas in infant feeding. Pediatrics 2008;121(5):1062–8.
59. Klemola T, Vanto T, Juntunen-Backman K, et al. Allergy to soy formula and to extensively hydrolyzed whey formula in infants with cow's milk allergy: a prospective, randomized study with a follow-up to the age of 2 years. J Pediatr 2002;140(2): 219–24.
60. Zeiger RS, Sampson HA, Bock SA, et al. Soy allergy in infants and children with IgE-associated cow's milk allergy. J Pediatr 1999;134(5):614–22.
61. David TJ. Anaphylactic shock during elimination diets for severe atopic eczema. Arch Dis Child 1984;59(10):983–6.
62. Awazuhara H, Kawai H, Maruchi N. Major allergens in soybean and clinical significance of IgG4 antibodies investigated by IgE- and IgG4-immunoblotting with sera from soybean-sensitive patients. Clin Exp Allergy 1997;27(3):325–32.
63. Shibasaki M, Suzuki S, Tajima S, et al. Allergenicity of major component proteins of soybean. Int Arch Allergy Appl Immunol 1980;61(4):441–8.
64. Holzhauser T, Wackermann O, Ballmer-Weber BK, et al. Soybean (glycine max) allergy in Europe: Gly m 5 (beta-conglycinin) and Gly m 6 (glycinin) are potential diagnostic markers for severe allergic reactions to soy. J Allergy Clin Immunol 2009;123(2):452–8.
65. L'Hocine L, Boye JI. Allergenicity of soybean: new developments in identification of allergenic proteins, cross-reactivities and hypoallergenization technologies. Crit Rev Food Sci Nutr 2007;47(2):127–43.
66. González R, Polo F, Zapatero L, et al. Purification and characterization of major inhalant allergens from soybean hulls. Clin Exp Allergy 1992;22(8):748–55.
67. Kalinski A, Weisemann JM, Matthews BF, et al. Molecular cloning of a protein associated with soybean seed oil bodies that is similar to thiol proteases of the papain family. J Biol Chem 1990;265(23):13843–8.
68. Kalinski A, Melroy DL, Dwivedi RS, et al. A soybean vacuolar protein (P34) related to thiol proteases is synthesized as a glycoprotein precursor during seed maturation. J Biol Chem 1992;267(17):12068–76.
69. Rihs HP, Chen Z, Ruëff F, et al. IgE binding of the recombinant allergen soybean profilin (rGly m 3) is mediated by conformational epitopes. J Allergy Clin Immunol 1999;104(6):1293–301.

70. van Zuuren EJ, Terreehorst I, Tupker RA, et al. Anaphylaxis after consuming soy products in patients with birch pollinosis. Allergy 2010;65(10):1348–9.
71. Kleine-Tebbe J, Vogel L, Crowell DN, et al. Severe oral allergy syndrome and anaphylactic reactions caused by a Bet v. 1- related PR-10 protein in soybean, SAM22. J Allergy Clin Immunol 2002;110(5):797–804.
72. Vissers YM, Jansen AP, Ruinemans-Koerts J, et al. IgE component-resolved allergen profile and clinical symptoms in soy and peanut allergic patients. Allergy 2011;66(8):1125–7.
73. Breiteneder H, Mills EN. Plant food allergens–structural and functional aspects of allergenicity. Biotechnol Adv 2005;23(6):395–9.
74. Burks AW, Williams LW, Helm RM, et al. Identification of soy protein allergens in patients with atopic dermatitis and positive soy challenges; determination of change in allergenicity after heating or enzyme digestion. Adv Exp Med Biol 1991;289:295–307.
75. Burks AW, Cockrell G, Connaughton C, et al. Identification of peanut agglutinin and soybean trypsin inhibitor as minor legume allergens. Int Arch Allergy Immunol 1994;105(2):143–9.
76. Ogawa T, Bando N, Tsuji H, et al. Alpha-subunit of beta-conglycinin, an allergenic protein recognized by IgE antibodies of soybean-sensitive patients with atopic dermatitis. Biosci Biotechnol Biochem 1995;59(5):831–3.
77. Beardslee TA, Zeece MG, Sarath G, et al. Soybean glycinin G1 acidic chain shares IgE epitopes with peanut allergen Ara h 3. Int Arch Allergy Immunol 2000;123(4):299–307.
78. L'Hocine L, Boye JI, Jouve S. Ionic strength and pH-induced changes in the immunoreactivity of purified soybean glycinin and its relation to protein molecular structure. J Agric Food Chem 2007;55(14):5819–26.
79. Piacentini GL, Benedetti M, Spezia E, et al. Anaphylactic sensitizing power of selected infant formulas. Ann Allergy 1991;67(4):400–2.
80. Osterballe M, Mortz CG, Hansen TK, et al. The prevalence of food hypersensitivity in young adults. Pediatr Allergy Immunol 2009;20(7):686–92.
81. Rozenfeld P, Docena GH, Añón MC, et al. Detection and identification of a soy protein component that cross-reacts with caseins from cow's milk. Clin Exp Immunol 2002;130(1):49–58.
82. Chruszcz M, Maleki SJ, Majorek KA, et al. Structural and immunologic characterization of Ara h 1, a major peanut allergen. J Biol Chem 2011;286(45): 39318–27.
83. Sicherer SH, Sampson HA, Burks AW. Peanut and soy allergy: a clinical and therapeutic dilemma. Allergy 2000;55(6):515–21.
84. Foucard T, Yman IM. A study on severe food reactions in Sweden–is soy protein an underestimated cause of food anaphylaxis? Allergy 1999;54(3):261–5.
85. Yunginger JW, Nelson DR, Squillace DL, et al. Laboratory investigation of deaths due to anaphylaxis. J Forensic Sci 1991;36(3):857–65.
86. Ballmer-Weber BK, Holzhauser T, Scibilia J, et al. Clinical characteristics of soybean allergy in Europe: a double-blind, placebo-controlled food challenge study. J Allergy Clin Immunol 2007;119(6):1489–96.
87. Pons L, Ponnappan U, Hall RA, et al. Soy immunotherapy for peanut-allergic mice: modulation of the peanut-allergic response. J Allergy Clin Immunol 2004;114(4): 915–21.
88. Bindslev-Jensen C, Briggs D, Osterballe M. Can we determine a threshold level for allergenic foods by statistical analysis of published data in the literature? Allergy 2002;57(8):741–6.

89. Cordle CT. Soy protein allergy: incidence and relative severity. J Nutr 2004;134(5): 1213S–9S.
90. Sicherer SH, Morrow EH, Sampson HA. Dose-response in double-blind, placebo-controlled oral food challenges in children with atopic dermatitis. J Allergy Clin Immunol 2000;105(3):582–6.
91. Amigo-Benavent M, Athanasopoulos V. Carbohydrate moieties on the in vitro immunoreactivity of soy [beta]-conglycinin. Food Research International 2009; 42(7):819–25.
92. Bando N, Tsuji H, Yamanishi R, et al. Identification of the glycosylation site of a major soybean allergen, Gly m Bd 30K. Biosci Biotechnol Biochem 1996; 60(2):347–8.
93. Kroghsbo S, Bøgh KL, Rigby NM, et al. Sensitization with 7S globulins from peanut, hazelnut, soy or pea induces IgE with different biological activities which are modified by soy tolerance. Int Arch Allergy Immunol 2011;155(3):212–24.
94. Müller U, Weber W, Hoffmann A, et al. Commercial soybean lecithins: a source of hidden allergens? Zschr für Lebensmittel-Untersuchung und –Forschung A 1998; 207:341–51.
95. Tsumura K, Kugimiya W, Bando N. Preparation of hypoallergenic soybean protein with processing functionality by selective enzymatic hydrolysis. Food Sci Tech Res 1999;5(2):171–5.
96. Tsuji H, Okada N, Yamanishi R. Fate of a major soybean allergen, Gly m Bd 30K, in rice-, barley-and soybean-koji miso (fermented soybean paste) during fermentation. Food Sci Tech Res 1997;3(2):145–9.
97. Kang J, Badger TM, Ronis MJ, et al. Non-isoflavone phytochemicals in soy and their health effects. J Agric Food Chem 2010;58(14):8119–33.
98. Masilamani M, Wei J, Bhatt S, et al. Soybean isoflavones regulate dendritic cell function and suppress allergic sensitization to peanut. J Allergy Clin Immunol 2011;128(6):1242.e1–50.e1.
99. Messina M. A brief historical overview of the past two decades of soy and iso-flavone research. J Nutr 2010;140(7):1350S–4S.
100. Kay AB. Allergy and allergic diseases. Second of two parts. N Engl J Med 2001; 344(2):109–13.
101. Kay AB. Allergy and allergic diseases. First of two parts. N Engl J Med 2001;344(1): 30–7.
102. Sampson HA. Food allergy. Part 2: diagnosis and management. J Allergy Clin Immunol 1999;103(6):981–9.
103. Sampson HA. Food allergy. Part 1: immunopathogenesis and clinical disorders. J Allergy Clin Immunol 1999;103(5 Pt 1):717–28.
104. Aalberse RC, Koshte V, Clemens JG. Immunoglobulin E antibodies that cross-react with vegetable foods, pollen, and Hymenoptera venom. J Allergy Clin Immunol 1981;68(5):356–64.
105. Kochuyt A, Hoeyveld EM, Stevens EA. Prevalence and clinical relevance of specific immunoglobulin E to pollen caused by sting- induced specific immuno-globulin E to cross-reacting carbohydrate determinants in Hymenoptera venoms. Clin Exp Allergy 2005;35(4):441–7.
106. van der Veen MJ, van Ree R, Aalberse RC, et al. Poor biologic activity of cross-reactive IgE directed to carbohydrate determinants of glycoproteins. J Allergy Clin Immunol 1997;100(3):327–34.
107. Ishihara H, Takahashi N, Oguri S, et al. Complete structure of the carbohydrate moiety of stem bromelain. An application of the almond glycopeptidase for structural studies of glycopeptides. J Biol Chem 1979;254(21):10715–9.

108. Bouwstra JB, Spoelstra EC, Waard PD, et al. Conformational studies on the N-linked carbohydrate chain of bromelain. Eur J Biochem 1990;190(1):113–22.
109. Wilson IB, Altmann F. Structural analysis of N-glycans from allergenic grass, ragweed and tree pollens: core alpha1,3-linked fucose and xylose present in all pollens examined. Glycoconj J 1998;15(11):1055–70.
110. Weber A, Schröder H, Thalberg K, et al. Specific interaction of IgE antibodies with a carbohydrate epitope of honey bee venom phospholipase A2. Allergy 1987;42(6):464–70.
111. Tretter V, Altmann F, Kubelka V, et al. Fucose alpha 1,3-linked to the core region of glycoprotein N-glycans creates an important epitope for IgE from honeybee venom allergic individuals. Int Arch Allergy Immunol 1993;102(3):259–66.
112. Aalberse RC, van Ree R. Cross-reactive carbohydrate determinants. Clin Rev Allergy Immunol 1997;15(4):375–87.
113. Mari A. IgE to cross-reactive carbohydrate determinants: analysis of the distribution and appraisal of the in vivo and in vitro reactivity. Int Arch Allergy Immunol 2002;129(4):286–95.
114. Commins SP, Platts-Mills TA. Anaphylaxis syndromes related to a new mammalian cross-reactive carbohydrate determinant. J Allergy Clin Immunol 2009;124(4):652–7.
115. Foetisch K, Westphal S, Lauer I, et al. Biological activity of IgE specific for cross-reactive carbohydrate determinants. J Allergy Clin Immunol 2003;111(4):889–96.
116. Fötisch K, Altmann F, Haustein D, et al. Involvement of carbohydrate epitopes in the IgE response of celery-allergic patients. Int Arch Allergy Immunol 1999;120(1):30–42.
117. Iacovacci P, Afferni C, Butteroni C, et al. Comparison between the native glycosylated and the recombinant Cup a1 allergen: role of carbohydrates in the histamine release from basophils. Clin Exp Allergy 2002;32(11):1620–7.
118. van Ree R, Aalberse RC. Specific IgE without clinical allergy. J Allergy Clin Immunol 1999;103(6):1000–1.
119. Lommerse JP, Kroon-Batenburg LM, Kamerling JP, et al. Conformational analysis of the xylose-containing N-glycan of pineapple stem bromelain as part of the intact glycoprotein. Biochemistry 1995;34(25):8196–206.
120. Galili U. The alpha-gal epitope and the anti-Gal antibody in xenotransplantation and in cancer immunotherapy. Immunol Cell Biol 2005;83(6):674–86.
121. Jin C, Hantusch B, Hemmer W, et al. Affinity of IgE and IgG against cross-reactive carbohydrate determinants on plant and insect glycoproteins. J Allergy Clin Immunol 2008;121(1):185–90.e2.
122. Chung CH, Mirakhur B, Chan E, et al. Cetuximab-induced anaphylaxis and IgE specific for galactose-alpha-1,3-galactose. N Engl J Med 2008;358(11):1109–17.
123. Commins SP, Satinover SM, Hosen J, et al. Delayed anaphylaxis, angioedema, or urticaria after consumption of red meat in patients with IgE antibodies specific for galactose-alpha-1,3-galactose. J Allergy Clin Immunol 2009;123(2):426–33.
124. Macher BA, Galili U. The Galalpha1,3Galbeta1,4GlcNAc-R (alpha-Gal) epitope: a carbohydrate of unique evolution and clinical relevance. Biochim Biophys Acta 2008;1780(2):75–88.
125. Spiro RG, Bhoyroo VD. Occurrence of alpha-D-galactosyl residues in the thyroglobulins from several species. Localization in the saccharide chains of the complex carbohydrate units. J Biol Chem 1984;259(15):9858–66.

126. Paschinger K, Fabini G, Schuster D, et al. Definition of immunogenic carbohydrate epitopes. Acta Biochim Pol 2005;52(3):629–32.
127. Galili U, Mandrell RE, Hamadeh RM, et al. Interaction between human natural anti-alpha-galactosyl immunoglobulin G and bacteria of the human flora. Infect Immun 1988;56(7):1730–7.
128. Springer GF, Horton RE. Blood group isoantibody stimulation in man by feeding blood group-active bacteria. J Clin Invest 1969;48(7):1280–91.
129. Koike C, Fung JJ, Geller DA, et al. Molecular basis of evolutionary loss of the alpha 1,3-galactosyltransferase gene in higher primates. J Biol Chem 2002; 277(12):10114–20.
130. Larsen RD, Rivera-Marrero CA, Ernst LK, et al. Frameshift and nonsense mutations in a human genomic sequence homologous to a murine UDP-Gal:beta-D-Gal(1,4)-D-GlcNAc alpha(1,3)-galactosyltransferase cDNA. J Biol Chem 1990; 265(12):7055–61.
131. Adédoyin J, Johansson SG, Grönlund H, et al. Interference in immunoassays by human IgM with specificity for the carbohydrate moiety of animal proteins. J Immunol Methods 2006;310(1–2):117–25.
132. Grönlund H, Adédoyin J, Commins SP, et al. The carbohydrate galactose-alpha-1,3-galactose is a major IgE-binding epitope on cat IgA. J Allergy Clin Immunol 2009;123(5):1189–91.
133. Wong KN, Wang X, Lee W, et al. Deglycosylation of meat extracts reduced the binding of cross-reactive antibodies to meat. XXV Congress of the European Academy of Allergology and Clinical Immunology. Vienna (Austria), June 10–14, 2006.
134. Commins SP, James HR, Kelly LA, et al. The relevance of tick bites to the production of IgE antibodies to the mammalian oligosaccharide galactose-α-1,3-galactose. J Allergy Clin Immunol 2011;127(5):1286–93.e6.

The Epidemiology of IgE-Mediated Food Allergy and Anaphylaxis

Katrina J. Allen, MBBS, FRACP, PhD[a,b,c,*], Jennifer J. Koplin, PhD[a]

KEYWORDS

- Epidemiology • Food allergy • Prevalence • Risk factors

The prevalence of IgE-mediated food allergy and anaphylaxis seems to have risen rapidly in developed countries[1,2] and is an evolving public health problem with emerging evidence that countries with rapid industrialization may follow suit.[3] Despite an increasing number of studies mounted to investigate the rise of allergic disease in general and food allergy in particular, the cause of the current epidemic of food allergy remains elusive.

It is estimated that about a quarter of the population will have an adverse reaction to food (of which food allergy is just one type) during their lifetime,[4] most of which occur during infancy and early childhood. An estimated 10% to 15% of children report symptoms of food allergy, although the prevalence of IgE-mediated food allergies (ie, symptoms of food allergy in the presence of food-specific IgE) is reported to be lower, at approximately 6% to 8% in children younger than 3 years and 3% to 4% of the adult population.[5] By contrast not much is known about the prevalence of non–IgE-mediated food allergies, although both eosinophilic esophagitis and celiac disease have been documented to be on the rise.[6,7]

More than 90% of IgE-mediated food allergies in children are caused by just eight food items: (1) cow's milk, (2) soy, (3) hen's egg, (4) peanuts, (5) tree nuts, (6) wheat, (7) fish, and (8) shellfish. Most children with cow's milk and egg allergy develop tolerance by late childhood, whereas allergies to peanut, sesame seeds, and tree nuts

Disclosure: None to declare.
[a] Murdoch Childrens Research Institute, The Royal Children's Hospital, Flemington Road, Parkville 3052, Melbourne, Victoria, Australia
[b] Department of Paediatrics, The University of Melbourne, The Royal Children's Hospital, Flemington Road, Parkville 3052, Melbourne, Victoria, Australia
[c] Department of Allergy and Immunology, The Royal Children's Hospital, Flemington Road, Parkville 3052, Victoria, Melbourne, Australia
* Corresponding author. Gastro and Food Allergy Research Group, Murdoch Childrens Research Institute, The Royal Children's Hospital, Flemington Road, Parkville 3052, Melbourne, Victoria, Australia.
E-mail address: katie.allen@rch.org.au

are more persistent, with less than 20% developing tolerance.[8] As a result, cow's milk and egg allergies are uncommon in adults and allergies to peanuts, tree nuts, fish, and shellfish predominate.[9] Much less is known about the natural history or population prevalence of non–IgE-mediated food allergy,[10] which is outside the scope of this article.

METHODOLOGIES FOR MEASURING FOOD ALLERGY PREVALENCE

Studies have shown that self-reported food allergy is an inaccurate measure of true food allergy.[9] There are multiple reasons why food allergy may be overreported by individuals, including inability to distinguish between food intolerance and allergy and incorrectly attributing symptoms to allergic reactions to food even where there is no evidence to support such contentions. It is also not possible to determine allergic status based on parent-report to foods that have not yet been introduced into an infant's diet. As such, any study on the prevalence of food allergy needs to be contextualized by the outcome used to define the condition.

The gold standard for the diagnosis of IgE-mediated food allergy is double-blind placebo-controlled food challenges. However, even this gold standard is limited by methodologic differences between studies in choice of food for challenges (eg, cooked vs raw eggs, which have different allergenicity) and criteria for defining a positive challenge because until recently criteria for the definition of a positive oral food challenge (OFC) have never been formalized.[11] Although most protocols state that a positive challenge is demonstrated by evidence of an immediate reaction consistent with IgE-mediated food allergy, such as urticaria, angioedema, or anaphylaxis, interpretation of more subjective symptoms, such as abdominal pain or nausea, or the more ubiquitous and less clearly defined sign of an eczema flare remains difficult. Differences in criteria for the definition of a positive OFC across different studies and different centers hinders the ability to compare food allergy prevalence estimates between studies and to identify risk factors for the development of food allergy (because phenotypes might vary across different study cohorts), and to assess the success of various treatment strategies (including oral immunotherapy).

A further limitation of even the small number of studies that have conducted formal graded food challenges is that most studies have not addressed the question of whether study participants are representative of the population from which they were sampled. The generalizability of their results to the general population may therefore be poor, particularly if families at high risk of allergic disease are overrepresented among participants. The extent to which this type of selection bias may affect results is rarely formally assessed, although recent cohort studies of food allergy have begun to address this using short questionnaires to assess prevalence of risk factors for allergy among those who do not wish to undergo testing for food allergy.[12]

Performing large-scale studies of challenge-proved food allergy is not always possible because of issues with compliance, risk to participants, and cost. As such, many population-based prevalence studies have relied on the detection of food-specific IgE antibodies as an indirect marker of food allergy, either alone or in conjunction with reported symptoms on ingestion of the food. The presence of IgE specific to food allergens can be detected using skin prick testing or in vitro measurement using the cap-fluoroenzyme immunoassay or radioallergosorbent test. Individuals are said to be "sensitized" to the food being studied if the size of the wheal (skin prick testing) or measured IgE level (cap-fluoroenzyme immunoassay or radioallergosorbent test) exceeds a prespecified threshold but confirmation of food allergy requires symptomatic ingestion of the food. Larger skin prick testing wheal sizes or higher measured IgE levels are associated with an increased likelihood that individuals are truly food allergic,[13,14] however this increase in specificity occurs with a corresponding loss of sensitivity.

THE MOST RECENT PREVALENCE ESTIMATES OF IGE-MEDIATED FOOD ALLERGY

Existing studies of food allergy incidence, prevalence, and natural history are difficult to compare because of inconsistencies and deficiencies in study design and variations in the definition of food allergy.[15] Rona and colleagues[9] assessed data from 51 publications and provided separate analyses for the prevalence of food allergy for five common foods (cow's milk, hen's egg, peanut, fish, and shellfish), stratified by whether the studies were in adults or children. The investigators report a pooled overall prevalence of self-reported food allergy for adults and children of 13% and 12%, respectively, to any of these five foods. However, pooled results are far lower (~3%) when food allergy is defined as either sensitization alone; sensitization with symptoms; or positive double-blind, placebo-controlled food challenge.

The prevalence of common food allergies as measured in recent population-based studies is illustrated in **Fig. 1**. Two recent cohort studies from the United Kingdom and Denmark reported that the foods most often responsible for symptoms of food allergy in infants and young children were egg, cow's milk, and peanuts. In the Danish study, the prevalence of egg and milk allergy reached a peak around 18 months of age, at 2.4% and 1% for egg and milk, respectively; with around 20% becoming tolerant to egg by 3 years; and 100% becoming tolerant to milk by 6 years of age.[16] Oral food challenges to peanut were not performed until the children reached 3 years of age; however, at 3 years of age the United Kingdom study reported a peanut allergy prevalence of 1.2%.[17]

Population data using challenge-proved outcomes is likely to represent the best quality data for prevalence estimates. Such data have been collected in the Health-Nuts study, which reports a prevalence of challenge-proved peanut allergy of 3% (95% confidence interval [CI], 2.4–3.8); egg allergy of 8.9% (95% CI, 7.8–10); and sesame allergy of 0.8% (95% CI, 0.5–1.1) in 1-year-old infants in Melbourne, Australia.[18] These figures were weighted to account for participation bias and represent the highest prevalence figures published to date. They reflect previous observations of a generally high prevalence of other allergic diseases in Australia and suggest that factors in Australia are primed for an evolving epidemic of allergic disease. The design strengths of the HealthNuts study include the use of a formal sampling frame to attain a representative population base, assessment of the degree of participation bias using short questionnaires administered to all nonparticipants, and use of oral food challenges to assess food allergy outcomes. In addition, oral food challenges were undertaken on all sensitized children irrespective of wheal size or previous history of ingestion reaction unless occurring in the previous 1 month for egg or 2 months for peanut and sesame.

Prevalence figures and the spectrum of food allergens seem to vary considerably between geographic regions,[9] and have been thought to predominantly reflect variations in diet among different cultures. Alternatively, some of the differences in food allergy prevalence between regions may be explained by either genetic variation across populations or variations in exposure to environmental factors, such as sunlight (ie, related to vitamin D levels) or factors related to the hygiene hypothesis (discussed later). Recent prevalence data from Chongqing, China, demonstrated a higher than expected rate of IgE-mediated food allergy,[3] with 2.5% reporting egg allergy and 1.3% cow's milk allergic, suggesting that increased urbanization might play a role in rising rates in countries undergoing rapid development.[19]

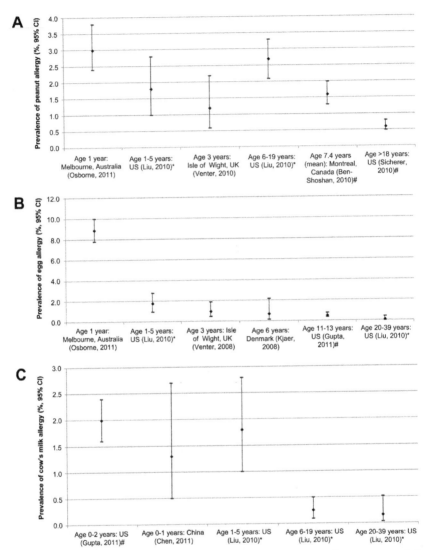

Fig. 1. Prevalence of common food allergies in different age groups in recent population-based studies: (A) peanut, (B) egg, (C) milk, (D) sesame, and (E) shellfish. Preference was given to those using oral food challenges to diagnose food allergy where available. * Based on specific IgE levels. # Self- or parent-reported food allergy. †Prevalence of SPT ≥3 mm. Note: Egg allergy in the Healthnuts study reflects raw egg challenge data - the most immunogenic form of egg.

FOOD-INDUCED ANAPHYLAXIS

Attempting to determine the population prevalence of anaphylaxis is made more difficult because of varying opinions on what constitutes anaphylaxis. Several classification systems have been used; however, a recent consensus document has defined anaphylaxis as a "serious allergic reaction that is rapid in onset and may cause death," and proposed diagnostic criteria for use in clinical care.[20] By these criteria, a diagnosis of anaphylaxis can be made if there is involvement of the respiratory or cardiovascular

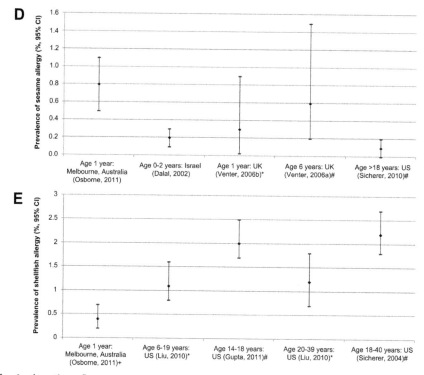

Fig. 1. (*continued*)

systems during an allergic reaction, or if a less severe reaction occurs in the setting of previously diagnosed allergy and likely exposure to the relevant allergen. In addition to the lack of consensus on the definition of anaphylaxis, the population prevalence of anaphylaxis has been difficult to accurately quantify because of analysis of different sample populations (eg, emergency department presentations, hospital admissions, general practitioner presentations, specialist allergist presentations), and the use of varying methodologies for data collection.[21]

Recent reports have found that the incidence of anaphylaxis is rising in Australia, the United Kingdom, and the United States.[2,22,23] In a recent study, Liew and colleagues[2] confirmed previous reports of an increasing world-wide incidence of hospital admissions for food-induced anaphylaxis, with an incidence in the Australian population of around 6 per 100,000 population reported in 2004 and 2005, an overall rise of 350% above the previous 11 years. Children younger than the age of 5 years had the highest rates of hospital admissions for food-induced anaphylaxis (9.4 per 100,000 population) and the rate of increase in hospital admissions over time was also greatest for this age group.

The spectrum of foods commonly responsible for causing allergic reactions including anaphylaxis varies between countries, although peanuts, tree nuts, and seafood were commonly implicated in hospitalizations and deaths from food-induced anaphylaxis in Australia, the United States, and the United Kingdom.[2,24,25] However, there are now increasing reports of anaphylaxis occurring to a wide range of foods including fruits and other foods not previously commonly associated with anaphylaxis, such as lupin.[26,27]

Attention has turned recently to identification of factors that may increase the risk of episodes of food-related anaphylaxis including clinical risk factors and modifiable lifestyle factors.[28] Recent studies confirm that individuals with asthma are at increased risk of anaphylaxis, including food-induced anaphylaxis, and that those with severe asthma are at the highest risk.[29,30] One of the most interesting recent lifestyle factors to be investigated is the relationship between vitamin D insufficiency and increased risk of food-induced anaphylaxis. There is now an emerging base of evidence demonstrating the relationship between latitude and anaphylaxis to support this contention.[31–34]

EPIDEMIOLOGY OF FATAL ANAPHYLAXIS

Data from national mortality reporting systems in the United Kingdom and Australia estimate the prevalence of anaphylaxis fatalities from all causes (including food, medication, insect sting, and idiopathic) to be 0.33 deaths per year per million population in the United Kingdom,[35] with Australia reporting the highest rate of 0.64 deaths per year per million population.[2] For as yet undetermined reasons in Australia only 6% of anaphylaxis deaths are ascribed to food-induced anaphylaxis compared with 31% in the United Kingdom.

Risk factors for a poor outcome from an episode of food-related anaphylaxis include age (risk is highest in adolescence and young adults); peanut or tree nut allergy; coexistent and poorly controlled asthma; posture (failure to be kept in the supine position); lack of access to self-injectable adrenaline; and failure to administer adrenaline in a timely manner. Although never formally investigated, hypothetical reasons for poorer outcomes in the adolescent and young adult age group include increased risk-taking behavior, issues of transition from parental locus of control, failure to adequately educate young people about the risks of anaphylaxis at the time that they are taking increased responsibility for their own health, and an increased prevalence of asthma and poorly managed asthma in these age-groups compared with those younger than 5 years of age.

WHAT IS THE EVIDENCE FOR A RISE IN INCIDENCE OF FOOD ALLERGY?

Food allergy is widely believed in the lay and scientific communities to be becoming increasingly common. Unfortunately, reports of an increasing prevalence of food allergy are difficult to substantiate because studies documenting the population prevalence of food allergy before the 1980s are not available to provide baseline data.

Recent studies have attempted to confirm anecdotal evidence of an increased incidence of peanut allergy. In a United Kingdom study, Venter and colleagues[36] found that peanut sensitization varied from 1.3%, to 3.3% to 2% in three sequential early childhood cohorts from the same geographic area, each surveyed 6 years apart, whereas reported peanut allergy increased from 0.5% to 1.4% then 1.2%. Although there was evidence that both peanut sensitization and allergy were significantly more common in the second cohort (born in 1994–1996) compared with the initial cohort (born in 1989), there was no evidence of a further increase in prevalence in the third cohort (born in 2001–2002).

Between three United States–wide telephone surveys conducted in 1997, 2002, and 2007, the prevalence of self-reported peanut or tree nut allergy increased from 0.6%, to 1.2% to 2.1% among children, although no change was observed for adults.[37] However, this increase in reported allergy was paralleled by a decreasing response rate across surveys (42% response rate in 2007), raising questions about whether these prevalence figures can be generalized to the wider population.

Further surveillance of allergy prevalence within populations using standardized methods is required to measure any future rise in allergy prevalence.

FACTORS ASSOCIATED WITH THE PRESUME RISE IN PREVALENCE

The cause of the presumed rise in food allergy and anaphylaxis prevalence is not known, but the short period over which the increase has occurred suggests that genetic factors alone cannot be causative because changes to the genome occur at an evolutionary pace. Environmental factors must therefore be central to the increase in prevalence, although these may be mediated through epigenetic modification (discussed later). Because food allergy is more common in developed than developing countries, and migrants seem to acquire the incident risk of allergy of their adopted country, it seems likely that the cause of the rise is linked to the "modern lifestyle." Although environmental factors including those associated with the hygiene hypothesis and dietary factors have been found to be associated with the development of eczema and atopy, there has been little investigation into whether they may also play a role in the development of food allergy. In addition to factors previously linked to allergic disease in general there may well be some factors that are specific to food allergy. These might include changing methods of food manufacturing and preparation, the advent of widespread use of antacids and proton pump inhibitors, use of medicinal creams containing food allergens, or later introduction of allergenic foods into the diet of infants.

THE ROLE OF GENETICS IN PREDISPOSITION TO FOOD ALLERGY

Although the rise in food allergy prevalence cannot be explained by genetic factors alone, there is strong evidence that susceptibility to food allergy is at least partly determined by genetics. Twin studies have shown that the concordance rate for peanut allergy was much higher among monozygotic (64.3%) than dizygotic (6.8%; $P<.0001$) twin pairs.[38] However, a recent study of familial aggregation observed the heritability of common food allergies (sesame, peanut, wheat, milk, egg white, soy, walnut, shrimp, and cod fish) to be between 0.15 and 0.35[39] suggesting genetic factors are not as important as other factors, such as environmental exposures, in the development of food allergies.

Eczema and food allergy seem to be closely linked, with eczematous infants having a greatly increased risk of food allergy.[40] There is increasing interest in the role of loss of function mutations in the filaggrin (FLG) gene, which lead to defects in skin barrier permeability, in the pathogenesis of eczema. Null mutations (R501X and 2282del4) in FLG are associated with an increased susceptibility to eczema.[41] Individuals with two null alleles in FLG have been shown to be four to seven times more likely to have eczema than those without.[42] One recent case-control study investigated whether FLG mutations were also associated with peanut allergy, reporting that those with peanut allergy were around five times more likely to have FLG loss-of-function mutations.[43] This result along with previous studies suggesting that peanut sensitization may occur through damaged skin[44–46] indicates that epithelial barrier dysfunction may play a role in the pathogenesis of peanut allergy.

ROLE OF RACE AND GENDER IN FOOD ALLERGY PREDISPOSITION

Gender disparities in the prevalence of some allergic disorders including allergic asthma have been well-described; however, the relationship between gender and food allergy is less clear.[47] Although asthma is more common in young boys, a gender switch occurs around the time of puberty with asthma being more common and more severe in women.[48,49] The reasons for this have yet to be elucidated but may relate to hormonal changes occurring during puberty.[48] Although this gender switch is also evident in clinical presentations with food allergy, this has not been formally explored at the population level.

Similarly, racial and ethnic differences in asthma prevalence have also been well described, whereas there have been few studies investigating the influence of ethnicity on the likelihood of developing food allergy. One United Kingdom study found that nonwhite infants were overrepresented in a pediatric food allergy clinic compared with general pediatric clinics.[50] In the United States, the 2007 National Health Interview Survey found that non-Hispanic children had higher rates of reported food allergy compared with Hispanic children.[51] Recently, the authors have found a higher rate of food-sensitized eczema among children of Asian descent in the HealthNuts cohort.[52] Interestingly, on examination of risk factors for eczema development (a closely associated infantile allergic disease) the authors found that Asian children were not only more likely to have eczema than their non-Asian counterparts but that their parents were less likely to have allergic disease than non-Asian parents. This was particularly so for Asian parents who had migrated to Australia less than 5 years previously, suggesting a strong gene–environment interaction even over and above that of a migrational generational effect (P. Martin, unpublished data, 2011).

MODIFIABLE ENVIRONMENTAL RISK FACTORS FOR FOOD ALLERGY DEVELOPMENT

Because the rise in food allergy has occurred more rapidly than changes to the genome would allow there has been more emphasis placed on what putative environmental factors might be associated with food allergy. Those that have changed most dramatically in the last half of the twentieth century and early part of the twenty-first century are under the most intense investigation. There are several hypotheses relating to modifiable environmental factors for an increased predisposition for food allergy. These include the "hygiene hypothesis," microbial diversity of the gastrointestinal tract, the "old friends" hypothesis, factors related to infant feeding, and the vitamin D hypothesis (**Fig. 2**).

There is now emerging evidence that at least some environmental exposures may exert their influence by "epigenetic" mechanisms of gene alteration. Animal models have demonstrated that environmental changes at critical times during development can alter the phenotype of genetically identical animals though epigenetic modification.[53] These include activating or silencing genes by altering DNA and histone methylation, histone acetylation, and chromatin structure. These epigenetic modifications determine the degree of DNA compaction and accessibility for gene transcription. The potential role of epigenetic variation in the cause of food allergy has recently been reviewed.[54]

The "Hygiene" Hypothesis

Microbial stimulation in early life plays a vital role in the development of the immune system[55] and the role of microbial exposures in allergic disease has been the subject of intense research since the development of the hygiene hypothesis in 1989.[56] Exposure to siblings and to other children through childcare, contact with pets, and delivery by caesarean section, all of which can occur in the early postnatal period before the introduction of food and expression of food allergy, have all been reported to affect the type or quantity of microbes (or their products) to which a child is exposed.[57–63] Further research is required to elucidate whether these factors play a role in the development of food allergy.

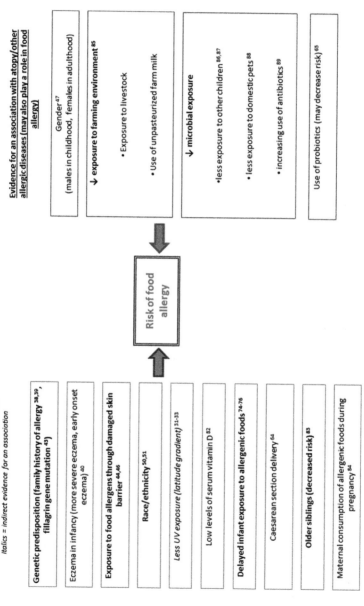

Evidence for an association with food sensitization or allergy

Bold = study shows an association with food allergy

Not bold = association with food sensitization only

Italics = indirect evidence for an association

Genetic predisposition (family history of allergy [38,39], fillagrin gene mutation [43])

Eczema in infancy (more severe eczema, early onset eczema) [40]

Exposure to food allergens through damaged skin barrier [44,46]

Race/ethnicity [50,51]

Less UV exposure (latitude gradient) [51-53]

Low levels of serum vitamin D [82]

Delayed infant exposure to allergenic foods [74-76]

Caesarean section delivery [64]

Older siblings (decreased risk) [83]

Maternal consumption of allergenic foods during pregnancy [84]

Evidence for an association with atopy/other allergic diseases (may also play a role in food allergy)

Gender [47] (males in childhood, females in adulthood)

↓ **exposure to farming environment** [85]

• Exposure to livestock

• Use of unpasteurized farm milk

↓ **microbial exposure**

• less exposure to other children [86,87]

• less exposure to domestic pets [88]

• increasing use of antibiotics [89]

Use of probiotics (may decrease risk) [65]

Risk of food allergy

Fig. 2. Factors that may increase the risk of IgE-mediated food allergy.

The Impact of Gastrointestinal Flora Composition

The composition of the gastrointestinal flora in infancy is affected by various factors, but because the fetal intestine is sterile the initial colonizing events in the infant are likely to be highly important in governing the type of commensal bacteria present in the first few days of life and possibly longer. The initial colonizing event is likely to be influenced by mode of delivery, with infants delivered by caesarean section having less contact with maternal flora, which acts a source of intestinal bacteria for the newborn. It has been hypothesized that differences in colonization might lead to an increased risk of allergy among infants born by caesarean section.[64] It is possible that commensural bacteria in the gastrointestinal tract may exert an immunomodulatory effect that leads to tolerance to both the commensural bacteria themselves and also to ingested food allergens.

The demonstrated importance of gastrointestinal flora in the development of the gut immune system has led to multiple studies of the impact of probiotics on the prevention and treatment of allergic disease. A recent review of these studies concluded that there is currently no evidence that probiotics are effective in the treatment of eczema, despite early studies in small numbers of infants and children showing promising results.[65,66] Few studies have investigated whether probiotic supplementation aids in the development of tolerance among food allergic individuals. Those that do exist have not shown any protective effect. In preventing allergic disease, there is some evidence that probiotic supplementation may reduce the risk of eczema in those with a family history of allergic disease. Again, food allergy was less often studied and there is currently little evidence for a protective effect of probiotic supplementation in the prevention of food allergy.

The "Old Friends" Hypothesis

After the initial colonizing events at birth, the infant immune system continues to be exposed to stimulus not only from the commensural bacteria in the infant gastrointestinal tract but also from external sources. The "old friends" hypothesis states that the immune system evolved at a time of constant exposure to certain organisms in the environment, such as helminths and environmental saprophytes, found in food and water.[67] These organisms needed to be tolerated, either because they were harmless and ubiquitous (environmental saprophytes, such as some species of mycobacteria) or because mounting an immune response would damage the host (some helminths). It is thought that continued exposure to these organisms might have caused down-regulation of the immune response not only to these organisms but also to self-antigens (autoimmunity) and food allergens (food allergy), possibly through the induction of regulatory T cells. Reduced exposure to these groups of organisms in the modern environment could therefore potentially explain the rise in allergic diseases and autoimmunity.

Other factors associated with a "modern lifestyle" include a myriad of changes to the level of public health including improved sanitation; secure water supplies (with associated decreased prevalence of *Helicobacter pylori* infection); widespread use of antibiotics and increasing rates of immunization; decreased helminthic infestation; improved food quality (and presumably less microbial load in the food chain); and generally improved nutrition and associated obesity. These factors might work individually or in concert to affect a failure in the development of oral immune tolerance in the first year of life when development of IgE-mediated food allergy is most likely to occur.

Evidence for Change in the Timing of Introduction of Solids and the Impact on Food Allergy Prevalence

Along with changes in food quality and a likely decrease in the microbial content of foods, there have also been significant changes in the age at which foods are introduced to infants. The age at which infants were typically introduced to solids has varied from extremely delayed introduction (after 1 year) before the 1920s to introduction in the first 3 months of life in the 1950s.[68] This was followed by recommendations in the 1980s to delay solids until 4 to 6 months of age.[69] By the late 1990s, expert bodies began to recommend delaying solids until after 6 months of age, with further delay in the introduction of allergenic foods, such as egg and nuts, until at least 2 years of age recommended for infants with a family history of allergy.[70] Recently revised guidelines from Europe, the United States, and Australia now state that there are no data to support the delay of introduction of allergenic solids in an infant's diet for the prevention of allergic disease.[71]

Recent attempts to study the relationship between timing of introduction of foods and food allergy have led to the suggestion that delayed introduction of allergenic foods may actually prevent the normal development of tolerance that occurs when foods are introduced during a "window of opportunity" in early infancy.[72] This was initially based on the observation that Israeli infants are introduced to peanut at a young age yet Israeli schoolchildren experience a low prevalence of peanut allergy, whereas the opposite is observed in the United Kingdom.[73] Early studies examining this issue were unable to rule out confounding factors as an explanation for the increased risk of food sensitization and allergy among infants with delayed introduction of foods.[74] As such these studies could be biased by "reverse causation," such that introduction of allergenic foods is preferentially delayed in infants who are already at increased risk of food allergy, either because of signs of allergy, such as eczema in the child, or because of a family history of allergy.

Recently, the relationship between timing of introduction of egg and risk of egg allergy was explored in the HealthNuts population-based study of infants. Those introduced to egg after 10 months of age were more likely to be egg allergic at 1 year compared with those introduced to egg at 4 to 6 months, even after controlling for family and personal history of allergy.[75] Consumption of cooked egg seemed to be more protective than consumption of egg in baked goods. This may suggest that dose and timing of introduction is important in the development of tolerance, an area that requires further investigation. The relationship between timing of introduction of cow's milk formula and risk of milk allergy has also been recently studied. In a study of 13,234 newborn infants in Israel, those introduced to cow's milk formula in the first 14 days of life were significantly less likely to develop symptoms of cow's milk allergy compared with infants first exposed to cow's milk formula between 15 and 194 days. However, the authors were unable to control for important potential confounding factors, such as socioeconomic status and atopic background.[76] Randomized controlled trials of early introduction of allergenic foods are currently underway exploring the relationship between timing of exposure and allergy.

Vitamin D Status

Recently, data have emerged demonstrating a latitude gradient in prevalence of food allergy, with those countries furthest from the equator recording the highest admissions to hospital for food allergy–related events,[33] prescriptions for adrenaline autoinjectors for the treatment of anaphylaxis,[31,32] and prescription of hypoallergenic infant formula.[77] These findings seem to be independent of longitude, physician density, or socioeconomic status. The authors have recently confirmed that Melbourne, the most southern major city in Australia, has the highest reported prevalence of infantile food allergy in the world with more than 10% of 1-year-old infants recruited from the general population having challenge-proved IgE-mediated food allergy.[18]

Because regions most distant from the equator are exposed to less ultraviolet radiation, one postulated explanation for the link between latitude and risk of food allergy is that low vitamin D levels in early life may be causing food allergy.[78] Further evidence to support this contention is the recent finding that children attending emergency departments in Boston with a food-related acute allergic reaction were more likely to be born in autumn and winter, when vitamin D levels reach their nadir, than in spring and summer.[79] This relationship between season of birth and food allergy has recently been confirmed in the Southern hemisphere.[80] Furthermore, the authors have recently demonstrated that the delayed introduction of egg, one of the richest sources of vitamin D in the infant diet,[81] in the first year of life increases the risk of developing egg allergy by at least fivefold independent of potential confounders.[75] One study has also reported that serum vitamin D deficiency is more common among children with peanut sensitization.[82]

SUMMARY

The last few years has seen an increased focus on better defining the prevalence of food allergy and studies are now emerging that attempt to understand the drivers of the rise in prevalence. As for other allergic diseases, the cause of the rise in food allergy is likely to be multifactorial. Improved precision about measurement of food allergy outcomes and epidemiologic exposures and the advent of improved epigenetic methodology is likely to accelerate the uncovering of putative causative factors.

REFERENCES

1. Sicherer SH, Munoz-Furlong A, Sampson HA. Prevalence of peanut and tree nut allergy in the United States determined by means of a random digit dial telephone survey: a 5-year follow-up study. J Allergy Clin Immunol 2003;112:1203–7.
2. Liew WK, Williamson E, Tang ML. Anaphylaxis fatalities and admissions in Australia. J Allergy Clin Immunol 2009;123:434–42.
3. Chen J, Hu Y, Allen KJ, et al. The prevalence of food allergy in infants in Chongqing, China. Pediatr Allergy Immunol 2011;22:356–60.
4. Schafer T, Bohler E, Ruhdorfer S, et al. Epidemiology of food allergy/food intolerance in adults: associations with other manifestations of atopy. Allergy 2001;56: 1172–9.
5. Sampson HA. Food allergy: accurately identifying clinical reactivity. Allergy 2005; 60(Suppl 79):19–24.
6. Prasad GA, Alexander JA, Schleck CD, et al. Epidemiology of eosinophilic esophagitis over three decades in Olmsted County, Minnesota. Clin Gastroenterol Hepatol 2009;7:1055–61.
7. Cook B, Oxner R, Chapman B, et al. A thirty-year (1970-1999) study of coeliac disease in the Canterbury region of New Zealand. N Z Med J 2004;117:U772.
8. Ho MH, Wong WH, Heine RG, et al. Early clinical predictors of remission of peanut allergy in children. J Allergy Clin Immunol 2008;121:731–6.
9. Rona RJ, Keil T, Summers C, et al. The prevalence of food allergy: a meta-analysis. J Allergy Clin Immunol 2007;120:638–46.

10. Allen KJ, Koplin JJ. The epidemiology of food allergy. In: Burks W, James JM, Eigenmenn P, editors. Food allergy. Edinburgh, London, New York, Oxford, Philadelphia, St Louis, Sydney, Toronto: Elsevier Saunders; 2012. p. 31–46.
11. Koplin JJ, Tang ML, Martin PE, et al. Predetermined challenge eligibility and cessation criteria for oral food challenges in the HealthNuts population-based study of infants. J Allergy Clin Immunol 2011. [Epub ahead of print].
12. Osborne NJ, Koplin JJ, Martin PE, et al. The HealthNuts population-based study of paediatric food allergy: validity, safety and acceptability. Clin Exp Allergy 2010; 40:1516–22.
13. Sporik R, Hill DJ, Hosking CS. Specificity of allergen skin testing in predicting positive open food challenges to milk, egg and peanut in children. Clin Exp Allergy 2000;30:1540–6.
14. Celik-Bilgili S, Mehl A, Verstege A, et al. The predictive value of specific immuno-globulin E levels in serum for the outcome of oral food challenges. Clin Exp Allergy 2005;35:268–73.
15. Chafen JJ, Newberry SJ, Riedl MA, et al. Diagnosing and managing common food allergies: a systematic review. JAMA 2010;303:1848–56.
16. Eller E, Kjaer HF, Host A, et al. Food allergy and food sensitization in early child-hood: results from the DARC cohort. Allergy 2009;64:1023–9.
17. Venter C, Pereira B, Voigt K, et al. Prevalence and cumulative incidence of food hypersensitivity in the first 3 years of life. Allergy 2008;63:354–9.
18. Osborne NJ, Koplin JJ, Martin PE, et al. Prevalence of challenge-proven IgE-mediated food allergy using population-based sampling and predetermined challenge criteria in infants. J Allergy Clin Immunol 2011;127:668–76.
19. Prescott S, Allen KJ. Food allergy: riding the second wave of the allergy epidemic. Pediatr Allergy Immunol 2011;22:155–60.
20. Sampson HA, Munoz-Furlong A, Campbell RL, et al. Second symposium on the definition and management of anaphylaxis: summary report. Second National Institute of Allergy and Infectious Disease/Food Allergy and Anaphylaxis Network symposium. J Allergy Clin Immunol 2006;117:391–7.
21. Tang ML, Osborne N, Allen K. Epidemiology of anaphylaxis. Curr Opin Allergy Clin Immunol 2009;9:351–6.
22. Gupta R, Sheikh A, Strachan DP, et al. Time trends in allergic disorders in the UK. Thorax 2007;62:91–6.
23. Decker WW, Campbell RL, Manivannan V, et al. The etiology and incidence of anaphylaxis in Rochester, Minnesota: a report from the Rochester Epidemiology Project. J Allergy Clin Immunol 2008;122:1161–5.
24. Bock SA, Munoz-Furlong A, Sampson HA. Fatalities due to anaphylactic reac-tions to foods. J Allergy Clin Immunol 2001;107:191–3.
25. Pumphrey RS, Gowland MH. Further fatal allergic reactions to food in the United Kingdom, 1999-2006. J Allergy Clin Immunol 2007;119:1018–9.
26. Asero R, Antonicelli L, Arena A, et al. Causes of food-induced anaphylaxis in Italian adults: a multi-centre study. Int Arch Allergy Immunol 2009;150:271–7.
27. Prieto A, Razzak E, Lindo DP, et al. Recurrent anaphylaxis due to lupin flour: primary sensitization through inhalation. J Investig Allergol Clin Immunol 2010; 20:76–9.
28. Koplin JJ, Martin PE, Allen KJ. An update on epidemiology of anaphylaxis in chil-dren and adults. Curr Opin Allergy Clin Immunol 2011;11:492–6.
29. Iribarren C, Tolstykh IV, Miller MK, et al. Asthma and the prospective risk of anaphylactic shock and other allergy diagnoses in a large integrated health care delivery system. Ann Allergy Asthma Immunol 2010;104:371–7.

30. Gonzalez-Perez A, Aponte Z, Vidaurre CF, et al. Anaphylaxis epidemiology in patients with and patients without asthma: a United Kingdom database review. J Allergy Clin Immunol 2010;125:1098–104.e1.
31. Mullins RJ, Clark S, Camargo CA Jr. Regional variation in epinephrine autoinjector prescriptions in Australia: more evidence for the vitamin D-anaphylaxis hypothesis. Ann Allergy Asthma Immunol 2009;103:488–95.
32. Camargo CA Jr, Clark S, Kaplan MS, et al. Regional differences in EpiPen prescriptions in the United States: the potential role of vitamin D. J Allergy Clin Immunol 2007;120:131–6.
33. Rudders SA, Espinola JA, Camargo CA Jr. North-south differences in US emergency department visits for acute allergic reactions. Ann Allergy Asthma Immunol 2010;104:413–6.
34. Sheehan WJ, Graham D, Ma L, et al. Higher incidence of pediatric anaphylaxis in northern areas of the United States. J Allergy Clin Immunol 2009;124:850–2.e2.
35. Pumphrey R. Anaphylaxis: can we tell who is at risk of a fatal reaction? Curr Opin Allergy Clin Immunol 2004;4:285–90.
36. Venter C, Hasan Arshad S, Grundy J, et al. Time trends in the prevalence of peanut allergy: three cohorts of children from the same geographical location in the UK. Allergy 2010;65:103–8.
37. Sicherer SH, Munoz-Furlong A, Godbold JH, et al. US prevalence of self-reported peanut, tree nut, and sesame allergy: 11-year follow-up. J Allergy Clin Immunol 2010;125:1322–6.
38. Sicherer SH, Furlong TJ, Maes HH, et al. Genetics of peanut allergy: a twin study. J Allergy Clin Immunol 2000;106:53–6.
39. Tsai H-J, Kumar R, Pongracicwz J, et al. Familial aggregation of food allergy and sensitization to food allergens: a family-based study. Clin Exp Allergy 2009;39:101–9.
40. Hill DJ, Hosking CS, de Benedictis FM, et al. Confirmation of the association between high levels of immunoglobulin E food sensitization and eczema in infancy: an international study. Clin Exp Allergy 2008;38:161–8.
41. Irvine A. Fleshing out filaggrin phenotypes. J Invest Dermatol 2007;127:504–7.
42. Marenholz I, Nickel R, Rüschendorf F, et al. Filaggrin loss-of-function mutations predispose to phenotypes involved in the atopic march. J Allergy Clin Immunol 2006;118:866–71.
43. Brown SJ, Asai Y, Cordell HJ, et al. Loss-of-function variants in the filaggrin gene are a significant risk factor for peanut allergy. J Allergy Clin Immunol 2011;127:661–7.
44. Lack G, Fox D, Northstone K, et al. Factors associated with the development of peanut allergy in childhood. N Engl J Med 2008;348:977–85.
45. Fox AT, Sasieni P, du Toit G, et al. Household peanut consumption as a risk factor for the development of peanut allergy. J Allergy Clin Immunol 2009;123:417–23.
46. Strid J, Hourihane J, Kimber I, et al. Epicutaneous exposure to peanut protein prevents oral tolerance and enhances allergic sensitization. Clin Exp Allergy 2005;35:757–66.
47. Chen W, Mempel M, Schober W, et al. Gender difference, sex hormones, and immediate type hypersensitivity reactions. Allergy 2008;63:1418–27.
48. Carey MA, Card JW, Voltz JW, et al. It's all about sex: gender, lung development and lung disease. Trends Endocrinol Metab 2007;18:308–13.
49. Almqvist C, Worm M, Leynaert B. Impact of gender on asthma in childhood and adolescence: a GA2LEN review. Allergy 2008;63:47–57.
50. Dias RP, Summerfield A, Khakoo GA. Food hypersensitivity among caucasian and non-caucasian children. Pediatr Allergy Immunol 2008;19:86–9.

51. Branum AM, Lukacs SL. Food allergy among children in the United States. Pediatrics 2009;124:1549–55.
52. Dharmage SC, Martin PE, Osborne NJ, et al. The Epidemiology of Food Sensitization-Associated Eczema in Infancy in HealthNuts, a population-based study. J Allergy Clin Immunol 2011;127(Suppl):AB35.
53. Martino DJ, Prescott SL. Silent mysteries: epigenetic paradigms could hold the key to conquering the epidemic of allergy and immune disease. Allergy 2010; 65:7–15.
54. Tan TH, Ellis JA, Saffery R, et al. The role of genetics and environment in the rise of childhood food allergy. Clin Exp Allergy 2011. [Epub ahead of print].
55. Holt PG, Upham JW, Sly PD. Contemporaneous maturation of immunologic and respiratory functions during early childhood: implications for development of asthma prevention strategies. J Allergy Clin Immunol 2005;116:16–24.
56. Strachan DP. Hay fever, hygiene, and household size. BMJ 1989;299:1259–60.
57. Celedon JC, Litonjua AA, Weiss ST, et al. Day care attendance in the first year of life and illnesses of the upper and lower respiratory tract in children with a familial history of atopy. Pediatrics 1999;104:495–500.
58. Koopman LP, Smit HA, Heijnen ML, et al. Respiratory infections in infants: interaction of parental allergy, child care, and siblings. The PIAMA study. Pediatrics 2001;108:943–8.
59. Heinrich J, Gehring U, Douwes J, et al. Pets and vermin are associated with high endotoxin levels in house dust. Clin Exp Allergy 2001;31:1839–45.
60. Waser M, Schierl R, von Mutius E, et al. Determinants of endotoxin levels in living environments of farmers' children and their peers from rural areas. Clin Exp Allergy 2004;34:389–97.
61. Adlerberth I, Lindberg E, Aberg N, et al. Reduced enterobacterial and increased staphylococcal colonization of the infantile bowel: an effect of hygienic lifestyle? Pediatr Res 2005;59:96–101.
62. Gronlund MM, Lehtonen OP, Eerola E, et al. Fecal microflora in healthy infants born by different methods of delivery: permanent changes in intestinal flora after cesarean delivery. J Pediatr Gastroenterol Nutr 1999;28:19–25.
63. Penders J, Thijs C, Vink C, et al. Factors influencing the composition of the intestinal microbiota in early infancy. Pediatrics 2006;118:511–21.
64. Koplin J, Allen K, Gurrin L, et al. Is caesarean delivery associated with sensitization to food allergens and IgE-mediated food allergy: a systematic review. Pediatr Allergy Immunol 2008;19:682–7.
65. Tang ML, Lahtinen SJ, Boyle RJ. Probiotics and prebiotics: clinical effects in allergic disease. Curr Opin Pediatr 2010;22:626–34.
66. Allen K. Probiotics in infant formulas. Paediatrics & Child Health in General Practice 2011;12(September):26.
67. Rook GA. Hygiene and other early childhood influences on the subsequent function of the immune system. Dig Dis 2011;29:144–53.
68. Committee on Nutrition. On the feeding of solid foods to infants. Pediatrics 1958; 21:685–92.
69. Barnes LA, Dallman PR, Anderson H, et al. American Academy of Pediatrics: Committee on Nutrition. On the feeding of supplemental foods to infants. Pediatrics 1980;65:1178–81.
70. American Academy of Pediatrics Committee on Nutrition. Hypoallergenic infant formulas. Pediatrics 2000;106:346–9.
71. Greer FR, Sicherer SH, Burks AW. Effects of early nutritional interventions on the development of atopic disease in infants and children: the role of maternal dietary

restriction, breastfeeding, timing of introduction of complementary foods, and hydrolyzed formulas. Pediatrics 2008;121:183–91.

72. Prescott SL, Smith P, Tang M, et al. The importance of early complementary feeding in the development of oral tolerance: concerns and controversies. Pediatr Allergy Immunol 2008;19:375–80.

73. Du Toit G, Katz Y, Sasieni P, et al. Early consumption of peanuts in infancy is associated with a low prevalence of peanut allergy. J Allergy Clin Immunol 2008;122: 984–91.

74. Poole JA, Barriga K, Leung DY, et al. Timing of initial exposure to cereal grains and the risk of wheat allergy. Pediatrics 2006;117:2175–82.

75. Koplin JJ, Osborne NJ, Wake M, et al. Can early introduction of egg prevent egg allergy in infants? A population-based study. J Allergy Clin Immunol 2010;126: 807–13.

76. Katz Y, Rajuan N, Goldberg MR, et al. Early exposure to cow's milk protein is protective against IgE-mediated cow's milk protein allergy. J Allergy Clin Immunol 2010;126:77–82.e1.

77. Mullins RJ, Clark S, Camargo CA Jr. Regional variation in infant hypoallergenic formula prescriptions in Australia. Pediatr Allergy Immunol 2010;21:e413–20.

78. Vassallo MF, Camargo CA Jr. Potential mechanisms for the hypothesized link between sunshine, vitamin D, and food allergy in children. J Allergy Clin Immunol 2010;126:217–22.

79. Vassallo MF, Banerji A, Rudders SA, et al. Season of birth and food-induced anaphylaxis in Boston. Allergy 2010;65:1492–3.

80. Mullins RJ, Clark S, Katelaris C, et al. Season of birth and childhood food allergy in Australia. Pediatr Allergy Immunol 2010;22:583–9.

81. Lowdon J. Getting bone health right from the start! Pregnancy, lactation and weaning. J Fam Health Care 2008;18:137–41.

82. Sharief S, Jariwala S, Kumar J, et al. Vitamin D levels and food and environmental allergies in the United States: results from the National Health and Nutrition Examination Survey 2005-2006. J Allergy Clin Immunol 2011;127:1195–202.

Can We Prevent Food Allergy by Manipulating the Timing of Food Exposure?

Kirsi M. Järvinen, MD, PhD[a],*, David M. Fleischer, MD[b]

KEYWORDS

- Peanut allergy • Cow's milk allergy • Egg allergy
- Food-specific IgE • Skin-prick test • Food introduction
- Food allergy • Diagnosis

Food allergy is defined as an adverse health effect arising from a specific immune response that is reproducible on exposure to a given food, and thus is an example of a defect in the development or a breakdown in the maintenance of oral tolerance. Little is known regarding which variables are important for the induction or failure of oral tolerance in the neonatal period. Investigations into the underlying mechanisms of neonatal oral tolerance in rodents have demonstrated that antigen administration directly after birth or within 5 to 7 days does not lead to suppression of systemic immunity but primes for subsequent humoral and delayed hypersensitivity responses.[1,2] Antigen transfer from breast milk induces tolerance in the young, although the antigen dose required for tolerance induction is 2 to 3 log steps lower.[3]

Clinically, the prevalence of food allergy has increased. Peanut allergy has dramatically increased in children within the last decade, with more than 1% of school children in the United States, United Kingdom, Canada, and Australia affected.[4–7] The previous advice by the American Academy of Pediatrics (AAP)[8] in 2000 was for breast-feeding mothers of high-risk infants to strictly avoid peanut and tree nuts and to consider elimination of cow's milk, egg, fish, and possibly other foods during lactation. The AAP went on to recommend that solid foods should not be started until 6 months of age, with dairy products not introduced until age 1 year, eggs until 2 years, and peanut, tree nuts, and fish until 3 years of age. These feeding guidelines were revised

[a] Division of Allergy and Immunology and Center for Immunology and Microbial Diseases, Albany Medical College, 47 New Scotland Avenue MC # 151, Albany, NY 12208, USA
[b] Division of Pediatric Allergy and Immunology, National Jewish Health, 1400 Jackson Street, J321, Denver, CO 80206, USA
* Corresponding author.
E-mail address: jarvink@mail.amc.edu

Immunol Allergy Clin N Am 32 (2012) 51–65
doi:10.1016/j.iac.2011.11.007   immunology.theclinics.com

in 2008 to avoid the strong recommendations on whether foods of high allergenic potential should be ingested during pregnancy, lactation, and infancy (**Table 1**).[9] The revision resulted from the controversy in the literature regarding the impact of maternal avoidance diets on food allergy prevention and the lack of information on what is the correct age to introduce foods of high allergenic potential to infants and toddlers.[10–13] This review provides a careful evaluation of the rationale and existing data on whether the manipulation of the timing of specific food exposures in the diet during pregnancy, lactation, and early childhood affects the development of food allergies in high-risk children.

BIOLOGICAL RATIONALE FOR TOLERANCE DEVELOPMENT ANTENATALLY AND POSTNATALLY

The normal development of immunologic tolerance is poorly understood. Most children become tolerant to common allergens, and a normal response to exposure is

Table 1
Summary of effects of nutritional interventions during pregnancy, lactation, and infancy on the development of atopy

Intervention	Evidence
Restriction diet during pregnancy	No evidence in prevention of atopic diseases
Restriction diet during lactation	No evidence in prevention of atopic diseases with the possible exception of atopic eczema
Length of exclusive breastfeeding	Exclusive breastfeeding for at least 4 months decreases the cumulative incidence of atopic dermatitis and cow's milk allergy in the first 2 years of life in infants at high risk of developing atopic disease Exclusive breastfeeding for at least 3 months protects against wheezing in early life
Use of hydrolyzed formulas	Modest evidence that atopic dermatitis may be delayed or prevented by the use of hydrolyzed formulas in early childhood in infants at high risk of developing atopic disease. Extensively hydrolyzed formulas may be more effective than partially hydrolyzed formulas in the prevention of atopic disease
Use of soy-based formulas	No evidence in allergy prevention
Timing of introduction of solid foods	No current convincing evidence that delaying introduction of solid food, including highly allergic foods such as fish, eggs, and foods containing peanut protein, beyond 4–6 months has a significant protective effect on the development of atopic disease. In infants after 4–6 months of age, there are insufficient data to support a protective effect of any dietary intervention for the development of atopic disease

Modified from Greer FR, Sicherer SH, Burks AW. American Academy of Pediatrics Committee on Nutrition, American Academy of Pediatrics Section on Allergy and Immunology. Effects of early nutritional interventions on the development of atopic disease in infants and children: the role of maternal dietary restriction, breastfeeding, timing of introduction of complementary foods, and hydrolyzed formulas. Pediatrics 2008;121(1):183–91.

production of immunoglobulin G (IgG) as opposed to IgE antibodies, reflecting a T-helper type 1 (Th1)-skewed immune response. Immunologic tolerance can develop during early T-cell development in the thymus during which T cells, which respond to self-antigens, are deleted by "negative selection" (central tolerance) or later in the circulation (peripheral tolerance). Inflammatory signals are required to elicit antigen-presenting cell (APC) activation and expression of costimulatory molecules to activate T cells, but in the absence of APC costimulation, potentially reactive T cells fail to respond and undergo clonal deletion by apoptosis.[14] However, the processes responsible for tolerance to food allergens are still poorly understood.

Initial immune responses to food allergens are detectable in fetal life, although their significance is still unclear. The ability of the fetus or newborn to respond to antigenic stimuli changes gradually with the maturation of the immune system. IgE production starts at 11 weeks of age,[15] but total IgE is still low (<1 kU/L) at birth[16]; cord blood–specific IgE can be detectable, but is also very low.[17] Most infants show early transient lymphoproliferation, and IgG antibody responses to food allergens are typically detected.[18,19] Also, a transient early IgE response is seen in many nonatopic children, whereas a prolonged, enhanced response is associated with atopy[20,21] and Th2 cytokine production.[21] The factors responsible for abrogation in some infants versus enhancement of IgE production in others are still not fully understood.

The current hypothesis is that the Th2-biased milieu of pregnancy[22] is typically redirected toward the Th1 (IgG) response postnatally in a normal situation. In those with an atopic predisposition the immune responses remain Th2 dominant (IgE).[23] After birth, maturation of Th1 immune function probably prevents persisting Th2 responses and subsequent allergic disease. Consistent with this, an association between neonatal Th1 immaturity, delayed production of interferon-δ and atopic risk has been reported.[24–26] Levels of soluble CD14, which may be responsible for downregulation of IgE production by B cells within the lymphoid follicles of the gastrointestinal tract, are lower in amniotic fluid in children who later develop atopic disease.[27] Soluble CD14, and therefore reduced soluble CD14, may predispose to a continued Th2 dominant balance. Food-specific cytokine and IgG antibody responses that are present in early infancy tend to persist,[21] which also speaks for a switch from Th2 (IgE) to Th1 (IgG) dominance.

Immaturity of APC function[28] results in low pro-Th1 cytokine (interleukin-12) production and thereby contributes to the Th2-skewed immune response in infants.[29] However, neonatal APCs are also less efficient in providing T-cell costimulation, which is more likely to contribute to development of tolerance.[30,31] Influence by bacteria and bacterial products has been proposed to promote the switch from Th2 responses at birth to balanced Th responses in normal infants. There is evidence in animal models that bacterial colonization is essential for maturation of Th1 function and induction of oral tolerance,[32] and that bacterial endotoxin exposure can prevent allergic sensitization.[33]

FACTORS AFFECTING TOLERANCE DEVELOPMENT

The factors influencing induction of oral tolerance include external factors such as nature of antigen, dose, duration and time of introduction, and host factors such as genetic background, host immaturity, commensal flora, and antigen uptake.[34] However, the proportional and combined effects of individual components on systemic immunity may vary.

In earlier animal studies of cow's milk hypersensitivity, Li and colleagues[35] found that whereas 5-week-old mice were susceptible to sensitization with peanut, they were unable to sensitize mice of the same age to cow's milk, even in the presence of cholera toxin. Oral feeding of milk to younger mice of 2 to 3 weeks of age, however, induced moderate levels of IgE and immediate skin reactions (itching) after oral feeding of sensitized mice. The nature of antigen indeed plays a role in sensitization and likely also affects the ease of tolerance development. When compared with cow's milk, peanut is a special antigen in that it has innate immunity and complement-activating mechanisms[36,37] in addition to its clinically evident greater allergenicity. For the investigation of neonatal oral tolerance in animal models, hen's egg albumin (ovalbumin [OVA]) and bovine serum albumin have been used the most.

Animal models have suggested that both repeated and single doses of antigen can induce tolerance, but with different conditions and mechanisms. Feeding with repeated doses of a low-dose antigen every other day for 2 weeks is effective for IgG and IgE suppression.[38,39] Multiple low doses (approximately <0.1 mg/g body weight) are likely to generate antigen-specific regulatory cells.[40,41] Continuous exposure of antigen in the drinking water may lead to an even more profound tolerance, even for when the administered total antigen dose has been corrected.[42] A single dose of 1 mg per mouse is suppressive for IgG and cell-mediated responses by direct inactivation of T cells (clonal anergy),[40,41] whereas a dose ten-fold less was not, and a dose approximately 100-fold less results in priming for systemic and local cell-mediated responses.[38,39] Furthermore, although priming was observed after a single feed, repeated antigen administrations after a sensitizing feed are capable of suppressing immune responses (delayed-type hyperreactivity more affected than IgG), and multiple feeds with the same total antigen dose as a single feed are more likely to overcome the initial priming effect.[1,43]

The genetic background of the host plays a role in tolerance development. Infants at high risk for allergy and a target for prevention include those with at least one first-degree relative (parent or sibling) with a documented allergic condition.[9,44] The problem with this approach is that such populations include children with varying levels of risk for developing food allergy, including from those with a sibling with food allergy and those with a parent with allergic rhinitis, in whom the impact of these interventions may differ. These populations have been investigated for development of allergic diseases in studies of primary allergy prevention, but unselected populations have been less studied.

Maternal rather than paternal atopic status has a greater effect on the atopic outcome of the progeny.[45,46] Eczema or perennial rhinitis in the mother is associated with elevated cord blood IgE.[47] In mice offspring, breastfeeding has been shown to have a crucial role in tolerance induction using adoptive nursing models.[48–50] This finding raises the question of whether maternal factors such as immunologic constituents of breast milk and dietary exposure in utero and during lactation play a role in tolerance induction.

The remainder of this article focuses on the effect of age on the introduction of food antigens in tolerance development.

EFFECT OF TIMING OF FOOD EXPOSURE: PREGNANCY AND LACTATION
Experimental Models

Maternal exposure to dietary antigen during pregnancy and lactation has generally shown to be protective against specific IgE sensitization in offspring.[3,51–55] It has been proposed that the protective effect during pregnancy and lactation is dependent on the age at which the offspring are sensitized.[52]

Although more numerous animal studies have assessed perinatal exposure to an inhaled antigen, few studies have assessed the effect of oral antigen exposure during pregnancy and lactation, and those studies have used mothers who are either naïve or sensitized to the food in question. Some of these studies have been performed in asthma models assessing the effect of inhaled (or oral in one study) OVA exposure during lactation on the development of OVA sensitization and asthma in the offspring. Using naïve mothers, Polte and Hansen[49] showed that high-dose exposure during pregnancy was protective against sensitization to OVA. Fusaro and colleagues[52] proposed that the effect of feeding is dependent on the dose and timing, with only low-dose exposure being protective in pregnancy, and showed in utero allergen priming to occur. In their model, exposure during lactation to a higher amount of OVA in naïve mothers was protective only when pups were sensitized during the first 3 days of life. This finding is in disagreement with that of another similar study, which showed protection via a small dose exposure during lactation.[51] However, humans are rarely naïve to a food antigen, and production of food-specific IgA and IgG is a normal physiologic phenomenon following ingestion of food proteins such as peanut and OVA,[56] which may be an important additional vehicle for transfer of vertical tolerance in food allergy.

Studies addressing the effect of maternal perinatal antigen exposure in immunized (nonallergic) mothers are fewer and have used doses of inhaled OVA antigen,[54] but have likewise demonstrated tolerance induction in the offspring by feeding during pregnancy or lactation. These studies may be particularly relevant to humans because food-specific immunoglobulins, including IgG and IgA, are commonly found in healthy, nonallergic subjects. One study assessed the effect of OVA exposure in OVA-sensitized mothers on the development of OVA sensitization in the progeny.[53] Using food-antigen exposure in mothers who are sensitized to the antigen in question also poses a problem for translation of the results into a human situation whereby patients with food allergy strictly avoid the allergen. Most of these studies assessed maternal exposure via inhalation and systemic sensitization via the intraperitoneal route in the offspring, although the oral route is the major route of exposure in food allergy. A further limitation is that although some studies have measured IgE sensitization as an outcome, it is known that it is a poor measure of true clinical food allergy. Only one model thus far has assessed anaphylactic allergy to peanut. It was shown that maternal perinatal exposure to peanut resulted in protection against peanut anaphylaxis in the offspring.[55] The mothers were fed peanut together with cholera toxin, a mucosal adjuvant, which may have effects different from feeding antigen alone.

Strobel[3] analyzed the effects of antigen dose during different time points on induction of neonatal tolerance by maternal antigen transfer from breast milk. Suckling mothers were fed for 3 days with a high dose of OVA at several time points between delivery and 18 days of lactation (before weaning). In offspring immunized at 4 weeks of age, feeding mothers during the first 3 days of life demonstrated a lack of tolerance induction. Whereas gavaged animals received 1 mg/g body weight, suckling animals received a smaller dose of antigen that was in a range typically associated with sensitization/priming.[39] The timing of immune responses observed after administration of antigen from breast milk were comparable with those after direct antigen administration.

Human Studies

The US Dietary Prevention Program[10,11] was a randomized, prospective study including 288 subjects with one parent with atopy and sensitization. Subjects were randomized to either prophylaxis or no prophylaxis. Prophylaxis included the following: avoidance of milk, egg, and peanut during the third trimester of pregnancy and lactation; supplementation with casein hydrolyzate; and introduction of solid food at 6 months, with introduction of cow's milk, wheat, and soy at 12 months, egg at

24 months, and peanut and fish at 36 months. Subjects were followed to the age of 7 years. There was a decrease in food allergy in the prophylaxis group; however, milk allergy was responsible for the difference seen. By age 7 years, however, food allergy occurred at similar rates in both groups.

Based on various studies, especially the one by Zeiger and colleagues,[10,11] as well as expert opinion, the AAP Committee on Nutrition[8] made recommendations in 2000 for prevention aimed at families with a history of atopic disease, although the wording of the recommendations reflected the limitations in the studies ("may consider," and so forth). A more recent meta-analysis and another review of the literature both concluded, however, that maternal avoidance diets during pregnancy were not effective in preventing allergic diseases (eczema, asthma, allergic sensitization) in children.[57,58] The data on maternal diets during lactation are too few to make conclusions, although they may reduce the risk of atopic dermatitis during the first 1 to 2 years of life, but this effect is lost in childhood. These and other reports led the AAP to change the recommendations in 2008.[9]

There is great controversy in the literature regarding the impact of maternal diets on peanut allergy, however.[11–13] A case-control study from South Africa[12] included a standardized questionnaire, which assessed maternal peanut consumption more or less than once a week on the infant's peanut-IgE in 25 children younger than 3 years with peanut sensitization (cases) or 25 without peanut sensitization (milk or egg allergic controls). Higher consumption during pregnancy (odds ratio [OR] 3.97, 95% confidence interval [CI] 0.73-24, $P = .063$) but not during lactation (OR 2.19, CI 0.39-13.47, $P = .47$) was found in peanut-sensitized cases, although the population studied was quite small. Another case-control study from the United Kingdom comprised a telephone survey that assessed maternal peanut consumption (yes or no) during pregnancy and lactation on peanut allergy development assessed by double-blind, placebo-controlled food challenge in 23 subjects with peanut allergy (cases), and in 70 atopic and 140 nonatopic controls. During pregnancy 65% of mothers with a child with peanut allergy consumed peanut compared with 71% atopic and 61% nonatopic controls (not significant); during lactation, 17% of mothers with cases consumed peanut compared with 5% of atopic or nonatopic controls ($P = .03$, but not significant after adjustment).

Since these reports, 2 larger observational studies have created even more controversy. Du Toit and colleagues[59] suggested that more frequent and larger consumption of peanut during breastfeeding and in infancy was associated with a low prevalence of peanut allergy as seen in Jewish Israeli children (0.17%) compared with Jewish children in the United Kingdom (1.85%). On the contrary, observational data from the United States support the concept that exposure to peanut in pregnancy and lactation may not be tolerogenic; this includes a human cohort of 503 high-risk infants with milk or egg sensitization in whom frequent maternal peanut ingestion during pregnancy predisposed infants to peanut sensitization.[60] As a limitation, all the studies possess potential recall bias and no controlled human clinical trials are available. Furthermore, infant diet, which is typically linked to maternal diet, may be a confounding factor.

EFFECT OF TIMING OF FOOD EXPOSURE: INFANCY
Experimental Models

Strobel and colleagues[1,2] investigated the immune responses of neonates after a timed and standardized feed of OVA and bovine serum albumin to see whether tolerance development was affected by age of introduction. Neonatal suckling mice within one litter were fed a single feed of either a high dose of antigen or saline by gavage feeds in utero 2 days before birth and at different times until 90 days of age.

Immunization was performed at 4 weeks of age. The investigators demonstrated that there is a transition from priming to tolerance induction at around 7 to 10 days of age, affecting antibody and cell-mediated responses.

At weaning there is a rapid change of intestinal morphologic parameters. In mice, feeding antigen close to the day of weaning (around 21 days) leads to a temporary reduction in the ease of tolerance induction in the young adult mouse.[1] It seems that this inability to induce tolerance is not merely a result of the immaturity of the digestive system or antigen-handling capacity of the neonatal gut, but that this regulatory imbalance can be partially restored with adult spleen cells.[61]

Human Studies

Length of breastfeeding

There are a few studies that have examined the effects of breastfeeding on the development of food allergies. The results are likely affected by variables including the length and exclusivity of breastfeeding and presence of other atopic disorders. One review of 132 studies with 56 deemed "conclusive" determined that breastfeeding is protective of atopic diseases (asthma, recurrent wheezing, atopic dermatitis), but not of food allergy.[62] A more recent review, however, found that exclusive breastfeeding for at least 4 months was associated with a lower cumulative incidence of cow's milk allergy until 18 months of age.[57] Since these meta-analyses and reviews, several additional studies, all of which suffer from certain biases, support or refute these conclusions.[63–65]

Cow's milk protein

Human milk is the optimal source of nutrition for term infants during the first 6 months of life. Cow's milk allergy (CMA) is typically the first manifestation of an atopic constitution, due to the fact that cow's milk protein, in the form of cow's milk–based infant formulas, often provides the first exposure to a foreign protein in large quantities via the gastrointestinal route.

The risk of developing CMA in infants exposed to cow's milk protein early in life has been assessed. A total of 6209 unselected healthy, full-term infants, of whom 5385 (87%) required supplementary milk while in the hospital, were randomly assigned to receive cow's milk formula (1789 infants), pasteurized human milk (1859 infants), or whey hydrolyzate formula (1737 infants).[66] The comparison group (824 infants) was composed of infants who were exclusively breastfed. The infants were followed for 18 to 34 months for symptoms suggestive of CMA. As a result, the cumulative incidence of CMA in the infants fed cow's milk formula was 2.4% compared with 1.7% in the pasteurized human milk group (OR 0.70, 95% CI 0.44-1.12) and 1.5% in the whey hydrolyzate group (OR 0.61, 95% CI 0.38-1.00). In the comparison group, CMA developed in 2.1% of the infants. These data indicate that feeding of cow's milk at maternity hospitals increases the risk of CMA when compared with feeding of other supplements, but exclusive breastfeeding does not eliminate the risk.

On the contrary, another more recent study showed that early exposure in infancy (<14 days of age) to cow's milk protein via formula as a supplement to breastfeeding might protect against IgE-mediated CMA.[67] This large prospective study of 13,019 infants in Israel investigated, by telephone interview, the association of age of introduction of cow's milk formula and the development of CMA. All mothers were encouraged to breastfeed. It was noticed that introduction between 4 and 6 months of age was associated with the highest risk for CMA and before 15 days of life with least risk (OR 19.3, 95% CI 6-62.1). In the study, feeding formula on a daily basis was qualified as introduction of formula. Sporadic exposures, such as in a nursery, were not counted toward formula introduction, which may be a confounding factor. Symptoms after the start of formula were questioned but symptoms before initiation of formula feeding were not, which may have influenced feeding decisions, raising issues of potential reverse causality. Also, the amount needed to prevent allergy was not determined from the study. Furthermore, the incidence of CMA in this Israeli cohort was surprisingly low in comparison with other studies from Westernized countries, suggesting differences in patient population, potentially based on different genetic backgrounds.

Studies have also been performed to assess the effects of hydrolyzed formulas for the prevention of CMA when compared with breast milk.[66,68] These studies only examined early and short-term exposure to hydrolyzed formula, which did not seem to have any impact on the development of allergic disease. From a biological standpoint this is logical, as the levels of cow's milk allergens in hydrolyzed formulas are similar to those in breast milk, and therefore the infant's level of exposure is equivalent on both regimens.

The protective effects of partially hydrolyzed formulas (pHFs) in comparison with cow's milk-based formulas in preventing CMA have been studied as well. Comparing a partial whey hydrolyzate with cow's milk–based formula in 2 relatively small studies, Vandenplas and colleagues[69,70] found significantly lower prevalence of cow's milk sensitivity at 6 months based on skin-prick test in pHF-fed infants. In the 5-year prospective study, however, there was no new statistical difference between the 2 groups after 6 months unless new cases of cow's milk sensitivity were considered, suggesting the primary effect of the pHF had occurred during the first 6 months of life. In both studies there was an overall high prevalence of cow's milk sensitivity, likely due to less strict diagnostic criteria and selection bias.

The feeding of high-risk infants with a pHF as opposed to an extensively hydrolyzed formula (eHF) to prevent food allergy has been compared.[71,72] The combined analysis of 2 of these studies, with a total of 352 infants, found no significant difference in the incidence of infant food allergy. However, other studies have identified some differences between feeding with pHFs and eHFs.

The German Infant Nutritional Study followed 945 high-risk newborn infants in a randomized trial investigating the effects of breastfeeding supplemented with partially hydrolyzed whey formula (pHF-W), extensively hydrolyzed whey formula (eHF-W), or extensively hydrolyzed casein formula (eHF-C) in the first 4 months of life.[73,74] Mothers were encouraged to breastfeed exclusively for 4 months; however, about two-thirds in each formula group introduced study formula during the first month. Clinician diagnosis of any allergic disease (atopic dermatitis, food allergy, allergic urticaria, asthma, and allergic rhinitis) was significantly lower in the eHF-C and pHF-W groups at 3 and 6 years of age (eHF-C: OR 0.76, 95% confidence interval [CI] 0.63–0.93 and OR 0.80, 95% CI 0.69–0.93, respectively; pHF-W: OR 0.78, 95% CI 0.64–0.95 and OR 0.82, 95% CI 0.70–0.96, respectively). However, rates of urticaria, food allergy, and asthma were not affected at 3 years of age for any of the formulas.[74,75]

Solid food introduction

Several recent studies, most of which are population-based, prospective birth cohorts, do not support delaying the introduction of solid foods beyond 4 to 6 months for the prevention of allergic disease.[59,76–78] In one of these cohorts, 642 children were followed to the age of 5.5 years.[76–78] Data on the introduction of solids were collected during the first year of life. Results were corrected for parental asthma and atopy. Sixty-two percent of the children were ever breastfed, with 3 months as the median duration of breastfeeding. Rice was the first solid food introduced at a median age of 3 months, and milk and egg were introduced at 6 and 8 months, respectively. A follow-up at age 6 years[76] showed that the introduction of solid foods after 4 to 6 months was not associated with a decreased OR for asthma, allergic rhinitis, or sensitization against food or inhalant allergens at 6 years of age. In fact, food sensitization was more frequent in children who began solids later.

Joseph and colleagues[79] recently explored the relationship between introduction of complementary food at younger than 4 months (by interviews) and sensitization to egg, milk, and peanut allergen at 2 years in 594 maternal-infant pairs. In multivariable analysis, early feeding reduced the risk of peanut sensitization (serum specific IgE >0.35 IU/mL) among children with a parental history (adjusted OR 0.2, 95% CI 0.1–0.7; $P = .007$), but only for children with a parental history of asthma or allergy. The relationship also became significant for egg when a cutoff for IgE of greater than 0.70 IU/mL was used (adjusted OR 0.5, 95% CI 0.3–0.9; $P = .022$). A major limitation is that only food sensitization was assessed with low specific IgE cutoffs.

A study of 1612 children followed to the mean age of 4.7 years examined the association between cereal grain exposures (wheat, barley, rye, oats) in the infant diet and the development of wheat allergy.[80] The data demonstrated that delaying the introduction of cereal until after 6 months did not protect against the development of parent-reported wheat allergy (4 cases with wheat-specific IgE), but may actually increase the child's risk, even after controlling for family history of allergy, breastfeeding duration, any food allergy, and introduction of rice cereal. Limitations to the study were a low number of subjects with wheat allergy (1%) and that the study was performed in a population with HLA predisposition to diabetes and celiac disease.

Another study compared 2 cohorts of children with similar ethnic backgrounds, 1 in Israel and 1 in the United Kingdom.[59] The prevalence of peanut allergy in primary

Table 2
Recommended practical advice for feeding infants at high risk for allergy (ie, those with at least one first-degree relative with a documented allergic condition, especially moderate to severe atopic dermatitis, food allergy, or asthma)

Breastfeeding	For the minimum first 4–6 months
Supplementation	With partially[a] or extensively[b] hydrolyzed formula for the first 6 months if unable to exclusively breastfeed
Solid food introduction	At 4–6 months starting with yellow/orange vegetables, fruits, and baby cereals; then advance to meats and different-stage foods as appropriate for feeding skills
Highly allergenic foods	Egg, dairy products other than cow's milk per se, peanut, tree nuts, fish, and shellfish can be gradually introduced to infants who have already tolerated the introduction of less allergenic foods (although cow's milk should be avoided until 1 year of age for reasons unrelated to allergy). If, however, an infant has an allergic reaction to a food, or develops moderate to severe atopic dermatitis, or has a sibling with peanut allergy, then evaluation by an allergist is suggested to determine a personalized plan for food introduction

Examples of hypoallergenic formulas available in the United States:
[a] Partially hydrolyzed whey (cow's milk protein): Good Start Supreme (Nestlé USA, Glendale, CA). Partially hydrolyzed whey/casein (cow's milk protein): Enfamil Gentlease Lipil (Mead Johnson Nutritionals, Evansville, IN).
[b] Extensively hydrolyzed casein (cow's milk protein): Enfamil Nutramigen Lipil (Mead Johnson Nutritionals); Enfamil Pregestimil (Mead Johnson Nutritionals); Similac Alimentum Advance (Ross Products, Columbus, OH).

school children was assessed by one validated questionnaire (approximately 5000 children in each country). Peanut consumption in infants was assessed by a second validated questionnaire (77 children in the United Kingdom and 99 in Israel). The prevalence of peanut allergy was 1.85% in the United Kingdom and 0.17% in Israel. Peanut was introduced earlier and consumed both more frequently and in larger quantities in Israel than in the United Kingdom. A randomized trial is under way to determine whether early introduction of peanut is protective of peanut allergy (www.leapstudy.co.uk).

The HealthNuts study, which is a population-based, cross-sectional study of 2589 infants in Australia, assessed the effect of age of egg introduction and development of egg allergy.[81] The risk of developing egg allergy increased when egg was introduced after 6 months when compared with before 6 months, and the risk further increased the later egg was introduced (adjusted ORs 1.6, 95% CI 1-2.6, and 3.4, 95% 1.8-6.5, for introduction at 10-12 and after 12 months, respectively). Effects were seen in high-risk and low-risk infants with introduction of cooked egg. The type of egg introduction was also important, as cooked egg as opposed to baked egg appeared to have the greatest effect. Results were adjusted for confounding factors, and egg allergy was confirmed by an oral food challenge.

Taken collectively, these studies do not support delaying the introduction of solid foods beyond 4 to 6 months for the prevention of allergic disease. In fact, this practice may even increase the risk of allergy. Thus, general guidelines for introducing solid foods to an infant's diet are also appropriate for infants at high risk for allergic disease (Table 2).

SUMMARY

Prevention of food allergies by the alteration of maternal and infant feeding practices serves as a simple and cost-effective approach to address the increasing prevalence of food allergy in children. Although antigen exposure during pregnancy and lactation has been shown to be protective in animal models, such studies have mostly been performed in OVA-induced asthma models with inhalation exposure. Few have used models of food allergy, including peanut allergy, and these have used mothers that are either naïve or sensitized to the antigen in question. However, humans are rarely naïve to a food antigen, and production of food-specific IgA and IgG is a normal physiologic phenomenon following ingestion of food proteins, making translation of most data from existing experimental models to humans challenging. In the few clinical trials available, the modification of maternal diets during pregnancy and/or lactation does not seem to influence the risk of food allergy, with the possible exception of peanut allergy. In infant diets, clinical data suggest that the use of certain hydrolyzed formulas rather than cow's milk formula may affect the development of CMA. The most recent and compelling data may be for a critical timeframe for introduction of the highly allergenic solid foods to infants' diet, as emerging studies are showing that earlier introduction may be better in preventing allergy.

REFERENCES

1. Strobel S, Ferguson A. Immune responses to fed protein antigens in mice. 3. Systemic tolerance or priming is related to age at which antigen is first encountered. Pediatr Res 1984;18(7):588-94.
2. Strobel S, Mowat AM, Ferguson A. Prevention of oral tolerance induction to ovalbumin and enhanced antigen presentation during a graft-versus-host reaction in mice. Immunology 1985;56(1):57-64.

3. Strobel S. Immunity induced after a feed of antigen during early life: oral tolerance v. sensitisation. Proc Nutr Soc 2001;60(4):437–42.
4. Grundy J, Matthews S, Bateman B, et al. Rising prevalence of allergy to peanut in children: data from 2 sequential cohorts. J Allergy Clin Immunol 2002;110(5):784–9.
5. Mullins RJ, Dear KB, Tang ML. Characteristics of childhood peanut allergy in the Australian capital territory, 1995 to 2007. J Allergy Clin Immunol 2009;123(3): 689–93.
6. Ben-Shoshan M, Harrington DW, Soller L, et al. A population-based study on peanut, tree nut, fish, shellfish, and sesame allergy prevalence in Canada. J Allergy Clin Immunol 2010;125(6):1327–35.
7. Sicherer SH, Munoz-Furlong A, Godbold JH, et al. US prevalence of self-reported peanut, tree nut, and sesame allergy: 11-year follow-up. J Allergy Clin Immunol 2010;125(6):1322–6.
8. American academy of pediatrics. Committee on nutrition. hypoallergenic infant formulas. Pediatrics 2000;106(2 Pt 1):346–9.
9. Greer FR, Sicherer SH, Burks AW. American Academy of Pediatrics Committee on Nutrition, American Academy of Pediatrics Section on Allergy and Immunology. Effects of early nutritional interventions on the development of atopic disease in infants and children: the role of maternal dietary restriction, breastfeeding, timing of introduction of complementary foods, and hydrolyzed formulas. Pediatrics 2008;121(1):183–91.
10. Zeiger RS, Heller S, Mellon MH, et al. Effect of combined maternal and infant food-allergen avoidance on development of atopy in early infancy: a randomized study. J Allergy Clin Immunol 1989;84(1):72–89.
11. Zeiger RS, Heller S. The development and prediction of atopy in high-risk children: follow-up at age seven years in a prospective randomized study of combined maternal and infant food allergen avoidance. J Allergy Clin Immunol 1995;95(6):1179–90.
12. Frank L, Marian A, Visser M, et al. Exposure to peanuts in utero and in infancy and the development of sensitization to peanut allergens in young children. Pediatr Allergy Immunol 1999;10(1):27–32.
13. Lack G, Fox D, Northstone K, et al. Avon Longitudinal Study of Parents and Children Study Team. Factors associated with the development of peanut allergy in childhood. N Engl J Med 2003;348(11):977–85.
14. Matzinger P. Tolerance, danger, and the extended family. Annu Rev Immunol 1994;12:991–1045.
15. Punnonen J, Aversa GG, Vandekerckhove B, et al. Induction of isotype switching and Ig production by CD5+ and CD10+ human fetal B cells. J Immunol 1992; 148(11):3398–404.
16. Kjellman NI, Croner S. Cord blood IgE determination for allergy prediction–a follow-up to seven years of age in 1,651 children. Ann Allergy 1984;53(2):167–71.
17. Host A, Husby S, Gjesing B, et al. Prospective estimation of IgG, IgG subclass and IgE antibodies to dietary proteins in infants with cow milk allergy. Levels of antibodies to whole milk protein, BLG and ovalbumin in relation to repeated milk challenge and clinical course of cow milk allergy. Allergy 1992;47(3):218–29.
18. Prescott SL, Holt PG, Jenmalm M, et al. Effects of maternal allergen-specific IgG in cord blood on early postnatal development of allergen-specific T-cell immunity. Allergy 2000;55(5):470–5.
19. Jenmalm MC, Bjorksten B. Development of immunoglobulin G subclass antibodies to ovalbumin, birch and cat during the first eight years of life in atopic and non-atopic children. Pediatr Allergy Immunol 1999;10(2):112–21.

20. Hattevig G, Kjellman B, Johansson SG, et al. Clinical symptoms and IgE responses to common food proteins in atopic and healthy children. Clin Allergy 1984;14(6):551–9.

21. Ng TW, Holt PG, Prescott SL. Cellular immune responses to ovalbumin and house dust mite in egg-allergic children. Allergy 2002;57(3):207–14.

22. Lin H, Mosmann TR, Guilbert L, et al. Synthesis of T helper 2-type cytokines at the maternal-fetal interface. J Immunol 1993;151(9):4562–73.

23. Holt PG. Development of sensitization versus tolerance to inhalant allergens during early life. Pediatr Pulmonol Suppl 1997;16:6–7.

24. Prescott SL, Macaubas C, Smallacombe T, et al. Reciprocal age-related patterns of allergen-specific T-cell immunity in normal vs. atopic infants. Clin Exp Allergy 1998;28(Suppl 5):39–44 [discussion: 50–1].

25. Holt PG, Clough JB, Holt BJ, et al. Genetic 'risk' for atopy is associated with delayed postnatal maturation of T-cell competence. Clin Exp Allergy 1992;22(12): 1093–9.

26. Prescott SL, Macaubes C, Yabuhara A, et al. Developing patterns of T cell memory to environmental allergens in the first two years of life. Int Arch Allergy Immunol 1997;113(1–3):75–9.

27. Jones CA, Holloway JA, Popplewell EJ, et al. Reduced soluble CD14 levels in amniotic fluid and breast milk are associated with the subsequent development of atopy, eczema, or both. J Allergy Clin Immunol 2002;109(5):858–66.

28. Taylor S, Bryson YJ. Impaired production of gamma-interferon by newborn cells in vitro is due to a functionally immature macrophage. J Immunol 1985;134(3):1493–7.

29. Jankovic D, Kullberg MC, Hieny S, et al. In the absence of IL-12, CD4(+) T cell responses to intracellular pathogens fail to default to a Th2 pattern and are host protective in an IL-10(-/-) setting. Immunity 2002;16(3):429–39.

30. Ridge JP, Fuchs EJ, Matzinger P. Neonatal tolerance revisited: turning on newborn T cells with dendritic cells. Science 1996;271(5256):1723–6.

31. Pohl D, Bockelmann C, Forster K, et al. Neonates at risk of atopy show impaired production of interferon-gamma after stimulation with bacterial products (LPS and SEE). Allergy 1997;52(7):732–8.

32. Sudo N, Sawamura S, Tanaka K, et al. The requirement of intestinal bacterial flora for the development of an IgE production system fully susceptible to oral tolerance induction. J Immunol 1997;159(4):1739–45.

33. Tulic MK, Knight DA, Holt PG, et al. Lipopolysaccharide inhibits the late-phase response to allergen by altering nitric oxide synthase activity and interleukin-10. Am J Respir Cell Mol Biol 2001;24(5):640–6.

34. Strobel S, Mowat AM. Immune responses to dietary antigens: oral tolerance. Immunol Today 1998;19(4):173–81.

35. Li XM, Kleiner G, Huang CK, et al. Murine model of atopic dermatitis associated with food hypersensitivity. J Allergy Clin Immunol 2001;107(4):693–702.

36. Shreffler WG, Castro RR, Kucuk ZY, et al. The major glycoprotein allergen from *Arachis hypogaea*, Ara h 1, is a ligand of dendritic cell-specific ICAM-grabbing nonintegrin and acts as a Th2 adjuvant in vitro. J Immunol 2006;177(6):3677–85.

37. Khodoun M, Strait R, Orekov T, et al. Peanuts can contribute to anaphylactic shock by activating complement. J Allergy Clin Immunol 2009;123(2):342–51.

38. Mowat AL. The regulation of immune responses to dietary protein antigens. Immunol Today 1987;8(3):93–8.

39. Lamont AG, Mowat AM, Parrott DM. Priming of systemic and local delayed-type hypersensitivity responses by feeding low doses of ovalbumin to mice. Immunology 1989;66(4):595–9.

40. Melamed D, Friedman A. In vivo tolerization of Th1 lymphocytes following a single feeding with ovalbumin: anergy in the absence of suppression. Eur J Immunol 1994;24(9):1974–81.

41. Garside P, Steel M, Worthey EA, et al. T helper 2 cells are subject to high dose oral tolerance and are not essential for its induction. J Immunol 1995;154(11): 5649–55.

42. Melamed D, Fishman-Lovell J, Uni Z, et al. Peripheral tolerance of Th2 lymphocytes induced by continuous feeding of ovalbumin. Int Immunol 1996;8(5): 717–24.

43. Strobel S. Neonatal oral tolerance. Ann N Y Acad Sci 1996;778:88–102.

44. Muraro A, Dreborg S, Halken S, et al. Dietary prevention of allergic diseases in infants and small children. part I: immunologic background and criteria for hypoallergenicity. Pediatr Allergy Immunol 2004;15(2):103–11.

45. Martinez FD, Wright AL, Taussig LM, et al. Asthma and wheezing in the first six years of life. The Group Health Medical Associates. N Engl J Med 1995;332(3): 133–8.

46. Liu CA, Wang CL, Chuang H, et al. Prenatal prediction of infant atopy by maternal but not paternal total IgE levels. J Allergy Clin Immunol 2003;112(5):899–904.

47. Bjerke T, Hedegaard M, Henriksen TB, et al. Several genetic and environmental factors influence cord blood IgE concentration. Pediatr Allergy Immunol 1994; 5(2):88–94.

48. Okamoto Y, Freihorst J, Ogra PL. Maternal determinants of neonatal immune response to ovalbumin: effect of breast feeding on development of anti-ovalbumin antibody in the neonate. Int Arch Allergy Appl Immunol 1989;89(1): 83–9.

49. Polte T, Hansen G. Maternal tolerance achieved during pregnancy is transferred to the offspring via breast milk and persistently protects the offspring from allergic asthma. Clin Exp Allergy 2008;38(12):1950–8.

50. Matson AP, Thrall RS, Rafti E, et al. Breastmilk from allergic mothers can protect offspring from allergic airway inflammation. Breastfeed Med 2009;4(3):167–74.

51. Verhasselt V, Milcent V, Cazareth J, et al. Breast milk-mediated transfer of an antigen induces tolerance and protection from allergic asthma. Nat Med 2008; 14(2):170–5.

52. Fusaro AE, de Brito CA, Taniguchi EF, et al. Balance between early life tolerance and sensitization in allergy: dependence on the timing and intensity of prenatal and postnatal allergen exposure of the mother. Immunology 2009;128(Suppl 1): e541–50.

53. Mosconi E, Rekima A, Seitz-Polski B, et al. Breast milk immune complexes are potent inducers of oral tolerance in neonates and prevent asthma development. Mucosal Immunol 2010;3(5):461–74.

54. Matson AP, Zhu L, Lingenheld EG, et al. Maternal transmission of resistance to development of allergic airway disease. J Immunol 2007;179(2):1282–91.

55. Lopez-Exposito I, Song Y, Jarvinen KM, et al. Maternal peanut exposure during pregnancy and lactation reduces peanut allergy risk in offspring. J Allergy Clin Immunol 2009;124(5):1039–46.

56. Tay SS, Clark AT, Deighton J, et al. Patterns of immunoglobulin G responses to egg and peanut allergens are distinct: ovalbumin-specific immunoglobulin responses are ubiquitous, but peanut-specific immunoglobulin responses are up-regulated in peanut allergy. Clin Exp Allergy 2007;37(10):1512–8.

57. Muraro A, Dreborg S, Halken S, et al. Dietary prevention of allergic diseases in infants and small children. part III: critical review of published peer-reviewed

observational and interventional studies and final recommendations. Pediatr Allergy Immunol 2004;15(4):291–307.

58. Kramer MS, Kakuma R. Maternal dietary antigen avoidance during pregnancy or lactation, or both, for preventing or treating atopic disease in the child. Cochrane Database Syst Rev 2006;3:CD000133.

59. Du Toit G, Katz Y, Sasieni P, et al. Early consumption of peanuts in infancy is associated with a low prevalence of peanut allergy. J Allergy Clin Immunol 2008; 122(5):984–91.

60. Sicherer SH, Wood RA, Stablein D, et al. Maternal consumption of peanut during pregnancy is associated with peanut sensitization in atopic infants. J Allergy Clin Immunol 2010;126(6):1191–7.

61. Peng HJ, Turner MW, Strobel S. Failure to induce oral tolerance to protein antigens in neonatal mice can be corrected by transfer of adult spleen cells. Pediatr Res 1989;26(5):486–90.

62. van Odijk J, Kull I, Borres MP, et al. Breastfeeding and allergic disease: a multidisciplinary review of the literature (1966-2001) on the mode of early feeding in infancy and its impact on later atopic manifestations. Allergy 2003;58(9):833–43.

63. Matheson MC, Erbas B, Balasuriya A, et al. Breast-feeding and atopic disease: a cohort study from childhood to middle age. J Allergy Clin Immunol 2007; 120(5):1051–7.

64. Kramer MS, Matush L, Vanilovich I, et al. Effect of prolonged and exclusive breast feeding on risk of allergy and asthma: cluster randomised trial. BMJ 2007; 335(7624):815.

65. Laubereau B, Brockow I, Zirngibl A, et al. Effect of breast-feeding on the development of atopic dermatitis during the first 3 years of life—results from the GINI-birth cohort study. J Pediatr 2004;144(5):602–7.

66. Saarinen KM, Juntunen-Backman K, Jarvenpaa AL, et al. Supplementary feeding in maternity hospitals and the risk of cow's milk allergy: a prospective study of 6209 infants. J Allergy Clin Immunol 1999;104(2 Pt 1):457–61.

67. Katz Y, Rajuan N, Goldberg MR, et al. Early exposure to cow's milk protein is protective against IgE-mediated cow's milk protein allergy. J Allergy Clin Immunol 2010;126(1):77–82.e1.

68. Juvonen P, Mansson M, Andersson C, et al. Allergy development and macromolecular absorption in infants with different feeding regimens during the first three days of life. A three-year prospective follow-up. Acta Paediatr 1996;85(9):1047–52.

69. Vandenplas Y, Hauser B, Van den Borre C, et al. The long-term effect of a partial whey hydrolysate formula on the prophylaxis of atopic disease. Eur J Pediatr 1995;154(6):488–94.

70. Vandenplas Y, Hauser B, Van den Borre C, et al. Effect of a whey hydrolysate prophylaxis of atopic disease. Ann Allergy 1992;68(5):419–24.

71. Halken S, Hansen KS, Jacobsen HP, et al. Comparison of a partially hydrolyzed infant formula with two extensively hydrolyzed formulas for allergy prevention: a prospective, randomized study. Pediatr Allergy Immunol 2000;11(3):149–61.

72. Oldaeus G, Anjou K, Bjorksten B, et al. Extensively and partially hydrolysed infant formulas for allergy prophylaxis. Arch Dis Child 1997;77(1):4–10.

73. von Berg A, Koletzko S, Grubl A, et al. The effect of hydrolyzed cow's milk formula for allergy prevention in the first year of life: the German Infant Nutritional Intervention Study, a randomized double-blind trial. J Allergy Clin Immunol 2003;111(3): 533–40.

74. von Berg A, Koletzko S, Filipiak-Pittroff B, et al. Certain hydrolyzed formulas reduce the incidence of atopic dermatitis but not that of asthma: three-year

results of the German Infant Nutritional Intervention Study. J Allergy Clin Immunol 2007;119(3):718–25.

75. von Berg A, Filipiak-Pittroff B, Kramer U, et al. Preventive effect of hydrolyzed infant formulas persists until age 6 years: long-term results from the German Infant Nutritional Intervention Study (GINI). J Allergy Clin Immunol 2008;121(6): 1442–7.

76. Zutavern A, Brockow I, Schaaf B, et al. Timing of solid food introduction in relation to eczema, asthma, allergic rhinitis, and food and inhalant sensitization at the age of 6 years: results from the prospective birth cohort study LISA. Pediatrics 2008; 121(1):e44–52.

77. Zutavern A, Brockow I, Schaaf B, et al. Timing of solid food introduction in relation to atopic dermatitis and atopic sensitization: results from a prospective birth cohort study. Pediatrics 2006;117(2):401–11.

78. Zutavern A, von Mutius E, Harris J, et al. The introduction of solids in relation to asthma and eczema. Arch Dis Child 2004;89(4):303–8.

79. Joseph CL, Ownby DR, Havstad SL, et al. Early complementary feeding and risk of food sensitization in a birth cohort. J Allergy Clin Immunol 2011;127(5). 1203–10.e5.

80. Poole JA, Barriga K, Leung DY, et al. Timing of initial exposure to cereal grains and the risk of wheat allergy. Pediatrics 2006;117(6):2175–82.

81. Koplin JJ, Osborne NJ, Wake M, et al. Can early introduction of egg prevent egg allergy in infants? A population-based study. J Allergy Clin Immunol 2010;126(4): 807–13.

Eosinophilic Esophagitis: Diagnosis and Management

Jay A. Lieberman, MD[a], Mirna Chehade, MD, MPH[a,b],*

KEYWORDS

- Eosinophilic esophagitis • Diagnosis • Diet • Treatment
- Fluticasone • Budesonide • Food allergy

Eosinophilic esophagitis (EoE) represents a diagnostic and therapeutic challenge to many allergists and gastroenterologists alike. This challenge is evidenced by a recent survey, which demonstrated that practicing physicians currently use a wide array of diagnostic criteria and therapeutic strategies when caring for patients with suspected EoE, many of which are admittedly not based on the published consensus guidelines at the time.[1] Because EoE is a disease characterized by tissue eosinophilia, and because most patients with EoE demonstrate sensitization to environmental or food allergens, many patients will end up in the care of an allergist. It is, therefore, important that practicing allergists be familiar with the presentation, diagnosis, and available treatment options for EoE so that they can effectively work in conjunction with gastroenterologists to optimize patient care. In this article, the authors review the clinical characteristics and endoscopic and histologic findings that define EoE and discuss various available therapies for EoE.

DIAGNOSIS

EoE is not simply a histologic diagnosis based on set number of eosinophils populating the esophageal mucosa. Rather, EoE is a chronic, immune-mediated disease that is defined by multiple criteria: (1) symptoms suggestive of esophageal dysmotility; (2) histologic evidence of eosinophilia is limited to the esophagus (and not in other

Disclosures: The authors have no conflict of interest to disclose.

[a] Division of Allergy and Immunology, Department of Pediatrics, Mount Sinai School of Medicine, One Gustave L. Levy Place, New York, NY 10029, USA

[b] Mount Sinai Center for Eosinophilic Disorders, Jaffe Food Allergy Institute, Mount Sinai School of Medicine, One Gustave L. Levy Place, New York, NY 10029, USA

* Corresponding author. Mount Sinai School of Medicine, Box 1198, One Gustave L. Levy Place, New York, NY 10029.

E-mail address: mirna.chehade@mssm.edu

parts of the gastrointestinal tract), where finding 15 esophageal intraepithelial eosinophils per high power field (HPF) is accepted as the minimum threshold for diagnosis; (3) the esophageal eosinophilia should remit with certain exclusion diets or topical corticosteroid therapy; and (4) the esophageal eosinophilia should not be responsive to proton pump inhibitor (PPI) therapy alone.[2] With these criteria established, one can now examine the typical presentation, endoscopic appearance, and histologic findings that are typically associated with EoE.

Clinical Presentation

The classic, on-paper case presentation for EoE is that of a Caucasian man in his second or third decade of life who presents with dysphagia or food impaction. The reality is that EoE has a diverse clinical presentation. Although there is a male predominance of 2:1 to 3:1, EoE can present in all age groups.[3,4] Racial disparity is also described, with most patients being white, non-Hispanic. It is not yet clear, however, if this finding is simply the result of referral patterns to various reporting centers or caused by a genetic predisposition to the disease. In fact, a relatively recent study conducted at a US-based military medical center revealed a larger percentage of African American patients with EoE than previously reported.[5] However, there is current evidence that EoE has a strong familial association.[3,6] Based on a population prevalence for EoE of 5 per 10,000 people, the sibling recurrence ratio for EoE is estimated at around 80. By comparison, the ratio is around 2 for other atopic diseases, such as asthma.[7]

Symptoms

Age-related differences in presenting symptoms are noticed with EoE. In the pediatric population, patients with EoE typically present with abdominal pain; gastroesophageal reflux symptoms, including nausea and vomiting; and, at times, failure to thrive.[4,8] Discerning EoE from acid-induced gastroesophageal reflux disease (GERD) by symptoms alone can be difficult, although dysphagia and early satiety/anorexia in children seem to be more commonly seen in EoE than in GERD.[9,10] In infants and younger children, symptoms can be hard to delineate, and the disease may simply manifest as feeding difficulties, such as food refusal and gagging with foods.[11]

In the adult population, symptoms are slightly better defined, with dysphagia and heartburn/chest pain being the most common presenting symptoms.[4,12] In fact, when examining a cohort of patients with refractory reflux-type symptoms, dysphagia was the lone symptom that predicted EoE rather than GERD.[13] When one looks at cohorts of patients referred for endoscopy for the complaint of dysphagia, 12% to 15% of those patients were eventually diagnosed with EoE.[14,15] Thus, in adult patients presenting with dysphagia, EoE should be strongly considered in the differential diagnosis.

Perhaps the most concerning, and clearly the most urgent, symptom of EoE is food impaction, which can be the presenting symptom for some adults. In studies examining cohorts of patients with solid food impaction requiring endoscopic removal, approximately 50% of these patients were later identified as having EoE.[16,17] Whether food impaction is a common long-term complication for all patients with EoE, however, is difficult to assess. A recent survey-based follow-up study of a large population of patients with histologic evidence consistent with EoE demonstrated that at least self-reported food impaction is common in these patients, with an incidence as high as 40% at a median follow-up of 15 years.[18]

Endoscopic Findings

Various esophageal endoscopic abnormalities exist in patients with EoE. These abnormalities include esophageal rings (resulting in an appearance referred to as esophageal trachealization), whitish exudates or plaques, linear furrows, edema, and esophageal narrowing or strictures (**Fig. 1**). When present, these findings can be predictive of EoE[10,12,19] but are not pathognomonic for the disease. In fact, in 2 studies examining endoscopy and biopsy results for all patients referred for dysphagia, only 34% to 38% of the patients with the previously mentioned endoscopic findings were found to have histologic evidence of EoE; and in one of the studies, 10% of those patients with histologic evidence of EoE had a normal-appearing esophagus on endoscopy.[14,15] Thus, although EoE will typically demonstrate characteristic findings of esophageal disease on endoscopy, these are not diagnostic alone.

Histologic Findings

Number of eosinophils

Given the range of symptoms and endoscopic findings in EoE, histologic examination of esophageal tissue must be performed before a diagnosis of EoE can be established (**Fig. 2**). A simple quantitative assessment of the number of eosinophils per HPF in hematoxylin-eosin–stained esophageal tissue sections is helpful in establishing the

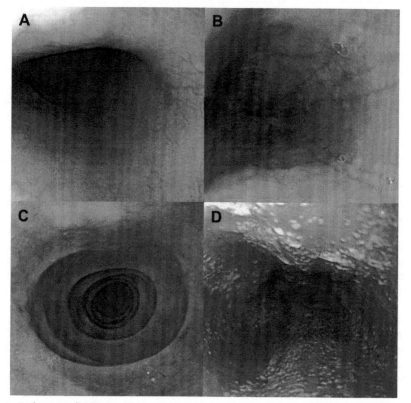

Fig. 1. Endoscopic findings in EoE. (*A*) Normal esophagus, (*B*) linear furrows, (*C*) esophageal rings, (*D*) white plaques.

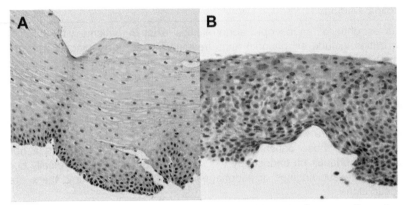

Fig. 2. Sections from endoscopically obtained esophageal biopsies (hematoxylin-eosin, original magnification × 200). (*A*) Esophageal epithelium in a healthy individual. (*B*) Esophageal epithelium in a patient with EoE.

diagnosis. The presence of at least 15 eosinophils per HPF in the maximally affected esophageal tissue samples is considered diagnostic.[2] This number, however, is not 100% specific for EoE because many other conditions can result in significant esophageal eosinophilia, especially severe GERD. Recent studies have shown that 39% to 75% of patients with esophageal eosinophilia (>15 per HPF) have resolution of their pathologic condition with PPI therapy alone.[20–22] Therefore, one needs to rule out PPI-responsive esophageal eosinophilia before diagnosing patients with EoE. This practice is typically done by an empiric therapy with a PPI at a high dose for 8 to 12 weeks before obtaining biopsies. An alternative to PPI therapy to rule out GERD is acid pH monitoring, but this procedure can be cumbersome and has limitations.[23]

When using the number of eosinophils as the histologic diagnostic criterion for EoE, one notices that a variety of methods have been used when establishing this value across studies and, therefore, not all data is comparable.[24,25] For example, using the average rather than the peak number of eosinophils per HPF may lead to a lower reported number of eosinophils per HPF. Variation in the number of endoscopic biopsies evaluated can also result in a different eosinophil count because EoE is a patchy disease, therefore, a lower number of biopsies may result in a lower sensitivity for diagnosis.[26] Finally, wide variations in the size of the high power field among microscopes have been reported, also affecting eosinophil counts.[24]

It should be noted that symptom severity does not seem to correlate with the extent of esophageal eosinophilia (ie, higher esophageal eosinophil counts do not translate to worse symptoms). Dysphagia is the only symptom that has been shown to have a positive correlation with the absolute number of esophageal eosinophils, although no validated symptom scores for EoE yet exist to evaluate this issue in depth.[9,27]

Other histologic markers

Given that quantitative assessment of eosinophils is not absolute in defining EoE, several studies have looked into additional histologic markers to better identify EoE. Pathologic changes, such as eosinophilic microabscesses and severe basal zone hyperplasia, are seen more often in tissue specimens from patients with EoE as compared with controls (including patients with GERD) and, therefore, can help distinguish EoE from other causes of esophageal eosinophilia.[28,29] Many studies have shown increases in extracellular staining of eosinophilic granules, such as major basic protein, eosinophil-derived neurotoxin, and eosinophil peroxidase, in patients with EoE as compared with healthy and GERD controls, suggesting that eosinophils may not merely be innocent bystanders in the disease process.[30–32] This eosinophilic degranulation likely plays a role in the development of subepithelial esophageal fibrosis, a long-term complication of EoE, and itself acting as a marker that, if present, also suggests a diagnosis of EoE over GERD.[33–35]

The examination of other cell types has shown that esophageal biopsies from patients with EoE have increased numbers of mast cells and increased tryptase staining in the esophageal epithelium[34,36–38] as well as increased lymphocytes.[39]

ALLERGY EVALUATION

It is thought that EoE is caused by multiple food allergens, based on several short-term studies resulting in disease remission in response to dietary eliminations.[40–42] The immunologic reaction underlying the role played by food antigens is thought to be a mix of immunoglobulin E (IgE)-mediated and non-IgE (cell mediated) hypersensitivity responses.[40] Results from skin prick testing (SPT) and atopy patch testing (APT) may help to identify foods that contribute to the disease process, and removal of identified foods can be an effective treatment,[43,44] although the sensitivity of these tests seems to be lower for foods not known to be common allergens (**Table 1**), rendering skin testing as a tool for guiding therapy no more effective than empiric elimination of common food allergens.[42,43]

In addition, prolonged avoidance of a food to which patients were sensitized but were previously ingesting without clinical reactions can result in the occurrence of systemic reactions on reintroduction of that food into the diet.[45,46] Therefore, if treating patients with an elimination or elemental diet, SPT or serum IgE testing may be advisable before reintroduction of foods to which sensitization was present, to better predict if patients are at risk for IgE-mediated clinical allergic reactions with the reintroduction of these foods.

Table 1						
Predictive values of SPT and APT in causing esophageal eosinophilia						
	SPT		**APT**		**SPT + APT**	
Food	**PPV (%)**	**NPV (%)**	**PPV (%)**	**NPV (%)**	**PPV (%)**	**NPV (%)**
Milk	96	58	83	59	92	41
Egg	85	75	78	83	85	88
Soy	70	69	67	87	74	93
Wheat	78	65	74	84	77	90
Corn	57	71	66	94	63	93
Beef	82	75	94	87	85	93
Chicken	50	83	67	96	63	99
Rice	50	86	59	97	61	100
Potato	60	90	54	95	61	97
Peanut	78	98	75	98	71	100
Oat	33	90	47	99	50	100
Barley	43	91	90	99	73	100

Abbreviations: NPV, negative predictive value; PPV, positive predictive value.
Data from Spergel JM, Brown-Whitehorn T, Beausoleil JL, et al. Predictive values for skin prick test and atopy patch test for eosinophilic esophagitis. J Allergy Clin Immunol 2007;119(2):509–11.

As for other allergic diatheses, most pediatric and adult patients with EoE have allergic rhinitis, asthma, atopic dermatitis, or food allergies and evidence of sensitization to multiple environmental or food allergens.[47,48] Although it is unclear if there is any causal effect of sensitization leading to EoE or vice versa, there at least seems to be a seasonality associated with EoE diagnosis, possibly suggesting some role for aeroallergens in the disease.[49-51] Because of the high incidence of concomitant allergic diatheses seen in patients with EoE, allergy evaluation to help manage these conditions is warranted in all patients with EoE.[2] Testing for respiratory allergies is not likely to alter the management or natural history of EoE, however, because treatment of allergic respiratory diseases has not been shown to effect EoE outcomes, although this has never been formally studied. This conclusion is in contrast to information obtained from food allergy testing, which may have an impact on EoE treatment and outcome.

TREATMENT

Current therapy goals in EoE include symptom improvement, improved quality of life, and resolution of esophageal eosinophilia. Although not all of these outcomes have been rigorously examined in well-designed trials, there are several reports on the outcomes of various therapies. When extrapolating the results of these studies into clinical practice, one should note that most data are generated from short-term studies, and there are very little data from long-term trials.

Dietary Therapy

Elemental diet
The first case series of patients displaying a clinical picture of non-GERD esophageal eosinophilia was so defined by the clinical and histologic response to an elemental diet (despite failure to respond to acid suppression therapy or Nissen fundoplication).[40] Applying the current definition of EoE, it is clear that the group of patients in that case series would be diagnosed with EoE. Subsequent, larger, retrospective studies in children confirmed that an elemental diet was effective in treating EoE in up to 97% of patients. The elemental diet consisted of complete elimination of dietary antigens and using an amino acid–based formula instead. Children were also allowed water and a single fruit, either grape or apple, and its juice.[3,41] This dietary regimen, although effective, can be difficult to adhere to given its obvious dietary restrictions and the requirement for ingestion of large volumes of formula to meet caloric needs. In fact, in some patients, nasogastric or gastrostomy tubes must be placed to allow for adequate caloric intake.

Elimination diet
Dietary elimination of certain food allergens is an alternative to an elemental diet that allows patients to consume a larger variety of foods and, thus, is more lenient in its restrictions and may be more attractive for older children and adults. In designing the elimination diet, one can either restrict proteins based on allergy testing or simply restrict the most common food allergens. No randomized, prospective trials yet exist comparing the two elimination methods. However, retrospective studies have generated data regarding both methods. With elimination of foods that test positive by SPT and APT, one could see improvement in esophageal eosinophilia in up to 77% of patients, whereas the elimination of the most common food allergens (cow's milk, soy, wheat, egg, peanut, tree nuts, and seafood) led to improvement in eosinophilia in 74% of patients in one report.[42,43] Although these elimination diets may offer a better lifestyle over an elemental diet, the elemental diet seems to have a greater success

rate in improving symptoms and esophageal eosinophil numbers in retrospective studies comparing both methods.[3,42]

When disease remission is achieved with a dietary restriction, it is advisable to gradually reintroduce foods into the diet of patients with EoE, keeping those that do not result in disease relapse in the patients' diet. This practice may contribute in improving the quality of life of patients with EoE and in preventing the rare possibility of loss of tolerance to those foods from an immediate reactivity standpoint, as previously explained. A report by Spergel and colleagues[44] provides some insight on the utility of testing in deciding which foods are likely to result in relapse of esophageal eosinophilia based on SPT and APT results (see **Table 1**). In sum, when food reintroduction is attempted, the likelihood of a food leading to an IgE-mediated reaction or relapse of esophageal eosinophilia, the nutritional value of the food, and the desirability of the food to patients need to be taken into account. Avoidance of some antigens may need to be continued indefinitely.

Given the complexity of dietary elimination diets and the possibility of caloric restriction and elimination of key nutrients, it is strongly recommended to consult with a dietitian with expertise in food allergies to supervise the process. The dietitian can provide patients with EoE with education on proper avoidance of food allergens, aid in dietary adherence, and prevent potential nutritional deficiencies.

Pharmacologic Therapy

Oral corticosteroids

As with most eosinophilic diseases, oral steroids improve esophageal eosinophilia and symptoms in patients with EoE.[3,52] Unfortunately, because disease relapse is common within less than 6 months following the cessation of the oral steroids and because of the established adverse effects of long-term treatment with systemic steroids, oral steroids are typically used only in severe cases. When required, the recommended dose is 1 to 2 mg/kg of prednisone equivalent.[2]

Topical corticosteroids

Topical corticosteroids were first reported as a treatment of EoE in a case series of 4 patients in 1998, and have since become a mainstay of treatment of EoE.[53] The first randomized, double-blind, placebo-controlled trial of topical steroids for EoE showed the superiority of swallowed fluticasone propionate over placebo in inducing histologic remission.[54] The treatment induced full remission in 50% of the patients in the active arm. The treatment effect of fluticasone was even more impressive in the only comparative trial to date of a topical steroid versus oral prednisone.[55] In that trial, 80 pediatric and adolescent subjects were randomized to either swallowed fluticasone (n = 40) or oral prednisone (n = 40) for 4 weeks. Histologic improvement was seen in 94% of the subjects in both groups, although to a greater degree in the prednisone group; symptom resolution was seen in all subjects in the prednisone group and in 97% of the subjects in the fluticasone group at week 4 of therapy.[55] In addition, one prospective trial examined both topical fluticasone and dietary therapy. In that study, fluticasone seemed to be more effective in resolving esophageal eosinophilia than dietary therapy.[56]

Swallowed budesonide, another form of topical corticosteroids, has also been shown to be effective in pediatric and adult patients with EoE using randomized, double-blind, placebo-controlled trials.[57,58] In the pediatric study,[57] budesonide suspension was mixed with sucralose to make a slurry termed oral viscous budesonide, which was swallowed. With this preparation, 87% of the subjects in the active arm achieved histologic resolution (defined as <7 eosinophils per HPF on follow-up esophageal biopsies), whereas none of the subjects in the placebo arm achieved resolution. Mean symptom scores and endoscopy scores also improved to a greater degree in those receiving viscous budesonide as compared with placebo. In the adolescent and adult study,[58] the budesonide suspension was nebulized and swallowed. Results from this trial showed at least some histologic response in 89% of the subjects and complete resolution in 72% in the active arm versus 11.1% disease resolution in the placebo arm. In addition to the resolution of eosinophilia and symptom improvement, topical steroid therapy has also been shown to reverse subepithelial fibrosis.[59]

Unfortunately, as seen with oral steroids, the therapeutic effect of topical steroids on the disease is abolished following cessation of treatment. In a 3-year follow-up study, 91% of patients reported recurrence of symptoms at an average of 9 months after receiving a 6-week treatment of swallowed fluticasone.[60] Even with a low-dosage (0.25 mg twice daily) maintenance regimen of budesonide, esophageal eosinophilia and associated symptoms can return.[61] Therefore, patients may have to continue on therapeutic dosages for an indefinite amount of time. Currently, ongoing trials continue to study fluticasone, budesonide, and beclomethasone. Published dosing for both topical steroids is outlined in **Table 2**.

Although not studied in depth, the observed adverse effects of topical steroids tend to be mild in general. In the one trial comparing topical fluticasone with prednisone,[55]

Table 2
Reported doses for topical corticosteroids for EoE from prospective studies

Study	Study Design and Number of Patients	Medication and Dosage[a]
Teitelbaum et al,[56] 2002	Open label, prospective N = 13	Fluticasone propionate 2 puffs twice daily: Age 2–4 y: 44 mcg/puff Age 5–10 y: 110 mcg/puff Age >10 y: 220 mcg/puff
Konikoff et al,[54] 2006	RDBPC N = 36	Fluticasone propionate 2 puffs twice daily: All subjects received 220 mcg/puff Ages ranged from 3–16 y
Schaefer et al,[55] 2008	Open label, randomized N = 80	Fluticasone propionate 2 puffs 4 times daily: Age 1–10 y: 110 mcg/puff Age >10 y: 220 mcg/puff
Dohil et al,[57] 2010	RDBPC N = 24	Oral viscous budesonide[b] Subjects <5 ft tall: 1 mg daily Subjects >5 ft tall: 2 mg daily Age range was 1–17 y
Straumann et al,[58] 2010	RDBPC N = 36	Swallowed nebulized budesonide All subjects received 1 mg twice daily All subjects were aged >16 y

Abbreviation: RDBPC, randomized, double blind, placebo controlled.
  [a] All subjects were instructed to swallow medications and not to eat/drink for 30 minutes after treatment.
  [b] Oral viscous budesonide = 10 g sucralose added per 1 mg budesonide suspension.

40% of the subjects in the prednisone arm developed systemic adverse effects of steroid therapy compared with none in the fluticasone arm. Topical fluticasone led, however, to candidal overgrowth in the esophagus in 15% of the fluticasone-treated subjects. A similar degree of candidal overgrowth was also seen in trials with budesonide (16.7%).[58] However, this may be a dose-related phenomenon, as in a long-term treatment study whereby patients treated with 0.5 mg of swallowed budesonide daily for 50 weeks did not show any evidence of fungal or viral esophageal infection.[61]

Other pharmacologic therapies

Because interleukin (IL)-5 is a known inducer of eosinophil proliferation and activation, and with the success of anti-IL-5 in lowering blood eosinophilia in other hypereosinophilic syndromes, it stands to reason that anti-IL-5 could be a useful therapy for patients with EoE. The first anecdotal evidence for this was published in 2004 in a case series of patients with various forms of eosinophilia, one of whom was an 18-year-old patient with EoE nonresponsive to steroid therapy.[62] In that case, mepolizumab led to a 10-fold decrease in the mean number of esophageal eosinophils with improvement in symptoms. This finding led to an open-label study 2 years later in 4 adult patients that once again showed a decrease in mean and maximum esophageal eosinophil numbers and an improvement in symptoms after 3 monthly infusions.[63] This study was followed by the first double-blind, placebo-controlled trial of mepolizumab, published in 2010.[64] In this study, 11 adult patients were randomized to mepolizumab (n = 5) or placebo (n = 6). Although the active treatment led to a greater decrease (54%) in mean esophageal eosinophil counts when compared with placebo (5%), the complete resolution of esophageal eosinophilia was not seen in any subject. In addition, no significant difference in symptom improvement was seen between the 2 groups. Larger multicenter trials using anti-IL-5 (mepolizumab and reslizumab) are currently ongoing, the final results of which are not yet published.

Other biologic agents that are currently under investigation for the treatment of EoE include anti–tumor necrosis factor (TNF) agents and anti-IgE therapy (omalizumab). There is currently one case series reporting the use of an anti-TNF agent (infliximab) in EoE in 3 adult patients refractory to steroids.[65] In this limited study, one patient had partial histologic response, another had no change, and the third had an increase in esophageal eosinophilia. There are currently no published studies to date using omalizumab; however, there is a single case report of 2 atopic patients with EoE who had symptom improvement with omalizumab but no improvement in endoscopic or histologic findings.[66]

Given that cysteinyl leukotrienes are known eosinophil chemoattractants, leukotriene antagonists seemed to be an attractive therapeutic option for EoE. One early study reported that montelukast at a dosage of 20 to 40 mg daily resolved symptoms in 6 out of 8 adult patients with EoE, but tissue eosinophilia remained.[67] Since that pilot study, studies examining cysteinyl leukotriene levels in esophageal biopsies have found them not to be increased in patients with EoE, and montelukast has recently been shown to be ineffective in maintaining histologic and clinical remission induced by fluticasone.[68,69]

Esophageal Dilation

Esophageal dilation can be an effective treatment of dysphagia, especially when this is caused by strictures. Although an in-depth review of the techniques, outcomes, and complications is beyond the scope and goal of this review, it is clear that the procedure can provide clinically significant symptomatic relief in up to 83% of patients, which can last for an average of 20 months.[70,71] Complications include chest pain

(~4%), deep mucosal tears (3%–9%), and rarely perforation (0%–1%).[70,72] The disadvantage of this therapy option is that it does not address the underlying esophageal inflammation, therefore, resulting in stricture recurrence.

SUMMARY AND KEY POINTS

EoE represents a clinicopathologic disease that is best managed by a team of health care providers, including gastroenterologists and allergists. With updated consensus recommendations available,[2] providers now have a resource to guide them in accurately diagnosing and effectively treating this disease. The following are some key points regarding this:

- The diagnosis of EoE should be made when there are symptoms suggestive of esophageal dysmotility in conjunction with evidence of esophageal eosinophilia despite adequate acid suppression (either with adequate PPI therapeutic trial or with evidence of a normal esophageal pH).
- A peak count of 15 intraepithelial eosinophils per HPF in an esophageal biopsy section is accepted as the minimum value to diagnose EoE.

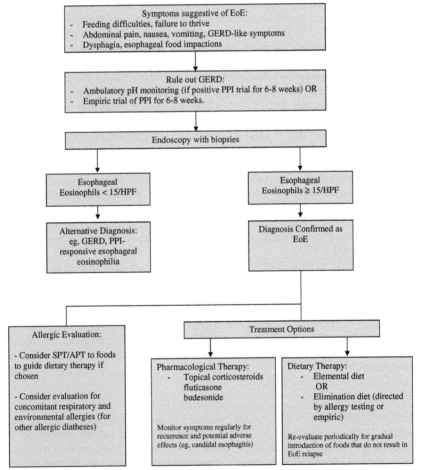

Fig. 3. Proposed approach for diagnosis and management of patients suspected to have EoE.

- Characteristic findings on endoscopy include esophageal rings, whitish exudates or plaques, linear furrows, edema, and esophageal narrowing. These findings, however, are not specific for EoE, and up to 10% of cases of EoE can have a normal-appearing endoscopy.
- Allergic evaluation is appropriate for all patients with EoE given the high prevalence of concomitant atopic disease. Although testing for food allergy may alter management decisions, there are no data to suggest that aeroallergen testing or treatment of respiratory allergy can alter disease.
- There are no Food and Drug Administration–approved treatments for EoE. However, various dietary therapies (amino acid–based formula, dietary restriction based on positive allergy testing, and empiric restriction of common food allergens) and topical corticosteroids have all been shown to be effective and are accepted therapies for the disease. Other therapies (eg, oral steroids and anti-IL-5) have been shown to be effective but should now be limited to refractory disease or investigational studies.
- A proposed algorithm for diagnosis and treatment of patients with EoE can be seen in **Fig. 3**.

REFERENCES

1. Spergel JM, Book WM, Mays E, et al. Variation in prevalence, diagnostic criteria, and initial management options for eosinophilic gastrointestinal diseases in the United States. J Pediatr Gastroenterol Nutr 2011;52(3):300–6.
2. Liacouras CA, Furuta GT, Hirano I, et al. Eosinophilic esophagitis: updated consensus recommendations for children and adults. J Allergy Clin Immunol 2011;128(1):3–20.e26; [quiz: 21–2].
3. Liacouras CA, Spergel JM, Ruchelli E, et al. Eosinophilic esophagitis: a 10-year experience in 381 children. Clin Gastroenterol Hepatol 2005;3(12):1198–206.
4. Kapel RC, Miller JK, Torres C, et al. Eosinophilic esophagitis: a prevalent disease in the United States that affects all age groups. Gastroenterology 2008;134(5):1316–21.
5. Veerappan GR, Perry JL, Duncan TJ, et al. Prevalence of eosinophilic esophagitis in an adult population undergoing upper endoscopy: a prospective study. Clin Gastroenterol Hepatol 2009;7(4):420–6, 426.e421–2.
6. Collins MH, Blanchard C, Abonia JP, et al. Clinical, pathologic, and molecular characterization of familial eosinophilic esophagitis compared with sporadic cases. Clin Gastroenterol Hepatol 2008;6(6):621–9.
7. Rothenberg ME. Biology and treatment of eosinophilic esophagitis. Gastroenterology 2009;137(4):1238–49.
8. Spergel JM, Brown-Whitehorn TF, Beausoleil JL, et al. 14 years of eosinophilic esophagitis: clinical features and prognosis. J Pediatr Gastroenterol Nutr 2009;48(1):30–6.
9. Aceves SS, Newbury RO, Dohil MA, et al. A symptom scoring tool for identifying pediatric patients with eosinophilic esophagitis and correlating symptoms with inflammation. Ann Allergy Asthma Immunol 2009;103(5):401–6.
10. Dellon ES, Gibbs WB, Fritchie KJ, et al. Clinical, endoscopic, and histologic findings distinguish eosinophilic esophagitis from gastroesophageal reflux disease. Clin Gastroenterol Hepatol 2009;7(12):1305–13 [quiz: 1261].
11. Mukkada VA, Haas A, Maune NC, et al. Feeding dysfunction in children with eosinophilic gastrointestinal diseases. Pediatrics 2010;126(3):e672–7.

12. Muller S, Puhl S, Vieth M, et al. Analysis of symptoms and endoscopic findings in 117 patients with histological diagnoses of eosinophilic esophagitis. Endoscopy 2007;39(4):339–44.
13. Garcia-Compean D, Gonzalez Gonzalez JA, Marrufo Garcia CA, et al. Prevalence of eosinophilic esophagitis in patients with refractory gastroesophageal reflux disease symptoms: a prospective study. Dig Liver Dis 2011;43(3):204–8.
14. Mackenzie SH, Go M, Chadwick B, et al. Eosinophilic oesophagitis in patients presenting with dysphagia–a prospective analysis. Aliment Pharmacol Ther 2008;28(9):1140–6.
15. Prasad GA, Talley NJ, Romero Y, et al. Prevalence and predictive factors of eosinophilic esophagitis in patients presenting with dysphagia: a prospective study. Am J Gastroenterol 2007;102(12):2627–32.
16. Desai TK, Stecevic V, Chang CH, et al. Association of eosinophilic inflammation with esophageal food impaction in adults. Gastrointest Endosc 2005;61(7):795–801.
17. Kerlin P, Jones D, Remedios M, et al. Prevalence of eosinophilic esophagitis in adults with food bolus obstruction of the esophagus. J Clin Gastroenterol 2007; 41(4):356–61.
18. DeBrosse CW, Franciosi JP, King EC, et al. Long-term outcomes in pediatric-onset esophageal eosinophilia. J Allergy Clin Immunol 2011;128(1):132–8.
19. Lai AL, Girgis S, Liang Y, et al. Diagnostic criteria for eosinophilic esophagitis: a 5-year retrospective review in a pediatric population. J Pediatr Gastroenterol Nutr 2009;49(1):63–70.
20. Molina-Infante J, Ferrando-Lamana L, Ripoll C, et al. Esophageal eosinophilic infiltration responds to proton pump inhibition in most adults. Clin Gastroenterol Hepatol 2011;9(2):110–7.
21. Rodrigo S, Abboud G, Oh D, et al. High intraepithelial eosinophil counts in esophageal squamous epithelium are not specific for eosinophilic esophagitis in adults. Am J Gastroenterol 2008;103(2):435–42.
22. Sayej WN, Patel R, Baker RD, et al. Treatment with high-dose proton pump inhibitors helps distinguish eosinophilic esophagitis from noneosinophilic esophagitis. J Pediatr Gastroenterol Nutr 2009;49(4):393–9.
23. Schlesinger PK, Donahue PE, Schmid B, et al. Limitations of 24-hour intraesophageal pH monitoring in the hospital setting. Gastroenterology 1985;89(4):797–804.
24. Sperry SL, Shaheen NJ, Dellon ES. Toward uniformity in the diagnosis of eosinophilic esophagitis (EoE): the effect of guidelines on variability of diagnostic criteria for EoE. Am J Gastroenterol 2011;106(5):824–32 [quiz: 833].
25. Dellon ES, Aderoju A, Woosley JT, et al. Variability in diagnostic criteria for eosinophilic esophagitis: a systematic review. Am J Gastroenterol 2007;102(10): 2300–13.
26. Gonsalves N, Policarpio-Nicolas M, Zhang Q, et al. Histopathologic variability and endoscopic correlates in adults with eosinophilic esophagitis. Gastrointest Endosc 2006;64(3):313–9.
27. Pentiuk S, Putnam PE, Collins MH, et al. Dissociation between symptoms and histological severity in pediatric eosinophilic esophagitis. J Pediatr Gastroenterol Nutr 2009;48(2):152–60.
28. Aceves SS, Newbury RO, Dohil R, et al. Distinguishing eosinophilic esophagitis in pediatric patients: clinical, endoscopic, and histologic features of an emerging disorder. J Clin Gastroenterol 2007;41(3):252–6.
29. Steiner SJ, Kernek KM, Fitzgerald JF. Severity of basal cell hyperplasia differs in reflux versus eosinophilic esophagitis. J Pediatr Gastroenterol Nutr 2006;42(5): 506–9.

30. Kephart GM, Alexander JA, Arora AS, et al. Marked deposition of eosinophil-derived neurotoxin in adult patients with eosinophilic esophagitis. Am J Gastroenterol 2010;105(2):298–307.
31. Mueller S, Neureiter D, Aigner T, et al. Comparison of histological parameters for the diagnosis of eosinophilic oesophagitis versus gastro-oesophageal reflux disease on oesophageal biopsy material. Histopathology 2008;53(6):676–84.
32. Protheroe C, Woodruff SA, de Petris G, et al. A novel histologic scoring system to evaluate mucosal biopsies from patients with eosinophilic esophagitis. Clin Gastroenterol Hepatol 2009;7(7):749–55.e711.
33. Aceves SS, Newbury RO, Dohil R, et al. Esophageal remodeling in pediatric eosinophilic esophagitis. J Allergy Clin Immunol 2007;119(1):206–12.
34. Chehade M, Sampson HA, Morotti RA, et al. Esophageal subepithelial fibrosis in children with eosinophilic esophagitis. J Pediatr Gastroenterol Nutr 2007;45(3):319–28.
35. Lee S, de Boer WB, Naran A, et al. More than just counting eosinophils: proximal oesophageal involvement and subepithelial sclerosis are major diagnostic criteria for eosinophilic oesophagitis. J Clin Pathol 2010;63(7):644–7.
36. Abonia JP, Blanchard C, Butz BB, et al. Involvement of mast cells in eosinophilic esophagitis. J Allergy Clin Immunol 2010;126(1):140–9.
37. Dellon ES, Chen X, Miller CR, et al. Tryptase staining of mast cells may differentiate eosinophilic esophagitis from gastroesophageal reflux disease. Am J Gastroenterol 2011;106(2):264–71.
38. Kirsch R, Bokhary R, Marcon MA, et al. Activated mucosal mast cells differentiate eosinophilic (allergic) esophagitis from gastroesophageal reflux disease. J Pediatr Gastroenterol Nutr 2007;44(1):20–6.
39. Lucendo AJ, Navarro M, Comas C, et al. Immunophenotypic characterization and quantification of the epithelial inflammatory infiltrate in eosinophilic esophagitis through stereology: an analysis of the cellular mechanisms of the disease and the immunologic capacity of the esophagus. Am J Surg Pathol 2007;31(4):598–606.
40. Kelly KJ, Lazenby AJ, Rowe PC, et al. Eosinophilic esophagitis attributed to gastroesophageal reflux: improvement with an amino acid-based formula. Gastroenterology 1995;109(5):1503–12.
41. Markowitz JE, Spergel JM, Ruchelli E, et al. Elemental diet is an effective treatment for eosinophilic esophagitis in children and adolescents. Am J Gastroenterol 2003;98(4):777–82.
42. Kagalwalla AF, Sentongo TA, Ritz S, et al. Effect of six-food elimination diet on clinical and histologic outcomes in eosinophilic esophagitis. Clin Gastroenterol Hepatol 2006;4(9):1097–102.
43. Spergel JM, Andrews T, Brown-Whitehorn TF, et al. Treatment of eosinophilic esophagitis with specific food elimination diet directed by a combination of skin prick and patch tests. Ann Allergy Asthma Immunol 2005;95(4):336–43.
44. Spergel JM, Brown-Whitehorn T, Beausoleil JL, et al. Predictive values for skin prick test and atopy patch test for eosinophilic esophagitis. J Allergy Clin Immunol 2007;119(2):509–11.
45. Flinterman AE, Knulst AC, Meijer Y, et al. Acute allergic reactions in children with AEDS after prolonged cow's milk elimination diets. Allergy 2006;61(3):370–4.
46. Larramendi CH, Martin Esteban M, Pascual Marcos C, et al. Possible consequences of elimination diets in asymptomatic immediate hypersensitivity to fish. Allergy 1992;47(5):490–4.

47. Erwin EA, James HR, Gutekunst HM, et al. Serum IgE measurement and detection of food allergy in pediatric patients with eosinophilic esophagitis. Ann Allergy Asthma Immunol 2010;104(6):496–502.

48. Roy-Ghanta S, Larosa DF, Katzka DA. Atopic characteristics of adult patients with eosinophilic esophagitis. Clin Gastroenterol Hepatol 2008;6(5):531–5.

49. Wang FY, Gupta SK, Fitzgerald JF. Is there a seasonal variation in the incidence or intensity of allergic eosinophilic esophagitis in newly diagnosed children? J Clin Gastroenterol 2007;41(5):451–3.

50. Almansa C, Krishna M, Buchner AM, et al. Seasonal distribution in newly diagnosed cases of eosinophilic esophagitis in adults. Am J Gastroenterol 2009; 104(4):828–33.

51. Moawad FJ, Veerappan GR, Lake JM, et al. Correlation between eosinophilic oesophagitis and aeroallergens. Aliment Pharmacol Ther 2010;31(4):509–15.

52. Liacouras CA, Wenner WJ, Brown K, et al. Primary eosinophilic esophagitis in children: successful treatment with oral corticosteroids. J Pediatr Gastroenterol Nutr 1998;26(4):380–5.

53. Faubion WA Jr, Perrault J, Burgart LJ, et al. Treatment of eosinophilic esophagitis with inhaled corticosteroids. J Pediatr Gastroenterol Nutr 1998;27(1):90–3.

54. Konikoff MR, Noel RJ, Blanchard C, et al. A randomized, double-blind, placebo-controlled trial of fluticasone propionate for pediatric eosinophilic esophagitis. Gastroenterology 2006;131(5):1381–91.

55. Schaefer ET, Fitzgerald JF, Molleston JP, et al. Comparison of oral prednisone and topical fluticasone in the treatment of eosinophilic esophagitis: a randomized trial in children. Clin Gastroenterol Hepatol 2008;6(2):165–73.

56. Teitelbaum JE, Fox VL, Twarog FJ, et al. Eosinophilic esophagitis in children: immunopathological analysis and response to fluticasone propionate. Gastroenterology 2002;122(5):1216–25.

57. Dohil R, Newbury R, Fox L, et al. Oral viscous budesonide is effective in children with eosinophilic esophagitis in a randomized, placebo-controlled trial. Gastroenterology 2010;139(2):418–29.

58. Straumann A, Conus S, Degen L, et al. Budesonide is effective in adolescent and adult patients with active eosinophilic esophagitis. Gastroenterology 2010; 139(5):1526–37, 1537.e1521.

59. Aceves SS, Newbury RO, Chen D, et al. Resolution of remodeling in eosinophilic esophagitis correlates with epithelial response to topical corticosteroids. Allergy 2010;65(1):109–16.

60. Helou EF, Simonson J, Arora AS. 3-yr-follow-up of topical corticosteroid treatment for eosinophilic esophagitis in adults. Am J Gastroenterol 2008;103(9):2194–9.

61. Straumann A, Conus S, Degen L, et al. Long-term budesonide maintenance treatment is partially effective for patients with eosinophilic esophagitis. Clin Gastroenterol Hepatol 2011;9(5):400–9.e401.

62. Garrett JK, Jameson SC, Thomson B, et al. Anti-interleukin-5 (mepolizumab) therapy for hypereosinophilic syndromes. J Allergy Clin Immunol 2004;113(1): 115–9.

63. Stein ML, Collins MH, Villanueva JM, et al. Anti-IL-5 (mepolizumab) therapy for eosinophilic esophagitis. J Allergy Clin Immunol 2006;118(6):1312–9.

64. Straumann A, Conus S, Grzonka P, et al. Anti-interleukin-5 antibody treatment (mepolizumab) in active eosinophilic oesophagitis: a randomised, placebo-controlled, double-blind trial. Gut 2010;59(1):21–30.

65. Straumann A, Bussmann C, Conus S, et al. Anti-TNF-alpha (infliximab) therapy for severe adult eosinophilic esophagitis. J Allergy Clin Immunol 2008;122(2):425–7.

66. Rocha R, Vitor AB, Trindade E, et al. Omalizumab in the treatment of eosinophilic esophagitis and food allergy. Eur J Pediatr 2011;170(11):1471–4.
67. Attwood SE, Lewis CJ, Bronder CS, et al. Eosinophilic oesophagitis: a novel treatment using montelukast. Gut 2003;52(2):181–5.
68. Gupta SK, Peters-Golden M, Fitzgerald JF, et al. Cysteinyl leukotriene levels in esophageal mucosal biopsies of children with eosinophilic inflammation: are they all the same? Am J Gastroenterol 2006;101(5):1125–8.
69. Lucendo AJ, De Rezende LC, Jimenez-Contreras S, et al. Montelukast was inefficient in maintaining steroid-induced remission in adult eosinophilic esophagitis. Dig Dis Sci 2011. [Epub ahead of print].
70. Dellon ES, Gibbs WB, Rubinas TC, et al. Esophageal dilation in eosinophilic esophagitis: safety and predictors of clinical response and complications. Gastrointest Endosc 2010;71(4):706–12.
71. Schoepfer AM, Gonsalves N, Bussmann C, et al. Esophageal dilation in eosinophilic esophagitis: effectiveness, safety, and impact on the underlying inflammation. Am J Gastroenterol 2010;105(5):1062–70.
72. Jung KW, Gundersen N, Kopacova J, et al. Occurrence of and risk factors for complications after endoscopic dilation in eosinophilic esophagitis. Gastrointest Endosc 2011;73(1):15–21.

Mental Health and Quality-of-Life Concerns Related to the Burden of Food Allergy

N.L. Ravid, BA[a], R.A. Annunziato, PhD[b,c], M.A. Ambrose, BA[b],
K. Chuang, MA[b], C. Mullarkey, BS[b], S.H. Sicherer, MD[d],
E. Shemesh, MD[b], A.L. Cox, MD[d,*]

KEYWORDS

• Food allergy • Distress • Bullying • Quality of life

Food allergy seems to be increasing. Based on data from the Centers for Disease Control in the United States, there was an 18% increase in prevalence of food allergy among children from 1997 to 2007, with prevalence estimates currently in the range of 4% to 8%.[1–3] Food allergy differs from other chronic diseases in that affected individuals are in generally good health, but their health may be episodically compromised by acute food-allergic reactions that may be severe or life-threatening. Management of this unpredictable condition may lead to significant distress for food-allergic children and their parents or caregivers. Several studies have examined the effect of food allergy on quality of life (QoL) and emotional impact in children and families, with a particular focus on measures of distress.[4,5] Food allergy has been shown to negatively impact parental, as well as patient, QoL.[5–8] Psychological distress, which includes anxiety, depression, social isolation, and stress, has been demonstrated in children and adolescents with food allergy, although there are variable findings with regard to whether distress is more prevalent among children with food allergy when compared with normative samples.[9]

Several studies have demonstrated a negative impact on health-related QoL, as well as increased distress among food-allergic children and families. However, making

---

[a] Mount Sinai School of Medicine, New York, NY, USA
[b] Division of Behavioral and Developmental Health, Department of Pediatrics, Mount Sinai Medical Center, 1468 Madison Avenue, New York, NY 10029, USA
[c] Department of Psychology, Fordham University, 441 East Fordham Road, Bronx, NY 10458, USA
[d] Division of Pediatric Allergy and Immunology, Mount Sinai Medical Center, One Gustave L Levy Place, New York, NY 10029, USA
* Corresponding author.
E-mail address: Amanda.cox@mssm.edu

Immunol Allergy Clin N Am 32 (2012) 83–95
doi:10.1016/j.iac.2011.11.005
0889-8561/12/$ – see front matter © 2012 Elsevier Inc. All rights reserved.

comparisons between studies is difficult because of the discrete populations studied, the differing study sizes and geographic locations, and the various methods or tools used to assess psychosocial effects of food allergy on children and their parents.[5] Applying the available findings to a therapeutic end poses an additional challenge in that there is a paucity of literature describing effective interventions. In addition, methods of assessing distress or changes in QoL that result from food allergy vary in the literature. Some studies focus only on parental evaluations,[10,11] while others survey both parents and children.[12] Several studies compared food-allergic children to nonallergic cohorts or to children with other chronic disease, such as diabetes.[13,14] Another study relates subjects' scores to normative scores for the applied tests in the larger population.[15] Moreover, individuals with food allergy often have other atopic conditions that may influence QoL and distress that may be underappreciated in these studies.

The broad range of ages studied should also be taken into consideration. Different developmental stages may influence the divergent manifestations of and means for assessing anxiety in children as opposed to adolescents. Types of questionnaires used and modes of administration also vary, with some studies relying on validated measures and others using modified and nonvalidated tests or qualitative measures such as interviews. Several tools to measure QoL, specifically in food-allergic patients or their families have been introduced and validated only recently.[5,7,8,16]

This article discusses recent information concerning the effects of food allergy on parent and child QoL, as well as distress. It notes the limitations of the available evidence and points out where further study is needed. There is a general movement in medicine toward focusing on QoL as an important outcome measure in health and disease.[17,18] The increasing number of articles about these effects in food allergy is an attestation to the growing importance that the field has started to ascribe to the QoL of affected patients and families.[5] However, our methods of assessment need refinement, especially with regard to the development of evidence-based interventions to improve QoL and reduce distress. Where there is an absence of solid data to back any specific recommendations, the authors provide impressions based on clinical experience with the understanding that, as more data are gathered, our understanding and recommendations will likely need modification.

THE CHILD'S PERSPECTIVE
Studies Examining the Emotional and QoL Consequences of Food Allergy Compared with Other Chronic Illnesses

Assessing the impact of food allergy on QoL requires a point of comparison. Groups evaluated have included children with no food allergy, children with different types or severities of food allergy, children with other allergic disorders, and children with other chronic health conditions. The effects of food allergy on QoL were recently reviewed and summarized.[5] This article offers a critical appraisal of some of the findings to date.

In a study conducted in England, both a self-reporting questionnaire designed by the researchers and an adapted allergy-specific questionnaire were used to survey 20 children with peanut allergy, ages 7 to 12 years, for their fear of adverse outcomes induced by potential or accidental consumption of peanuts.[13] The responses of these children were compared with those of 20 children with insulin-dependent diabetes mellitus. The percentage of children reporting anxiety and the level of anxiety (ranked from high to low) was significantly greater in children with food allergy when compared with children with insulin-dependent diabetes mellitus. In a comparison of food allergy and chronic disease performed in the Netherlands, 98 individuals with various food allergies were surveyed within a larger group of 758, ages 12 to 25 years, with chronic acquired digestive diseases, including inflammatory bowel diseases, chronic liver diseases, congenital disorders, and celiac disease.[14] The survey included a self-reporting questionnaire and the Hospital and Anxiety Depression Scale to probe for burden of disease as measured by leisure activity, sexuality, education, work, and finances. The study found that individuals with food allergy experienced daily disease burden with an impact on school and leisure activities, comparable in several categories to other chronic digestive disorders.

In another study performed in the Netherlands, QoL of food-allergic individuals was compared with that of the general population, as well as to patients with other chronic diseases.[15] Generic QoL questionnaires were completed by food-allergic children (8–12 years), adolescents (13–17 years), and adults (≥18 years). QoL scores were compared with published scores for individuals with irritable bowel syndrome, diabetes mellitus, and rheumatoid arthritis. Food-allergic children and adolescents reported poorer QoL than patients with diabetes mellitus, but had better QoL scores than patients with rheumatoid arthritis, asthma, or irritable bowel syndrome. In addition, food-allergic adolescents and adults showed impairments in QoL compared with the general population. Children, however, demonstrated the least QOL impairment due to food allergy.

Comparisons of these studies are interesting but have limitations due to their differing methodologies and study subjects. Although the findings of Avery and colleagues[13] relate to anxiety while those of Flokstra-de Blok and colleagues[15] relate to QoL, both groups found that food-allergic individuals scored worse than diabetic patients did in these respective psychosocial domains. On the other hand, Calsbeek and colleagues[14] found that comparison of food allergy to a chronic, high somatic-impact disease such as inflammatory bowel disease revealed a lesser social impairment in food allergy. This is consistent with Flokstra-de Blok and colleagues'[15] report of better QoL in food-allergic patients compared with patients with irritable bowel syndrome, asthma, and rheumatoid arthritis. The findings of these studies collectively suggest that the emotional effects seen in patients with food allergy are not easily comparable to those encountered in other disease processes. The clinical manifestations of food allergy are largely episodic in that the disorder is generally not apparent unless or until an allergic reaction occurs. This distinctive characteristic of food allergy may contribute to features of increased anxiety (about the development of acute reactions) but may also result in a lesser impact on socialization when compared with a less episodic, chronic illness such as diabetes. More comparative data are needed before further conclusions can be made.

Studies that Primarily Investigate Children with Food Allergy

Studies comparing food-allergic children to each other, rather than to non–food-allergic cohorts, have suggested additional factors affecting food allergy-related distress and QoL, including epinephrine prescription, history of anaphylaxis, and perception of competence in managing personal health.

In a British study, 41 children (ages 6–16 years) with peanut and tree nut allergies and their mothers completed questionnaires to assess perceived stress and QoL.[12] Children who were not prescribed epinephrine showed greater distress. Distress was not, however, associated with whether or not the child actually carried the prescribed autoinjector. Of note, prior severity of allergic reaction, including anaphylaxis, did not significantly influence child and maternal levels of distress.

Another study, also conducted in England, focused on the impact of awareness and negative-versus-positive perceptions of food allergy on anxiety.[19] Of 162 young adults (ages 15–20 years) who were surveyed at a university, 24 self-reported allergy to certain foods. All completed a Perceived Health Competence Scale and a State-Trait Anxiety Inventory (STAI). As expected, allergic patients were more anxious than those who did not report having allergy. Interestingly, within the small group of 24 food-allergic individuals, those who reported feeling more competent in handling their illness had higher anxiety levels compared with those who reported less competence. Objective assessment of patient levels of "perceived health competence" revealed that most patients who self-reported themselves as "highly competent" did not know the meaning of the term "anaphylaxis." This suggests that self-reported levels of "perceived health competence" in this study were unreliable and unlikely to signify true proficiency in disease management. Nonetheless, the investigators speculated that the association between participants' reported feelings of better competency in managing their illness, as well as increased anxiety, could be attributed to the fact that an increased understanding of food allergy could contribute to a heightened awareness of its risks.[15]

An alternate explanation for the association between anxiety and perceived health competence may be that anxiety prompts patients to inquire more about their illness and thus leads to self-reported higher competence. Based on this conjecture, anxiety among the adolescents surveyed may have contributed to a report of higher competence, rather than competence leading to a report of anxiety, even in cases where patients misjudged or overestimated their knowledge about food allergy. Thus, anxious patients may be more motivated to learn about their disorder, and educating them to become truly competent in managing their food allergy could perhaps decrease their anxiety. On the other hand, as inferred from these findings, patients with food allergy may develop increased anxiety as they learn more about their illness. These seemingly contradictory interpretations would lead to entirely different approaches to patients with food allergy. Accordingly, conclusions derived from cross-sectional studies involving self-reported symptoms or attitudes must be considered cautiously because self-reports do not always faithfully or completely represent the real attitudes, knowledge, or symptoms of the reporting individuals.

Although distress or anxiety are usually perceived as negative emotions that lead to suffering, in fact, some level of anxiety may be adaptive and can lead to better disease management and reduce risk-taking behaviors. Indeed, risk-taking behaviors, such as knowingly ingesting unsafe foods or not carrying prescribed epinephrine, have been noted in adolescents and young adults. In a survey of 13- to 21-year-old food-allergic patients in the United States, alarmingly high rates of risk-taking were reported (ie, 54% reported purposely ingesting unsafe foods and only 61% reported always carrying epinephrine).[20] Those who reported more unsafe behaviors also reported being less concerned about their allergy, and reported feeling "different" more often than those who took fewer risks.

The QoL of children with food allergy and the QoL of their parents has been the focus of several recent studies, as reviewed by Lieberman and Sicherer.[5] QoL of teenagers living with food allergy has been evaluated in the context of developing a specific questionnaire to assess QoL in this group of patients.[7] Teenagers identified limitations on social activities, not being able to eat what others were eating, and limited choice of restaurants as the areas with most adverse impact on their QoL.

Overall, these studies suggest that food-allergic individuals and their families may be more anxious and distressed, and have a lower QoL, when compared with the general population. Increased self-reported "competence" in managing the illness is not necessarily associated with reduced anxiety, although these outcomes may be different if patients cultivate true disease-related competence. Being more anxious, however, is not always problematic, as anxiety can be adaptive and protective against risky behaviors. These findings should be considered when developing therapeutic interventions to improve distress or QoL in patients with food allergy and their families.

THE FAMILY PERSPECTIVE

Awareness of the emotional impact of food allergy has been extended to include the families living with this condition and has led to research on the distress that family members experience and potentially project on one another. The constant fear of anaphylaxis, as well as the consistent vigilance necessary to prevent accidental allergen exposures, can place significant strain on those caring for children with food allergy. Furthermore, parents have the added burden of communicating the risks to others involved in the child's care.

A study of more than 1000 parents of food-allergic children in the United States found overall QoL for caregivers to be variable, although caregivers consistently reported being troubled by social limitations resulting from their child's food allergy.[10] Poor QoL was significantly more likely among caregivers with more knowledge about food allergy and among caregivers whose children had been to the emergency department for food allergy within the preceding year, had multiple food allergies, or were allergic to specific foods (milk, egg, or wheat). In another United States survey of 253 families of food-allergic children, which used a validated, self-administered, children's health questionnaire (CHQ-PF50), parents scored significantly lower (worse) on general health perception, parental emotional impact, and limitation on family activities compared with established norms.[6]

In a study aimed at exploring the challenges faced by parents of young children with food allergy, Rouf and colleagues[21] interviewed a small group of British mothers of food-allergic children and identified themes of parental acclimation to the diagnosis, efforts toward normalizing living with the risks posed by food allergy, and parental concern about their child's identity and inclusion in social life. The study identified that there was a readjustment period to the diagnosis for these mothers that, in different subjects, elicited grief, anxiety, and hope. The study also identified maternal concern over parental responsibility in transferring care of the child to others, teaching others, and cultivating a "normalized" sense of identity in food-allergic children. Another United States study surveyed 2495 parents and found that their children's food allergies adversely affected the parent's personal relationships with the community as well as within the family.[22] Moreover, as reviewed by Klinnert and Robinson,[23] there is concern that parents with extreme levels of anxiety, especially those for whom social interactions with others are also affected, may adopt maladaptive coping strategies. For instance, parents may impose unreasonable social restrictions on the food-allergic child that can interfere with the child's age-appropriate development.

Parental gender may influence the responses and behavioral changes related to food allergy. In one British study of 46 families in which there was a peanut-allergic child, responses of mothers were compared with fathers. Mothers reported greater anxiety and stress than fathers.[24] Importantly, mothers rated the anxiety of their children higher (worse) than the children rated their own anxiety levels. The discrepancy between child and parent reporting of anxiety underscores the importance of directly assessing the child himself or herself for impact of food allergy. This is consistent with the findings of parental reporting of the psychosocial impact of other illnesses on children.[25]

The burden of managing the risks posed to children with food allergy lies with parents or primary caregivers. QoL assessments within families where there is a food-allergic child may show a greater impact on parents than on the children. The influence of a child's food allergy on child and parent QoL were examined in a study comparing QoL for 30 food-allergic children to 15 comparative normal children, as well as QoL between their respective caregivers.[11] The findings indicated that, although food allergy influenced QoL for some children, their parent's QoL was hindered to a greater extent. Furthermore, parents report a better QoL for their food-allergic children than children do when asked directly about themselves, suggesting that direct evaluation of child QoL is necessary.[26]

Comparison of adult and child perspectives on food allergy may reveal specific factors that contribute to child distress from food allergy. LeBovidge and colleagues[9] surveyed 69 children ages 8 to 17 years with food allergy and 141 mothers of food-allergic children ages 2 to 17 years to investigate the influence of maternal anxiety and negative attitudes toward food allergy on the development of child distress using several validated non–disease-specific questionnaires. Scores for anxiety, depression and social stress symptoms in children with food allergy were comparable to average normative child distress scores. The results of this study highlight resilience among children with food allergy. Greater distress was found only in children with a negative approach to food allergy and in younger children of mothers with greater anxiety.

Herbert and Dahlquist[27] examined food allergy as it relates to anxiety, depression, and the impact on autonomy and the influence of parental behavior for 86 food-allergic young adults ages 18 to 22 years. Responses were compared with 344 healthy individuals of the same age. Three nonstandardized questionnaires and several standardized ones were administered. The investigators found that food-allergic participants and healthy participants scored similarly with regard to social self-confidence, autonomy, depression, and anxiety. The subgroup of food-allergic individuals who had a perceived experience of anaphylaxis described greater anxiety about their condition and rated their parents as more overprotective in comparison with food-allergic individuals without a perceived experience of anaphylaxis. The investigators proposed that anaphylaxis in food-allergic patients is a predictor of psychological distress. Conversely, an experience of anaphylaxis may result in reduced distress if individuals are able to manage and master the allergic reaction; thus, the relationship between anaphylaxis and long-term distress requires further investigation.[12]

It is evident from the publications cited above that QoL is negatively affected in families of children who suffer from food allergy. Furthermore, several studies suggest that there is a greater impact on QoL of parents than on the QoL of food-allergic children themselves, at least in the younger age groups. It has not yet been well established whether anxiety is more prevalent among families of children with food allergy than in the general population or compared with families coping with other illnesses. When anxiety is substantially increased, it is likely to be high in both the caretaker and the child. Parental anxiety levels, patient perceptions of food allergy, and coping mechanisms all likely have marked effects on the anxiety and adaptive behaviors of children with food allergy.

The Impact of Oral Food Challenges

Management of pediatric food allergy often involves supervising oral food challenges to either confirm the diagnosis of a food allergy (by positive oral food challenge), or to determine tolerance or resolution of a particular food allergy (by negative oral food challenge). An intervention such as an oral food challenge may result in health-related QoL changes over time for patients and families affected by food allergy.

A few studies have attempted to determine parental anxiety levels related to the performance of oral food challenges.[28–31] Anxiety levels were evaluated in parents of 57 Dutch children with suspected peanut or hazelnut allergy who underwent double-blind placebo-controlled food challenges (DBPCFC) using the Spielberger STAI.[28] Results were compared with Dutch normative values, as well as with parents who refused DBPCFC. The investigators found that parents of children with suspected peanut or hazelnut allergy had high levels of STAI anxiety compared with normal. However, after DBPCFC, state anxiety was significantly lower, regardless of whether their children passed or failed the oral food challenge. Lower state anxiety was maintained even 1 year after food challenge.

In another study, a questionnaire was completed by parents of children with egg allergy. Parents of children who did not undergo food challenge were compared with parents of children who did undergo an open oral food challenge to egg, including 27 who had positive challenges and 57 who had negative challenges to egg. Similar to the above findings among parents of peanut or hazelnut-allergic children, Kemp and colleagues[29] found that performance of an egg oral challenge was associated with reduced adverse parental concerns for most parameters related to expectations about their children's egg allergy, regardless of challenge outcome. These investigators concluded that the experience of an oral food challenge provided parents with greater certainty about their child's food allergy. DunnGalvin and colleagues[30] found comparable results for parental food-allergy QoL using the Food Allergy Quality of Life–Parent Form in a sample of children 0 to 12 years of age undergoing oral food challenges. Scores did improve after oral food challenges for parents of children who had negative challenges, as well as for those whose children had positive challenges.

The studies so far do suggest that oral food challenges may be one area where an intervention may influence or reduce parental anxiety, alleviate distress, and have a positive effect on QoL. However, none of these studies included a random allocation of patients, which precludes any assumption of cause-and-effect relationship between the performance of the food challenge and the apparent association with improved outcomes. It is possible that patients who choose to undergo a food challenge procedure are less anxious then those who do not choose to do it. If so, the difference between anxiety scores in the studied groups could simply reflect a characteristic of those families who tend to proceed with a challenge versus those who do not. The food challenge itself may not be an important factor in relieving anxiety. Although additional research in this area should be conducted before any conclusions or firm recommendations are made, it is possible that, for those who choose to do the challenge, the ensuing information about the child's allergy leads to lesser anxiety. Future studies in this field should be conducted with validated instruments and should assess similar QoL and distress measures among food-allergic children themselves.

FOOD ALLERGY AND BULLYING: AN EMERGING ISSUE

Bullying has devastating effects on children. A study conducted in the United States showed that youth subjected to multiple victimizations experienced more psychological distress and performed worse in school compared with their peers.[32] Another study has shown a clear association between bullying and psychological distress among middle-school boys.[33] In Finland, being bullied in childhood is a predictor of becoming a teenage mother and teen pregnancy has been proposed as one of many long-term outcomes of bullying.[34] School bullying is typically targeted at children that are more vulnerable. A child with food allergy may experience separation from his or her peers during certain social situations, and may have an underlying increased level of anxiety and social stress. These factors may make food-allergic children more susceptible to bullying and its psychological effects.

In a recent study by Lieberman and colleagues,[35] the bullying experience was examined in food-allergic children. A questionnaire designed to assess the nature of teasing, harassment, or bullying of food-allergic patients was distributed to attendees at several regional Food Allergy & Anaphylaxis Network conferences. Most of the surveys were completed by parents of food-allergic children. Of the 353 responses, 24% reported being bullied directly because of food allergy and, of these, most (86%) had experienced multiple episodes of bullying. Most bullying experiences (82%) occurred at school where bullies were mainly classmates. Bullying included teasing or verbal or physical harassment. Of those who experienced bullying, 57% described physical harassment, including being purposely touched with a food allergen. It was also found that 79% of those bullied perceived that they were bullied exclusively because of their food allergy. Furthermore, the respondents cited feelings of sadness, depression, embarrassment, and humiliation because of being bullied; 42.3% felt that the food-allergic child would be harassed or teased again in the future.

Other studies of parent-reported assessment of childhood QoL and anxiety have shown that parents may overestimate child anxiety with respect to food allergy and may not be reliable sources of information regarding their child's experience of food allergy.[24] The findings in the above study on bullying were largely based on parent-completed questionnaires; thus, on parent perception of the food-allergic child's experience. Future studies should directly question the food-allergic child about bullying. Nonetheless, this preliminary study clearly suggests that bullying of food-allergic children does occur and is likely prevalent in the school setting. The extent and correlates of bullying related to food allergy should be further investigated with the aims of raising awareness about this phenomenon and developing interventions to reduce or prevent bullying.

INTERVENTIONS THAT ATTEMPT TO IMPROVE EMOTIONAL OUTCOMES AND QOL

No published studies have evaluated the impact of any intervention on food-allergic children themselves. Studies evaluating the efficacy of educational interventions in other pediatric chronic diseases, including diabetes and asthma, have shown limited improvement in measurable clinical outcomes. For example, in one study of a brief, intensive diabetes educational intervention, patient satisfaction and empowerment improved whereas measures of diabetes such as hemoglobin A1c remained unchanged.[36] Similarly, in a meta-analysis of 37 studies investigating whether asthma self-management education affects children's use of acute care services, emergency department visits and number of hospitalizations decreased, whereas the likelihood of hospitalization and urgent physician visits for asthma remained the same.[37]

To date, only one study has evaluated the impact of an intervention on constructs related to QoL and distress on families who have children with food allergy; however, this study did not use validated measures of those constructs. Lebovidge[38] and colleagues report that a group intervention, consisting of an educational workshop presented to 61 families with food-allergic children, was well accepted. Parents' pre-intervention and postintervention self-reports indicated increased perception of competence in coping with food allergy and reduced perceived burden of coping with the illness. This study provides preliminary justification for further investigation of group interventions in this population. However, because the study design lacked controls, outcomes were self-reported and not based upon validated instruments, and child-specific assessments were not performed, the authors cannot conclude that the intervention was effective until further studies are performed.

CONCLUSIONS AND FUTURE DIRECTIONS

Box 1 presents a summary of the reviewed articles concerning findings related to QoL, anxiety, and distress in food-allergic patients and their families. Although QoL is invariably reported to be adversely affected, there are discrepancies among reports with regard to the impact of food allergy on distress and anxiety in children. Some articles demonstrate a clear correlation between the two, although others find no significant association. The use of qualitative as opposed to quantitative methods of study, as well as general as opposed to food allergy-specific instruments, may partially account for the variance in findings. Of note, the sample sizes are generally too small to merit definitive conclusions about the rate or level of distress in food-allergic children compared with children who do not have food allergy. The authors also observe that many of the patient populations recruited for these studies come from backgrounds of high education or income, are already attending an advocacy conference, or are in the care of highly focused allergists. Increasing the diversity of participating subjects with respect to income, health care access, ethnicity, and advocacy awareness will yield more information.

In addition, even when anxiety scales are used, investigators do not use "event-specific" anxiety but rather anxiety traits or states. Those may be less relevant constructs in this population because anxiety in food allergy is frequently related to a specific event, or to a fear about an event, and should be evaluated as such. In addition, the mere demonstration of increased distress in food-allergic children does not

Box 1 Reviewed articles categorized by construct and outcome		
Construct	**Parents and Family**	**Patients**
QoL	*Decreased* • Lieberman and Sicherer,[5] 2011 • Gupta et al,[22] 2010 *Variable* • Springston et al,[10] 2010	*Decreased* • Resnick et al,[7] 2010 • Flokstra-de Blok et al,[15] 2010
Anxiety	*Increased* • Rouf et al,[21] 2011 • Klinnert et al,[23] 2008 • King et al,[24] 2009	*Increased* • Avery et al,[13] 2003 • Calsbeek et al,[14] 2006 *No change* • Lebovidge et al,[9] 2009 • Herbert and Dahlquist,[27] 2008
Distress	—	*Increased* • Cummings et al,[12] 2010

imply a pathologic reaction to the illness. Evaluation of correlates of event-specific distress in larger samples, with QoL and other constructs as the outcome variable, would enable an understanding of a threshold of distress in this group of patients. Only beyond that threshold could distress be considered maladaptive. Conversely, levels of distress below that threshold could be desirable. Finally, a total lack of distress may be maladaptive and a cause for concern in the food-allergic population because it could lead to excessive risk-taking.

The experience of being bullied has only recently been studied in the context of food allergy. Additional studies of patients, and potentially of those involved in bullying, are needed to explore the association between bullying and food allergy, as well as whether fear of being bullied contributes to anxiety in children with food allergy. Other considerations might include whether the type and severity of food allergy has an impact on the frequency and form of bullying. Additional research is needed to distinguish between outcomes found via parental reporting versus child reporting of the influence of food allergy on the experiences of being bullied. Of particular interest would be whether parents are aware of most cases of bullying and how bullying is managed when parents are aware.

Parents undoubtedly have a major influence on children's psychological response to their food allergy, and this deserves further exploration. Another unresolved inquiry is whether food allergy and anxiety are organically associated via a genetic link (eg, manifestations of an altered sympathetic nervous system), or whether anxiety develops because of learning patterns, as reviewed recently.[4] Concerning learning patterns, in some patients it may be that increased perceived competency in managing food allergy will lead to increased anxiety.[19] However, it may be that patients who are anxious at baseline are more likely to seek further knowledge about their illness. A cause-and-effect relationship between disease knowledge and distress in food allergy has not yet been substantiated. One pilot study indicated that educational workshops might increase perceived competence in parents.[38] Additional well-designed studies are needed to further examine the outcomes of educational interventions on QoL and distress, as well as to clarify the relationship between knowledge about food allergy and patient or parent anxiety.

SUMMARY

The study of food allergy-related mental health and QoL is truly in its infancy, thus further research is desired in each area reviewed. Based on findings from the available studies in the field, the authors propose the following recommendations with the caveat that, as understanding of the psychosocial impact of food allergy evolves, these recommendations may need to be modified or completely changed.

1. It is important to evaluate event-related anxiety in children with food allergy and their parents as a part of routine clinical visits, because anxiety can affect QoL and illness perception. Both very little and very marked anxiety in either the patient or parent should be of concern.
2. Age-appropriate, validated, food allergy-specific assessments of QoL are available and should be used to evaluate the QoL concerns of food-allergic children and their parents. Food allergy decreases QoL owing to its restrictive effects on diet patterns, social activities, and the need to avoid certain circumstances in which there may be a risk of an accidental exposure to a food.
3. It is not yet clear how to improve QoL in affected patients and families, but several opportunities do exist. To name just a few, a diagnostic test such as a food

challenge may improve QoL by confirming persistence versus tolerance of a food allergen, demonstrating appropriate management of an allergic reaction, or reaffirming the extent of avoidance that is needed to protect the patient.[29,30] The provision of more focused information may achieve a similar goal as suggested recently.[39]

4. Some understanding of food allergy is important for patients so that they can manage their illness; however, more knowledge may be associated with increased anxiety and decreased QoL. Thus, it is important to impart knowledge about the illness in a supportive and reassuring way, and to emphasize that successful management of food allergy is possible and, under most circumstances, should not lead to significant disability.

5. Bullying is an emerging concern. Clinicians should inquire about bullying at routine visits.

6. Potentially promising targets for intervention include specific QoL concerns, distress (if excessive), increased knowledge about the illness, and education about coping.

7. Schools are where children socialize most, so a child's safety and comfort in school lunch settings are crucial. In addition, schools are the sites of most bullying in this population.[35] Therefore, the arrangements made by schools to accommodate the child's needs should be of interest to practitioners who may be called on to advocate for a food-allergic child's specific needs.[39,40]

8. When there is a concern about excessive distress or anxiety, allergists and primary care providers should consider referral to a mental health provider or suggest the use of integrated centers that have a psychiatrist or psychologist on staff.

REFERENCES

1. Branum AM, Lukacs SL. Food allergy among children in the United States. Pediatrics 2009;124(6):1549–55.
2. Gupta RS, Springston EE, Warrier MR, et al. The prevalence, severity, and distribution of childhood food allergy in the United States. Pediatrics 2011;128(1):e9–17.
3. Sicherer SH. Epidemiology of food allergy. J Allergy Clin Immunol 2011;127(3): 594–602.
4. Cummings AJ, Knibb RC, King RM, et al. The psychosocial impact of food allergy and food hypersensitivity in children, adolescents and their families: a review. Allergy 2010;65(8):933–45.
5. Lieberman JA, Sicherer SH. Quality of life in food allergy. Curr Opin Allergy Clin Immunol 2011;11(3):236–42.
6. Sicherer SH, Noone SA, Munoz-Furlong A. The impact of childhood food allergy on quality of life. Ann Allergy Asthma Immunol 2001;87(6):461–4.
7. Resnick ES, Pieretti MM, Maloney J, et al. Development of a questionnaire to measure quality of life in adolescents with food allergy: the FAQL-teen. Ann Allergy Asthma Immunol 2010;105(5):364–8.
8. Cohen BL, Noone S, Munoz-Furlong A, et al. Development of a questionnaire to measure quality of life in families with a child with food allergy. J Allergy Clin Immunol 2004;114(5):1159–63.
9. Lebovidge JS, Strauch H, Kalish LA, et al. Assessment of psychological distress among children and adolescents with food allergy. J Allergy Clin Immunol 2009; 124(6):1282–8.
10. Springston EE, Smith B, Shulruff J, et al. Variations in quality of life among caregivers of food allergic children. Ann Allergy Asthma Immunol 2010;105(4):287–94.

11. Valentine AZ, Knibb RC. Exploring quality of life in families of children living with and without a severe food allergy. Appetite 2011;57(2):467–74.
12. Cummings AJ, Knibb RC, Erlewyn-Lajeunesse M, et al. Management of nut allergy influences quality of life and anxiety in children and their mothers. Pediatr Allergy Immunol 2010;21(4 Pt 1):586–94.
13. Avery NJ, King RM, Knight S, et al. Assessment of quality of life in children with peanut allergy. Pediatr Allergy Immunol 2003;14(5):378–82.
14. Calsbeek H, Rijken M, Bekkers MJ, et al. School and leisure activities in adolescents and young adults with chronic digestive disorders: impact of burden of disease. Int J Behav Med 2006;13(2):121–30.
15. Flokstra-de Blok BM, Dubois AE, Vlieg-Boerstra BJ, et al. Health-related quality of life of food allergic patients: comparison with the general population and other diseases. Allergy 2010;65(2):238–44.
16. Flokstra-de Blok BM, DunnGalvin A, Vlieg-Boerstra BJ, et al. Development and validation of a self-administered Food Allergy Quality of Life Questionnaire for children. Clin Exp Allergy 2009;39(1):127–37.
17. Tyedin K, Cumming TB, Bernhardt J. Quality of life: an important outcome measure in a trial of very early mobilisation after stroke. Disabil Rehabil 2010; 32(11):875–84.
18. Ganz PA, Land SR, Geyer CE Jr, et al. Menstrual history and quality-of-life outcomes in women with node-positive breast cancer treated with adjuvant therapy on the NSABP B-30 trial. J Clin Oncol 2011;29(9):1110–6.
19. Lyons AC, Forde EM. Food allergy in young adults: perceptions and psychological effects. J Health Psychol 2004;9(4):497–504.
20. Sampson MA, Munoz-Furlong A, Sicherer SH. Risk-taking and coping strategies of adolescents and young adults with food allergy. J Allergy Clin Immunol 2006; 117(6):1440–5.
21. Rouf K, White L, Evans K. A qualitative investigation into the maternal experience of having a young child with severe food allergy. Clin Child Psychol Psychiatry 2011. [Epub ahead of print].
22. Gupta RS, Springston EE, Smith B, et al. Food allergy knowledge, attitudes, and beliefs of parents with food-allergic children in the United States. Pediatr Allergy Immunol 2010;21(6):927–34.
23. Klinnert MD, Robinson JL. Addressing the psychological needs of families of food-allergic children. Curr Allergy Asthma Rep 2008;8(3):195–200.
24. King RM, Knibb RC, Hourihane JO. Impact of peanut allergy on quality of life, stress and anxiety in the family. Allergy 2009;64(3):461–8.
25. Shemesh E, Newcorn JH, Rockmore L, et al. Comparison of parent and child reports of emotional trauma symptoms in pediatric outpatient settings. Pediatrics 2005;115(5):e582–9.
26. van der Velde JL, Flokstra-de Blok BM, Dunngalvin A, et al. Parents report better health-related quality of life for their food-allergic children than children themselves. Clin Exp Allergy 2011;41(10):1431–9.
27. Herbert LJ, Dahlquist LM. Perceived history of anaphylaxis and parental overprotection, autonomy, anxiety, and depression in food allergic young adults. J Clin Psychol Med Settings 2008;15(4):261–9.
28. Zijlstra WT, Flinterman AE, Soeters L, et al. Parental anxiety before and after food challenges in children with suspected peanut and hazelnut allergy. Pediatr Allergy Immunol 2010;21(2 Pt 2):e439–45.
29. Kemp AS, Allen CW, Campbell DE. Parental perceptions in egg allergy: does egg challenge make a difference? Pediatr Allergy Immunol 2009;20(7):648–53.

30. DunnGalvin A, Cullinane C, Daly DA, et al. Longitudinal validity and responsiveness of the Food Allergy Quality of Life Questionnaire–Parent Form in children 0-12 years following positive and negative food challenges. Clin Exp Allergy 2010; 40(3):476–85.

31. Strinnholm A, Brulin C, Lindh V. Experiences of double-blind, placebo-controlled food challenges (DBPCFC): a qualitative analysis of mothers' experiences. J Child Health Care 2010;14(2):179–88, 32.

32. Holt MK, Finkelhor D, Kantor GK. Multiple victimization experiences of urban elementary school students: associations with psychosocial functioning and academic performance. Child Abuse Negl 2007;31(5):503–15.

33. Dao TK, Kerbs JJ, Rollin SA, et al. The association between bullying dynamics and psychological distress. J Adolesc Health 2006;39(2):277–82.

34. Lehti V, Sourander A, Klomek A, et al. Childhood bullying as a predictor for becoming a teenage mother in Finland. Eur Child Adolesc Psychiatry 2011; 20(1):49–55.

35. Lieberman JA, Weiss C, Furlong TJ, et al. Bullying among pediatric patients with food allergy. Ann Allergy Asthma Immunol 2010;105(4):282–6.

36. George JT, Valdovinos AP, Russell I, et al. Clinical effectiveness of a brief educational intervention in Type 1 diabetes: results from the BITES (Brief Intervention in Type 1 diabetes, Education for Self-efficacy) trial. Diabet Med 2008;25(12): 1447–53.

37. Coffman JM, Cabana MD, Halpin HA, et al. Effects of asthma education on children's use of acute care services: a meta-analysis. Pediatrics 2008;121(3): 575–86.

38. LeBovidge JS, Timmons K, Rich C, et al. Evaluation of a group intervention for children with food allergy and their parents. Ann Allergy Asthma Immunol 2008; 101(2):160–5.

39. Sicherer SH, Mahr T. American Academy of Pediatrics Section on Allergy and Immunology. Management of food allergy in the school setting. Pediatrics 2010; 126(6):1232–9.

40. Young MC, Munoz-Furlong A, Sicherer SH. Management of food allergies in schools: a perspective for allergists. J Allergy Clin Immunol 2009;124(2):175–82, 182.e1–4 [quiz: 183–4].

Beyond Skin Testing: State of the Art and New Horizons in Food Allergy Diagnostic Testing

Jean-Christoph Caubet, MD[a], Hugh A. Sampson, MD[b],*

KEYWORDS

- Allergy • Food • IgE-mediated • Diagnosis • Microarray
- Molecular • Component-resolved diagnosis • Basophils

Food allergy represents a major health problem in infants and children, with an increasing prevalence. Recent epidemiologic studies based on objective diagnostic methods estimate that 1% to 10.8% of the general population suffer from food allergy.[1] The term "food allergy" refers to adverse immunologic reactions to food and should be distinguished from food intolerances that do not have an immune basis, such as a lactase deficiency. However, up to 35% of the population in Western countries self-report food allergy, indicating the magnitude of the problem and the need for appropriate diagnostic methods.[1,2] Accurate diagnosis of food allergy is important not only to prevent serious or even life-threatening reactions but also to avoid unnecessary dietary restrictions that could place individuals at risk for nutritional deficiencies and growth deficits.

In the diagnosis of food allergy no single investigation is fully reliable, and a stepwise approach is recommended by the international guidelines.[3] After a detailed history and physical examination, the allergy workup may be completed by in vivo and/or in vitro allergy tests, that is, skin-prick tests and/or measurement of food-specific immunoglobulin E (IgE) antibodies. Diagnostic cutoff values have been proposed to predict the likelihood of reactivity to various specific foods (**Table 1**). However, none of these diagnostic parameters have achieved sufficiently high predictive values, and thus most patients still need to undergo clinician-supervised oral food challenges

Potential conflicts of interest–none.

[a] Division of Pediatric Allergy and Immunology, Department of Pediatrics, Mount Sinai School of Medicine, One Gustave L. Levy Place, New York City, NY 10029-6574, USA
[b] Division of Allergy and Immunology, Department of Pediatrics, Mount Sinai School of Medicine, One Gustave L. Levy Place, Box 1198, New York City, NY 10029-6574, USA
* Corresponding author.
E-mail address: hugh.sampson@mssm.edu

Immunol Allergy Clin N Am 32 (2012) 97–109
doi:10.1016/j.iac.2011.11.002
0889-8561/12/$ – see front matter © 2012 Elsevier Inc. All rights reserved.

immunology.theclinics.com

Table 1
Laboratory tests to assess the likelihood of obtaining a positive or negative oral food challenge in young children

| Food | Serum Food-IgE (kU$_A$/L)[a] | |
	≈95% Positive	≈50% Negative[b]
Cow's milk	≥15[89] ≥5 if younger than 1 y[91]	≤2[90]
Egg white	≥7[89] ≥2 if younger than 2 y[92]	≤2[90]
Peanut	≥14[89]	≤2 with and ≤5 without history of peanut reaction[93]
Fish	≥20[89]	

[a] Phadia ImmunoCAP.
[b] In the authors' experience, children with about 50% chance of experiencing a negative challenge are the optimal candidates for an office-based oral food challenge. However, serum levels of food-specific IgE antibodies are not absolute indications or contraindications to performing an oral food challenge. Laboratory test results have to be always interpreted in the context of clinical history.
Modified from Nowak-Wegrzyn A, Assa'ad AH, Bahna SL, et al. Work Group report: oral food challenge testing. J Allergy Clin Immunol 2009;123(Suppl 6):S365–83; with permission.

(OFC). However, OFC are resource consuming and are associated with a risk for severe anaphylaxis. New testing methodologies are required to assess the presence and severity of a food allergy, as well as the resolution of the disease. At present, research efforts focus on improving diagnostic tests and on developing new tools that provide better prognostic performance. This review discusses several promising novel approaches for the diagnosis of IgE-mediated food allergy and their potential clinical applications.

MOLECULAR DIAGNOSIS IN FOOD ALLERGY

Current tests used to diagnose IgE-mediated food allergy perform relatively poorly in differentiating asymptomatic sensitization from true allergic reactions because they are typically performed with crude allergen extracts. Indeed, these extracts are difficult to standardize and consist of a mixture of allergenic and nonallergenic components, some of them cross-reacting with homologous proteins from other sources (ie, cross-reactive carbohydrate determinants) (**Table 2**).[4,5] Molecular diagnostic technologies have been recently introduced into allergy research as promising tools. Instead of measuring the IgE response to complex allergen extracts, specific responses at the level of individual allergenic proteins (component-resolved diagnosis [CRD]) or the IgE-binding epitopes of those allergens (epitope mapping or profiling) are evaluated.

Component-Resolved Diagnosis

The term "component-resolved diagnosis" has been used to designate diagnostic tests based on pure allergen proteins, which are either produced by recombinant expression of allergen-encoding complementary DNA or by purification from natural allergen sources.[6] For the most common foods, many allergenic proteins have been identified, sequenced, and cloned. Recent advances in proteomics research, including 2-dimensional gel electrophoresis, mass spectrometry, protein arrays, and improved bioinformatics, have largely expanded the library of known food components, although identification of new allergens is increasing steadily.[7,8] The benefits and problems of the different allergen preparations available are outlined in **Table 2**.

Table 2
Benefits and problems of allergen preparations used for in vitro diagnostics

	Natural Extracts	Native Allergens	Recombinant Proteins
Advantages	Easy to prepare Ideally, all allergenic proteins are present	Enabling of CRD Native protein structures are mostly preserved Presence of all natural isoforms and posttranslational modifications	Enabling of CRD and application of a single isoform Lack of impurities with other food proteins Standardization of amount and structural characteristics
Disadvantages	Standardization problems caused by the natural variability of active ingredients and endogenous degradation that also can cause low assay sensitivity Complex mixtures of allergenic and nonallergenic components sometimes resulting in low assay specificity	Laborious preparation Yield depends on composition of source material Risk of variable batch composition caused by different copurification yields of isoforms Risk of low-level contamination with other allergens from the same source and purification artifacts	Laborious preparation Proteins can be unfolded or partially unfolded and might not be properly modified after translation Risk of low-level contamination with components of the expression system and purification artifacts

Abbreviation: CRD, component-resolved diagnosis.
Reproduced from Steckelbroeck S, Ballmer-Weber BK, Vieths S. Potential, pitfalls, and prospects of food allergy diagnostics with recombinant allergens or synthetic sequential epitopes. J Allergy Clin Immunol 2008;121(6):1323–30; with permission.

Potential Clinical Application of CRD

Studies comparing diagnostic performances of CRD to traditional allergy tests, that is, skin-prick tests and specific IgE, suggest that component testing could improve specificity for several foods. For example, a recent study evaluated the effectiveness of CRD to distinguish between patients allergic to peanuts and those sensitized but clinically tolerant.[9] By using specific IgE to the component protein, Ara h 2, with a cutoff point of 0.35 kU$_A$/L, 97.5% of the population was correctly classified, and all patients allergic to peanut were correctly identified. The misclassification rate using a whole peanut-specific IgE level of 15 kU$_A$/L was about 18% in this study.

Similarly, the value of specific IgE antibodies to omega-5-gliadin (Tri a 19) has been evaluated in the diagnosis of wheat allergy. Although Tri a 19 was previously identified as a major allergen in wheat-dependent exercise-induced anaphylaxis,[10] recently it has been shown to be a significant allergen in young children with immediate allergic reactions to wheat.[11,12] In a recent study, the level of specific IgE to Tri a 19 was related to the challenge outcome in wheat-sensitized children and to the severity of the reaction.[12] Moreover, specific IgE to Tri a 19 had superior performance to that of wheat-specific IgE for the prediction of clinical reactivity to wheat. However, not all investigators have found it specific.[13]

Measurement of specific IgE to individual components may also provide important additional information to identify different clinical phenotypes of food allergy. In children allergic to egg, greater levels of ovomucoid-specific IgE were found in those reacting to baked egg than in those tolerant to baked egg and regular egg.[14] Low levels of IgE against ovomucoid indicated a low risk of reaction to baked egg. Likewise, the authors found that casein-specific IgE has superior accuracy for predicting baked milk reactivity compared with cow's milk–specific IgE. (Caubet JC, Nowak-Węgrzyn A, Moshier E, et al. Utility of casein-specific IgE levels in predicting reactivity to baked milk. Submitted for publication.)

Furthermore, CRD may be useful in predicting the severity and/or persistence of the disease. High levels of casein-specific IgE antibodies have been identified as a risk factor for persistence of cow's milk allergy[15,16] and for more severe allergic reactions, especially in asthmatic children.[17] Similarly, it has been shown in 2 different studies that children with persistent egg allergy had significantly higher ovomucoid-specific IgE levels than those who outgrew their egg allergy.[18,19] A favorable prognosis was associated with the absence or a decline in ovomucoid-specific IgE titers.[18]

Determining allergen sensitization profiles could help to assess the risk of cross-reactive allergies to other food sources and to avoid unnecessary exclusion diets. The most illustrative example is patients with fish allergy. Because of a high degree of cross-reactivity between parvalbumin from different fish species,[20] patients sensitized to a fish parvalbumin (eg, Gad c 1 from cod[21] and Cyp c 1 from carp[22]) are likely to react to a range of different fish species. However, some patients allergic to fish can tolerate some fish species while being allergic to others.[23] A recent study suggests that the different expression level of parvalbumin in specific species might explain tolerance to some species such as swordfish.[24] The differences in clinical response to fish species might also be explained by reactivity to allergens other than parvalbumins.[25] A better understanding of the allergenic characteristics of different fish species helps to better predict cross-reactivity[26,27] and improve the management of patients allergic to fish.

In addition, component testing may help to differentiate between sensitization caused by cross-reactivity with pollens and systemic clinical allergy (**Table 3**). In peanut allergy, for example, the presence of specific IgE antibodies to Ara h 8 (a Bet v 1 homolog) is a marker for birch-pollen–related reactions to peanut. For example,

Table 3
Plant food allergens classified according to their cross-reactive potential

Food	Pollen Cross-Reactive Components[a]	Lipid Transfer Protein	Pollen Non–Cross-Reactive Components[b]
Peanut	Ara h 8[c] Ara h 5[d]	Ara h 9	Ara h 1; Ara h 2; Ara h 3 Ara h 4; Ara h 6; Ara h 7
Hazelnut	Cor a 1[c] Cor a 2[d]	Cor a 8	Cor a 9 Cor a 11
Soybean	Gly m 4[c] Gly m 3[d]	Gly m 1	Gly m 5 Gly m 6
Wheat	Tri a 12[d]	Tri a 14	Tri a 19 (ω-5 gliadin) Tri a 21 (α gliadin) Tri a 26 (high–molecular weight glutenin) Tri a 28 (α-amylase inhibitor dimer 0.19)

[a] Birch-tree pollen, Timothy grass pollen for wheat.
[b] Storage seed proteins, albumins, and globulins.
[c] PR10 proteins.
[d] Profilin.

among children selected from a large birth cohort, peanut allergy symptoms were reported in 87% of the children with IgE reactivity to pollen-unrelated Ara h 1, 2, or 3, but not to Ara h 8 (n = 46), compared with 17% of children with IgE reactivity to Ara h 8, but not to Ara h 1, 2, or 3 (n = 23).[28] Moreover, patients sensitized to Ara h 1, 2, or 3 have been shown to have more severe symptoms.[29]

Like peanut allergy, IgE-mediated allergy to soy may be the result of primary sensitization to soy but could also result from cross-reactivity to birch-related tree pollen and a variety of legumes.[30–34] The presence of Gly m 5–specific and Gly m 6–specific IgE is a marker of primary sensitization associated with a higher risk of severe reactions.[31,32] Sensitization to Gly m 4 is common in patients allergic to birch pollen and is often associated with local reactions, although systemic reactions may also occur.[33,34]

Allergen Components on Microarray

In the United States, the allergen components are commercially available using the ImmunoCAP system (Phadia AB, Uppsala, Sweden). In Europe, protein microarray has recently been introduced for measuring specific IgE and is commercialized in the form of the ImmunoCAP-ISAC, Immuno Solid-phase Allergen Chip (VBC Genomics, Vienna, Austria; Phadia, Uppsala, Sweden).[35,36] It currently has 112 native/recombinant component allergens from 51 allergenic sources. This technology has 2 main advantages: it simultaneously assesses specific IgE to different components and requires very small amounts of sera, which is especially relevant in children. Moreover, ImmunoCAP-ISAC can be considered a cost-efficient approach because it delivers results for more than 100 components.

Ott and colleagues[37] evaluated the clinical performance characteristics of this assay regarding the outcome of the OFC for suspected allergy to cow's milk (n = 85) and eggs (n = 60), and found no advantage over the usual diagnostic tests, that is, skin-prick test and whole protein–based specific IgE. Although the diagnostic capability was not enhanced with the use of CRD, the investigators recommended the use of microarrayed allergen components as a minimally invasive tool because of the low quantity of serum required for analysis.

Using a customized version of the ISAC microarray, D'Urbano and colleagues[38] also investigated children with suspected cow's milk allergy and egg allergy, comparing allergen components with OFC. The results indicated that serial testing of specific IgE and microarray components had a clinical performance very close to that of the OFC. These investigators proposed to use the microarray as a second-level assay if the level of specific IgE is above 95% of the positive predictive value.[39] This approach could lead to a decrease in the number of the OFC to be performed.

Recent studies have also provided interesting results on microarray testing for the diagnosis of peanut,[9] wheat,[40] and milk allergy,[41] as well as for the diagnosis of oral allergy syndrome to apple.[42]

Using the same platform, more significant information could be obtained. For example, it is theoretically feasible that by spotting different concentrations of allergens on the chip, relative IgE antibody affinity can be determined.[43] Moreover, the parallel determination of different antibody isotypes (IgA, IgM, IgG, and IgE) using microarrays seems to offer promising results,[44] even when attachment to the microarray is achieved using whole food extracts.[45] A drawback of CRD microarrays is the risk of overdiagnosis and misinterpretation of the complex results of such tests.[46] Well-designed large-scale studies from different geographic areas are needed to evaluate the practical use of allergenic components in food-allergic patients.

Role of Epitope Mapping in the Diagnosis of Food Allergy

Food allergens must at least partially survive digestion and absorption from the gastrointestinal tract to be immunogenic, which has led to the hypothesis that individuals who generate IgE antibodies recognizing a greater number or a specific pattern of sequential epitopes (eg, those not easily destroyed by denaturation and partial digestion) are more likely to have clinical allergy rather than asymptomatic IgE sensitization.[47] Furthermore, the importance of recognizing sequential IgE-binding epitopes in the persistence and severity of allergy has been highlighted in several studies on milk,[48–50] peanut,[51,52] egg,[19,53] and wheat allergens.[54] For example, Vila and colleagues[55] found higher levels of IgE antibodies to specific sequential epitopes from casein in children who have persistent cow's milk allergy in comparison with those who were to develop tolerance.

In the past, epitope mapping was mainly performed using SPOT membrane-based immunoassays[48,49,56] whereby peptides were synthesized on a nitrocellulose membrane and then incubated with the patients' sera. However, synthesis of large numbers of peptides is relatively error prone, time consuming, labor intensive, and expensive and has limitations because of the specific chemistry of the method. A large volume of serum is required, and there is also a limitation of the number of targeted peptides. With the development of microarray technology and evolution in peptide synthesis techniques, peptide microarray-based immunoassays for epitope mapping of allergens may be the next step. Recently, several clinical studies on milk,[57,58] peanut,[51,52] and shrimp allergy[59] provided promising results, demonstrating that greater IgE epitope diversity and/or higher affinity were associated with clinical phenotype and/or severity of allergy. In the future, this assay might be useful for predicting the outcome of food allergy and for identifying patients at risk for persistent allergy as potential candidates for proactive treatment. However, technical issues and limitations need to be addressed before clinical use is attempted.

FUNCTIONAL ASSAYS
Basophil Activation Testing

Basophils represent a significant effector population in allergic pathogenesis. Because they can be stimulated ex vivo, they provide the theoretical potential of measuring a biological allergic response, more so than specific IgE.[60,61] The first approach to basophil functional responses was the histamine release test, but this has remained controversial due to its insufficient sensitivity and specificity.[62,63] Several groups proposed using flow cytometry to identify the population of basophils and measure their activation based on upregulation of cell-surface molecules (eg, CD63 and CD203c).[64–66] The basophil activation test (BAT) is increasingly under investigation.[67]

Recently, based on 36 prospectively recruited patients, Rubio and colleagues[68] showed that BAT was a better predictor of milk allergy using challenge outcomes as the gold standard. It was also observed that children with clinical sensitivity to milk-containing baked products had greater basophil reactivity than tolerant children.[66] Another recent study examined the performance of BAT for predicting challenge outcome in a group of 71 children with egg or milk allergy previously diagnosed by challenge outcomes or convincing history.[69] These investigators found that assessment of food antigen–induced CD203c expression on basophils is useful to determine whether children will outgrow food allergy as well as to make decisions regarding whether or not to perform OFC. Other studies suggest that BAT is comparable to skin-prick tests or specific IgE levels in its ability to distinguish clinical allergy from sensitization in patients with food-pollen allergy syndrome.[70–73]

Recently a few papers have been published in which the BAT is activated using purified or recombinant components.[74–77] For example, Erdmann and colleagues[72] investigated the diagnostic value of BAT with recombinant allergens (Mal d 1, Dau c 1, and Api g 1) for the diagnosis of apple, carrot, or celery allergy in patients allergic to birch. The investigators found high specificities that were comparable to those of specific IgE to apple, carrot, and celery, but the sensitivities were lower in comparison with prick-to-prick testing using fresh fruits or vegetables. In the future, in analogy to CRD, the BAT as functional test may be used to define a patient's sensitization profile, using purified or recombinant allergen components, facilitating the discrimination between true allergy and clinically irrelevant sensitization to cross-reactive molecules.

Evaluation of T-Cell Responses

T-cell responses to food allergens have also been evaluated in the diagnosis of food allergy. Food-allergic patients in general have higher proliferative responses than sensitized patients or healthy controls, suggesting an intrinsic excessive reactivity of the T cells in food-allergic patients.[78] However, lymphocyte proliferation assays are neither diagnostic nor predictive of clinical reactivity in individual patients with food allergy.[79,80]

More specific analysis of allergen-specific T-cell responses may be useful to distinguish between sensitization and clinically relevant allergy. Recently, Flinterman and colleagues[81] used the CRD approach to characterize peanut-specific T-cell responses in patients allergic to peanuts (n = 18), peanut-sensitized patients (n = 7), and nonallergic control patients (n = 11). The T-cell response to crude peanut extract was stronger in children with peanut allergy than in those with peanut sensitization or without peanut allergy. Only the children with peanut allergy had detectable interleukin-13 production in response to major peanut allergens (Ara h 1, Ara h 3, and Ara h 6). Although T-cell subset CRD is unlikely to displace OFC as the gold standard, if reproduced these results could open a new perspective on the diagnosis of food allergy.

OTHER ASSESSMENT
Serum-Specific IgG Antibodies

Based on studies from the 1980s indicating that antigen-specific IgG_4 could induce histamine release from basophils,[82] testing for blood IgG_4 has been increasingly performed with screening for hundreds of food items in patients with suspected food allergy and intolerance. Testing for food-specific IgG typically yields multiple positive results, which often represents a normal immune response to food. Indeed, specific IgG_4 antibodies are not predictive of food allergy,[83] and national and international guidelines do not recommend testing of IgG_4 to food in the allergy workup.[3]

On the other hand, emerging data from immunotherapy trials suggest that the IgG_4 immunoglobulin class may play a protective role, serving as blocking antibodies, in tolerance development.[84,85] Because the balance between allergen-specific IgE and IgG_4 production may affect whether clinical allergy or tolerance develops, the determination of the ratio of specific IgE/IgG_4 may be more useful than the absolute amount of IgG_4 for assessing the ongoing status of food sensitization. For example, measurement of the specific ratios IgE/IgG_4 to ovalbumin and/or ovomucoid has been shown to be useful in following the development of tolerance and outgrowing egg allergy in research studies.[86,87] These data need to be confirmed in further studies.

Other Nonvalidated Tests

Several other methods have been evaluated for the diagnosis of food allergy, including facial thermography, gastric juice analysis, endoscopic allergen provocation, hair analysis, applied kinesiology, provocation neutralization, electrodermal test (Vega), and mediator release assay (lifestyle, eating, and performance diet). However, there is a lack of evidence demonstrating that any of the tests have diagnostic value in food allergy.

SUMMARY

Improved interpretation of allergic testing facilitates the diagnosis of food allergy and eliminates unnecessary OFCs. Research efforts are focused on improving diagnostic tests and on developing tests that have a better prognostic performance. Molecular diagnostic assays are especially promising and could significantly improve the management of food allergic patients by providing a more individualized medical approach to care. However, these methods still need to be validated against OFCs, considered the gold standard, in large-scale studies and in different geographic regions. Functional assays, such as BATs, particularly in combination with allergen components, might also be useful and need to be further investigated. In the future, coupling the diversity of a microarray approach with the potential functionality and biological activity of a cell-based test may result in a new system to improve the diagnosis of food allergy.[88]

ACKNOWLEDGMENTS

We thank Dr Anna Nowak-Węgrzyn for kindly providing **Table 3**.

REFERENCES

1. Rona RJ, Keil T, Summers C, et al. The prevalence of food allergy: a meta-analysis. J Allergy Clin Immunol 2007;120(3):638–46.
2. Woods RK, Stoney RM, Raven J, et al. Reported adverse food reactions overestimate true food allergy in the community. Eur J Clin Nutr 2002;56(1):31–6.
3. NIAID-Sponsored Expert Panel, Boyce JA, Assa'ad A, et al. Guidelines for the diagnosis and management of food allergy in the United States: report of the NIAID-sponsored expert panel. J Allergy Clin Immunol 2010;126(Suppl 6):S1–58.

4. Guilloux L, Morisset M, Codreanu F, et al. Peanut allergy diagnosis in the context of grass pollen sensitization for 125 patients: roles of peanut and cross-reactive carbohydrate determinants specific IgE. Int Arch Allergy Immunol 2009;149(2): 91–7.

5. van der Veen MJ, van Ree R, Aalberse RC, et al. Poor biologic activity of cross-reactive IgE directed to carbohydrate determinants of glycoproteins. J Allergy Clin Immunol 1997;100(3):327–34.

6. Valenta R, Vrtala S. Recombinant allergens for specific immunotherapy. Allergy 1999;54(Suppl 56):43–4.

7. Sancho AI, Hoffmann-Sommergruber K, Alessandri S, et al. Authentication of food allergen quality by physicochemical and immunological methods. Clin Exp Allergy 2010;40(7):973–86.

8. Beyer K. Characterization of allergenic food proteins for improved diagnostic methods. Curr Opin Allergy Clin Immunol 2003;3(3):189–97.

9. Nicolaou N, Murray C, Belgrave D, et al. Quantification of specific IgE to whole peanut extract and peanut components in prediction of peanut allergy. J Allergy Clin Immunol 2011;127(3):684–5.

10. Matsuo H, Dahlstrom J, Tanaka A, et al. Sensitivity and specificity of recombinant omega-5 gliadin-specific IgE measurement for the diagnosis of wheat-dependent exercise-induced anaphylaxis. Allergy 2008;63(2):233–6.

11. Palosuo K, Varjonen E, Kekki OM, et al. Wheat omega-5 gliadin is a major allergen in children with immediate allergy to ingested wheat. J Allergy Clin Immunol 2001;108(4):634–8.

12. Ito K, Futamura M, Borres MP, et al. IgE antibodies to omega-5 gliadin associate with immediate symptoms on oral wheat challenge in Japanese children. Allergy 2008;63(11):1536–42.

13. Beyer K, Chung D, Schulz G, et al. The role of wheat omega-5 gliadin IgE antibodies as a diagnostic tool for wheat allergy in childhood. J Allergy Clin Immunol 2008;122(2):419–21.

14. Ando H, Moverare R, Kondo Y, et al. Utility of ovomucoid-specific IgE concentrations in predicting symptomatic egg allergy. J Allergy Clin Immunol 2008;122(3):583–8.

15. Sicherer SH, Sampson HA. Cow's milk protein-specific IgE concentrations in two age groups of milk-allergic children and in children achieving clinical tolerance. Clin Exp Allergy 1999;29(4):507–12.

16. Garcia-Ara MC, Boyano-Martinez MT, Diaz-Pena JM, et al. Cow's milk-specific immunoglobulin E levels as predictors of clinical reactivity in the follow-up of the cow's milk allergy infants. Clin Exp Allergy 2004;34(6):866–70.

17. Boyano-Martinez T, Garcia-Ara C, Pedrosa M, et al. Accidental allergic reactions in children allergic to cow's milk proteins. J Allergy Clin Immunol 2009;123(4):883–8.

18. Bernhisel-Broadbent J, Dintzis HM, Dintzis RZ, et al. Allergenicity and antigenicity of chicken egg ovomucoid (Gal d III) compared with ovalbumin (Gal d I) in children with egg allergy and in mice. J Allergy Clin Immunol 1994;93(6):1047–59.

19. Jarvinen KM, Beyer K, Vila L, et al. Specificity of IgE antibodies to sequential epitopes of hen's egg ovomucoid as a marker for persistence of egg allergy. Allergy 2007;62(7):758–65.

20. Van Do T, Elsayed S, Florvaag E, et al. Allergy to fish parvalbumins: studies on the cross-reactivity of allergens from 9 commonly consumed fish. J Allergy Clin Immunol 2005;116(6):1314–20.

21. Van Do T, Hordvik I, Endresen C, et al. Characterization of parvalbumin, the major allergen in Alaska pollack, and comparison with codfish Allergen M. Mol Immunol 2005;42(3):345–53.

22. Swoboda I, Bugajska-Schretter A, Verdino P, et al. Recombinant carp parvalbumin, the major cross-reactive fish allergen: a tool for diagnosis and therapy of fish allergy. J Immunol 2002;168(9):4576–84.

23. Bernhisel-Broadbent J, Scanlon SM, Sampson HA. Fish hypersensitivity. I. In vitro and oral challenge results in fish-allergic patients. J Allergy Clin Immunol 1992; 89(3):730–7.

24. Griesmeier U, Vazquez-Cortes S, Bublin M, et al. Expression levels of parvalbumins determine allergenicity of fish species. Allergy 2010;65(2):191–8.

25. Das Dores S, Chopin C, Romano A, et al. IgE-binding and cross-reactivity of a new 41 kDa allergen of codfish. Allergy 2002;57(Suppl 72):84–7.

26. Pascual C, Martin Esteban M, Crespo JF. Fish allergy: evaluation of the importance of cross-reactivity. J Pediatr 1992;121(5 Pt 2):S29–34.

27. Kobayashi A, Tanaka H, Hamada Y, et al. Comparison of allergenicity and allergens between fish white and dark muscles. Allergy 2006;61(3):357–63.

28. Asarnoj A, Moverare R, Ostblom E, et al. IgE to peanut allergen components: relation to peanut symptoms and pollen sensitization in 8-year-olds. Allergy 2010;65(9):1189–95.

29. Astier C, Morisset M, Roitel O, et al. Predictive value of skin prick tests using recombinant allergens for diagnosis of peanut allergy. J Allergy Clin Immunol 2006; 118(1):250–6.

30. L'Hocine L, Boye JI. Allergenicity of soybean: new developments in identification of allergenic proteins, cross-reactivities and hypoallergenization technologies. Crit Rev Food Sci Nutr 2007;47(2):127–43.

31. Holzhauser T, Wackermann O, Ballmer-Weber BK, et al. Soybean (*Glycine max*) allergy in Europe: Gly m 5 (beta-conglycinin) and Gly m 6 (glycinin) are potential diagnostic markers for severe allergic reactions to soy. J Allergy Clin Immunol 2009;123(2):452–8.

32. Ito K, Sjolander S, Sato S, et al. IgE to Gly m 5 and Gly m 6 is associated with severe allergic reactions to soybean in Japanese children. J Allergy Clin Immunol 2011;128(3):673–5.

33. Kleine-Tebbe J, Vogel L, Crowell DN, et al. Severe oral allergy syndrome and anaphylactic reactions caused by a Bet v 1-related PR-10 protein in soybean, SAM22. J Allergy Clin Immunol 2002;110(5):797–804.

34. Mittag D, Vieths S, Vogel L, et al. Soybean allergy in patients allergic to birch pollen: clinical investigation and molecular characterization of allergens. J Allergy Clin Immunol 2004;113(1):148–54.

35. Hiller R, Laffer S, Harwanegg C, et al. Microarrayed allergen molecules: diagnostic gatekeepers for allergy treatment. FASEB J 2002;16(3):414–6.

36. Jahn-Schmid B, Harwanegg C, Hiller R, et al. Allergen microarray: comparison of microarray using recombinant allergens with conventional diagnostic methods to detect allergen-specific serum immunoglobulin E. Clin Exp Allergy 2003;33(10):1443–9.

37. Ott H, Baron JM, Heise R, et al. Clinical usefulness of microarray-based IgE detection in children with suspected food allergy. Allergy 2008;63(11):1521–8.

38. D'Urbano LE, Pellegrino K, Artesani MC, et al. Performance of a component-based allergen-microarray in the diagnosis of cow's milk and hen's egg allergy. Clin Exp Allergy 2010;40(10):1561–70.

39. Sampson HA, Ho DG. Relationship between food-specific IgE concentrations and the risk of positive food challenges in children and adolescents. J Allergy Clin Immunol 1997;100(4):444–51.

40. Constantin C, Quirce S, Poorafshar M, et al. Micro-arrayed wheat seed and grass pollen allergens for component-resolved diagnosis. Allergy 2009;64(7):1030–7.

41. Hochwallner H, Schulmeister U, Swoboda I, et al. Microarray and allergenic activity assessment of milk allergens. Clin Exp Allergy 2010;40(12):1809–18.
42. Ebo DG, Bridts CH, Verweij MM, et al. Sensitization profiles in birch pollen-allergic patients with and without oral allergy syndrome to apple: lessons from multiplexed component-resolved allergy diagnosis. Clin Exp Allergy 2010;40(2):339–47.
43. Hamilton RG, Saito H. IgE antibody concentration, specific activity, clonality, and affinity measures from future diagnostic confirmatory tests. J Allergy Clin Immunol 2008;122(2):305–6.
44. Renault NK, Gaddipati SR, Wulfert F, et al. Multiple protein extract microarray for profiling human food-specific immunoglobulins A, M, G and E. J Immunol Methods 2011;364(1–2):21–32.
45. Noh G, Ahn HS, Cho NY, et al. The clinical significance of food specific IgE/IgG4 in food specific atopic dermatitis. Pediatr Allergy Immunol 2007;18(1):63–70.
46. Knol EF, Knulst AC. Application of multiplexed immunoglobulin E determination on a chip in component-resolved diagnostics in allergy. Clin Exp Allergy 2010; 40(2):190–2.
47. Sampson HA. Improving in-vitro tests for the diagnosis of food hypersensitivity. Curr Opin Allergy Clin Immunol 2002;2(3):257–61.
48. Chatchatee P, Jarvinen KM, Bardina L, et al. Identification of IgE- and IgG-binding epitopes on alpha(s1)-casein: differences in patients with persistent and transient cow's milk allergy. J Allergy Clin Immunol 2001;107(2):379–83.
49. Chatchatee P, Jarvinen KM, Bardina L, et al. Identification of IgE and IgG binding epitopes on beta- and kappa-casein in cow's milk allergic patients. Clin Exp Allergy 2001;31(8):1256–62.
50. Jarvinen KM, Chatchatee P, Bardina L, et al. IgE and IgG binding epitopes on alpha-lactalbumin and beta-lactoglobulin in cow's milk allergy. Int Arch Allergy Immunol 2001;126(2):111–8.
51. Shreffler WG, Beyer K, Chu TH, et al. Microarray immunoassay: association of clinical history, in vitro IgE function, and heterogeneity of allergenic peanut epitopes. J Allergy Clin Immunol 2004;113(4):776–82.
52. Flinterman AE, Knol EF, Lencer DA, et al. Peanut epitopes for IgE and IgG4 in peanut-sensitized children in relation to severity of peanut allergy. J Allergy Clin Immunol 2008;121(3):737.e10–743.e10.
53. Cooke SK, Sampson HA. Allergenic properties of ovomucoid in man. J Immunol 1997;159(4):2026–32.
54. Battais F, Mothes T, Moneret-Vautrin DA, et al. Identification of IgE-binding epitopes on gliadins for patients with food allergy to wheat. Allergy 2005;60(6):815–21.
55. Vila L, Beyer K, Jarvinen KM, et al. Role of conformational and linear epitopes in the achievement of tolerance in cow's milk allergy. Clin Exp Allergy 2001;31(10): 1599–606.
56. Frank R. The SPOT-synthesis technique. Synthetic peptide arrays on membrane supports—principles and applications. J Immunol Methods 2002;267(1):13–26.
57. Wang J, Lin J, Bardina L, et al. Correlation of IgE/IgG4 milk epitopes and affinity of milk-specific IgE antibodies with different phenotypes of clinical milk allergy. J Allergy Clin Immunol 2010;125(3):695–702, 702.e1–702.e6.
58. Savilahti EM, Rantanen V, Lin JS, et al. Early recovery from cow's milk allergy is associated with decreasing IgE and increasing IgG4 binding to cow's milk epitopes. J Allergy Clin Immunol 2010;125(6):1315.e9–1321.e9.
59. Ayuso R, Sanchez-Garcia S, Lin J, et al. Greater epitope recognition of shrimp allergens by children than by adults suggests that shrimp sensitization decreases with age. J Allergy Clin Immunol 2010;125(6):1286.e3–1293.e3.

60. Ocmant A, Mulier S, Hanssens L, et al. Basophil activation tests for the diagnosis of food allergy in children. Clin Exp Allergy 2009;39(8):1234–45.
61. Shreffler WG. Evaluation of basophil activation in food allergy: present and future applications. Curr Opin Allergy Clin Immunol 2006;6(3):226–33.
62. Hamilton RG, Franklin Adkinson N Jr. In vitro assays for the diagnosis of IgE-mediated disorders. J Allergy Clin Immunol 2004;114(2):213–5 [quiz: 226].
63. Demoly P, Lebel B, Messaad D, et al. Predictive capacity of histamine release for the diagnosis of drug allergy. Allergy 1999;54(5):500–6.
64. Ebo DG, Sainte-Laudy J, Bridts CH, et al. Flow-assisted allergy diagnosis: current applications and future perspectives. Allergy 2006;61(9):1028–39.
65. De Weck AL, Sanz ML, Gamboa PM, et al. Nonsteroidal anti-inflammatory drug hypersensitivity syndrome. A multicenter study. I. Clinical findings and in vitro diagnosis. J Investig Allergol Clin Immunol 2009;19(5):355–69.
66. Wanich N, Nowak-Wegrzyn A, Sampson HA, et al. Allergen-specific basophil suppression associated with clinical tolerance in patients with milk allergy. J Allergy Clin Immunol 2009;123(4):789.e20–794.e20.
67. Sturm GJ, Kranzelbinder B, Sturm EM, et al. The basophil activation test in the diagnosis of allergy: technical issues and critical factors. Allergy 2009;64(9):1319–26.
68. Rubio A, Vivinus-Nebot M, Bourrier T, et al. Benefit of the basophil activation test in deciding when to reintroduce cow's milk in allergic children. Allergy 2011;66(1):92–100.
69. Sato S, Tachimoto H, Shukuya A, et al. Basophil activation marker CD203c is useful in the diagnosis of hen's egg and cow's milk allergies in children. Int Arch Allergy Immunol 2010;152(Suppl 1):54–61.
70. Ebo DG, Hagendorens MM, Bridts CH, et al. Flow cytometric analysis of in vitro activated basophils, specific IgE and skin tests in the diagnosis of pollen-associated food allergy. Cytometry B Clin Cytom 2005;64(1):28–33.
71. Erdmann SM, Heussen N, Moll-Slodowy S, et al. CD63 expression on basophils as a tool for the diagnosis of pollen-associated food allergy: sensitivity and specificity. Clin Exp Allergy 2003;33(5):607–14.
72. Erdmann SM, Sachs B, Schmidt A, et al. In vitro analysis of birch-pollen-associated food allergy by use of recombinant allergens in the basophil activation test. Int Arch Allergy Immunol 2005;136(3):230–8.
73. Moneret-Vautrin DA, Sainte-Laudy J, Kanny G, et al. Human basophil activation measured by CD63 expression and LTC4 release in IgE-mediated food allergy. Ann Allergy Asthma Immunol 1999;82(1):33–40.
74. Hauswirth AW, Natter S, Ghannadan M, et al. Recombinant allergens promote expression of CD203c on basophils in sensitized individuals. J Allergy Clin Immunol 2002;110(1):102–9.
75. Kahlert H, Cromwell O, Fiebig H. Measurement of basophil-activating capacity of grass pollen allergens, allergoids and hypoallergenic recombinant derivatives by flow cytometry using anti-CD203c. Clin Exp Allergy 2003;33(9):1266–72.
76. Sanz ML, Garcia-Aviles MC, Tabar AI, et al. Basophil activation test and specific IgE measurements using a panel of recombinant natural rubber latex allergens to determine the latex allergen sensitization profile in children. Pediatr Allergy Immunol 2006;17(2):148–56.
77. Gamboa PM, Sanz ML, Lombardero M, et al. Component-resolved in vitro diagnosis in peach-allergic patients. J Investig Allergol Clin Immunol 2009;19(1):13–20.
78. Hourihane JO, Dean TP, Warner JO. Peanut allergic subjects' peripheral blood mononuclear cell proliferative responses to crude peanut protein. Clin Exp Allergy 1998;28(2):163–8.

79. Hoffman KM, Ho DG, Sampson HA. Evaluation of the usefulness of lymphocyte proliferation assays in the diagnosis of allergy to cow's milk. J Allergy Clin Immunol 1997;99(3):360–6.
80. Thottingal TB, Stefura BP, Simons FE, et al. Human subjects without peanut allergy demonstrate T cell-dependent, TH2-biased, peanut-specific cytokine and chemokine responses independent of TH1 expression. J Allergy Clin Immunol 2006;118(4):905–14.
81. Flinterman AE, Pasmans SG, den Hartog Jager CF, et al. T cell responses to major peanut allergens in children with and without peanut allergy. Clin Exp Allergy 2010;40(4):590–7.
82. Fagan DL, Slaughter CA, Capra JD, et al. Monoclonal antibodies to immunoglobulin G4 induce histamine release from human basophils in vitro. J Allergy Clin Immunol 1982;70(5):399–404.
83. Stapel SO, Asero R, Ballmer-Weber BK, et al. Testing for IgG4 against foods is not recommended as a diagnostic tool: EAACI Task Force Report. Allergy 2008; 63(7):793–6.
84. Wachholz PA, Durham SR. Mechanisms of immunotherapy: IgG revisited. Curr Opin Allergy Clin Immunol 2004;4(4):313–8.
85. Uermosi C, Beerli RR, Bauer M, et al. Mechanisms of allergen-specific desensitization. J Allergy Clin Immunol 2010;126(2):375–83.
86. Lemon-Mule H, Sampson HA, Sicherer SH, et al. Immunologic changes in children with egg allergy ingesting extensively heated egg. J Allergy Clin Immunol 2008;122(5):977.e1–983.e1.
87. Tomicic S, Norrman G, Falth-Magnusson K, et al. High levels of IgG4 antibodies to foods during infancy are associated with tolerance to corresponding foods later in life. Pediatr Allergy Immunol 2009;20(1):35–41.
88. Lin J, Renault N, Haas H, et al. A novel tool for the detection of allergic sensitization combining protein microarrays with human basophils. Clin Exp Allergy 2007; 37(12):1854–62.
89. Sampson HA. Utility of food-specific IgE concentrations in predicting symptomatic food allergy. J Allergy Clin Immunol 2001;107(5):891–6.
90. Perry TT, Matsui EC, Kay Conover-Walker M, et al. The relationship of allergen-specific IgE levels and oral food challenge outcome. J Allergy Clin Immunol 2004;114(1):144–9.
91. Garcia-Ara C, Boyano-Martinez T, Diaz-Pena JM, et al. Specific IgE levels in the diagnosis of immediate hypersensitivity to cows' milk protein in the infant. J Allergy Clin Immunol 2001;107(1):185–90.
92. Boyano-Martinez T, Garcia-Ara C, Diaz-Pena JM, et al. Prediction of tolerance on the basis of quantification of egg white-specific IgE antibodies in children with egg allergy. J Allergy Clin Immunol 2002;110(2):304–9.
93. Sicherer SH, Morrow EH, Sampson HA. Dose-response in double-blind, placebo-controlled oral food challenges in children with atopic dermatitis. J Allergy Clin Immunol 2000;105(3):582–6.

Oral Immunotherapy and Anti-IgE Antibody-Adjunctive Treatment for Food Allergy

Kari C. Nadeau, MD, PhD[a,1], Arunima Kohli, BS[b,1],
Shuba Iyengar, MD[c], Rosemarie H. DeKruyff, PhD[d],
Dale T. Umetsu, MD, PhD[d],*

KEYWORDS

- Food allergy • Immunotherapy • Anti-IgE antibody/omalizumab
- Desensitization

Food allergy is an immune-based disorder in which patients develop acquired immunity to foods, resulting in gastrointestinal, respiratory, or dermatologic reactions on reexposure to food allergens.[1,2] Food allergy is a significant health concern, with prevalence rates rising dramatically over the past decade. Several recent comprehensive reviews of food allergy in Europe, Asia, and the United States estimate that food allergy affects 3% to 5% of adults and 3% to 8% of children.[3–6] Food allergy is also responsible for the greatest proportion of anaphylaxis cases seen in hospital and emergency departments, with approximately one-third of anaphylaxis cases caused by food allergy.[7] Although any food can cause anaphylaxis, peanut and tree nut allergies are the most dangerous, accounting for most fatal or near-fatal cases of anaphylaxis.[8,9]

Currently, the clinically recommended method of treating food allergy is strict food avoidance, supplemented with rapid emergency care of acute symptoms (eg, anaphylaxis) that may occur with accidental ingestion.[10] Unfortunately, food allergen avoidance is difficult, because food allergens are often hidden or undeclared in commercially prepared foods; this results in frequent accidental ingestions, making

[1] Co first authors.
[a] Stanford Food Allergy Program, Division of Immunology and Allergy, Stanford University, 300 Pasteur Drive, Stanford, CA 94305, USA
[b] Division of Immunology and Allergy, Department of Pediatrics, Stanford University, 300 Pasteur Drive, Stanford, CA 94305, USA
[c] Division of Pulmonary Medicine, Massachusetts General Hospital, Boston, MA 02114, USA
[d] Division of Immunology, Children's Hospital, Harvard Medical School, Karp Laboratories, One Blackfan Circle, Boston, MA 02115, USA
* Corresponding author.
E-mail address: dale.umetsu@childrens.harvard.edu

Immunol Allergy Clin N Am 32 (2012) 111–133
doi:10.1016/j.iac.2011.11.004   immunology.theclinics.com
0889-8561/12/$ – see front matter © 2012 Elsevier Inc. All rights reserved.

the management of food allergy challenging and stressful for patients and their families.[11] To address this problem, several investigators have attempted to develop effective therapies for food allergy, either to reduce the severity of allergic reactions associated with accidental food exposure or to eliminate reactions when the food is added to the patient's diet. These approaches involve use of both food allergen–specific and food allergen–nonspecific methods. Food allergen–nonspecific methods include treatment with monoclonal antibodies (mAb) to neutralize IgE (eg, omalizumab) or with herbal mixtures suggested by traditional Chinese medicine. Food allergen–specific methods include oral immunotherapy (OIT), sublingual immunotherapy, and epicutaneous immunotherapy with both native and recombinant food allergens as antigens.[12] This article focuses on OIT, one of the most promising current therapies.

FOOD OIT

The ultimate goal of food allergy therapies is to achieve tolerance to food allergens, which might be equivalent to a cure. Under the conditions of tolerance, patients with food allergy can safely consume food without following a daily oral food regimen to maintain clinical nonreactivity.[13] In most OIT protocols, small amounts of allergen are administered orally to patients in gradually increasing amounts, with the immediate goal to induce desensitization, achieving the first step toward tolerance. With desensitization, the treated patient manifests a decreased response to the ingested food allergens but must continue to take daily food doses to maintain nonreactivity.[13] Allergens are usually given to patients in the form of a protein powder mixed with a safe vehicle.[1] Initial doses and dose escalations are typically administered in a controlled setting, such as a clinic or hospital, to monitor for adverse effects. Each successful dose escalation is followed by the daily consumption of the tolerated dose at home.[1,12] Before and at the end of OIT, a double-blind placebo-controlled food challenge (DBPCFC) is often performed to measure the improvement in the amount of the food allergen tolerated.[13]

Major OIT Studies

Although the first successful use of OIT was reported in 1908,[12] it did not generate much clinical attention until approximately 25 years ago, when a 1984 study by Patriarca and colleagues[14] showed that an OIT protocol could successfully treat various food allergies. This was followed by a 1999 case study of a 12-year-old girl with milk allergy, in which investigators described successful desensitization with an OIT rush protocol, in which doses were elevated rapidly over a period of days instead of weeks or months.[15] Over the past 10 years, there has been a great number of additional OIT studies performed, most of which have been conducted in children (summarized in **Table 1**).[1,12]

Patriarca and colleagues, 2003

In a study published in 2003, Patriarca and colleagues[16] performed OIT in children and adults using milk, egg, fish, orange, and a variety of fruits and vegetables. The control group comprised 16 patients following a strict elimination diet. The OIT protocol consisted of administering progressively increasing doses of the food allergen, with initial doses diluted in water and later doses undiluted. Dose elevation occurred over a period of 4 to 6 months, with duration depending on the specific allergen. Of the 59 patients enrolled in the study, 47 received a total of 54 oral desensitization courses. Of the 54 treatments, 45 resulted in successful desensitization, representing an 83% success rate. No difference was found between adults and children. Several immunologic changes accompanied successful completion of OIT therapy: food-specific IgE levels decreased ($P<.01$), food-specific IgG_4 levels increased ($P<.01$), and skin prick test (SPT) responses, initially positive, became negative after 18 months. None of these changes was observed in the control group. However, several patients (51%) experienced side effects, such as urticaria, emesis, angioedema, diarrhea, and abdominal pain, with 9 patients (17%) stopping the treatment entirely because of the severity of side effects.[1,12,16]

Meglio and colleagues, 2004

In 2004, Meglio and colleagues[17] reported the results of OIT in 21 children (mean age, 6 years 11 months) with IgE-mediated cow's milk allergy. The OIT protocol consisted of increasing doses of cow's milk, initially diluted (administration of undiluted doses began on day 49 of the desensitization protocol), which were administered to patients over a period of 6 months. Of the 21 patients, 15 (71%) completed the treatment, reaching the target tolerated daily intake goal of 200 mL of cow's milk by the end of the 6 months, and an additional 3 children showed incomplete desensitization, tolerating an increased daily intake of cow's milk of 40 to 80 mL by the end of the trial. Three patients (14%) were unable to be desensitized and stopped the desensitization protocol after the first doses. SPT responses decreased significantly ($P<.001$) in patients who showed desensitization, but no significant change in milk-specific IgE levels was seen (mean, pre–milk-specific IgE, 17.1 kU/L and post–milk-specific IgE, 12.7 kU/L; $P>.1$). Of the 21 patients, 13 (62%) developed side effects of varying severity during the treatment, including rhinitis, abdominal pain, temporary throat pruritus, angioedema, and asthma.[12,17]

Buchanan and colleagues, 2007

In 2007, Buchanan and colleagues[18] published the results of a 24-month pilot study examining the use of OIT to treat egg allergy in children. Seven subjects were enrolled (mean age, 4 years); patients with a history of egg-induced anaphylaxis were excluded. The OIT protocol consisted of three phases: modified rush desensitization, buildup, and maintenance. In the modified rush phase, increasing doses were administered approximately every half hour. If a dose caused severe symptoms, the modified rush phase was concluded and the highest tolerated dose was used as the initial daily dose. The maintenance phase began when patients reached a daily dose of 300 mg, which they were then instructed to take for the rest of the study.[18]

All seven subjects completed the study. All subjects experienced mild side effects during the modified rush phase; one subject experienced significant side effects at the start of the build-up phase.[1,12,18] Four of the subjects (57%) shows desensitization during the DBPCFC that followed the study. All subjects were able to tolerate higher levels of egg during the post-study DBPCFC than during the pre-study food challenge.[18] However, two of these subjects reacted to a second DBPCFC that was administered 3 months after the study, and therefore no conclusions were made regarding long-term tolerance. Egg-specific IgG levels increased significantly over the 24 months of the study ($P = .002$). Egg-specific IgE levels decreased in five of the seven subjects, but the mean change was not statistically significant.

Staden and colleagues, 2007

In 2007, Staden and colleagues[19] reported the results of a study in which 45 children were randomly assigned to either OIT (n = 25) or an elimination diet (control; n = 20) for the treatment of cow's milk and egg allergies. The OIT protocol consisted of an induction phase, in which patients were administered fresh cow's milk or egg protein daily at home, with doses increasing progressively to established maximum doses (250 mL cow's milk, 2800 mg egg protein), and a maintenance phase, with minimum daily maintenance doses (100 mL cow's milk, 1600 mg egg protein) in addition to deliberate intake.[19] In the OIT group, all patients experienced side effects. Of the 25

Table 1
Summary of major OIT studies in the past decade

Year	Study	Allergen(s)	Age	Completed Study	Completed Food Challenge	Immunologic Changes	Side Effects	Doses
2003	Patriarca et al[16] Clinical trial Gradual dose escalation 4–6 mo	Milk (n = 29) Egg (n = 15) Fish (n = 11) Albumin (n = 3) Orange (n = 2) Other (n = 6) Control: elimination (n = 16)	3–55 y	38/59 (64%) 45/54 doses (83.3%)	n/a	After 18 mo: ↓ IgE ↑ IgG$_4$ SPT: positive → negative (78%)	51.1%: urticaria, emesis, diarrhea, angioedema, abdominal pain; 9 (16.7%): dropped out because of severity of side effects	*Maintenance:* Milk: 120 mL Egg: 50 mL Fish: 160 mg
2004	Meglio et al[17] Gradual dose escalation 6 mo	Milk (n = 21)	5–10 y (mean, 6 y 10 m)	15/21 (71%) Note: 3 subjects increased tolerance, but did not reach maintenance dose	n/a	After 6 mo: SPT: significant ↓ IgE: no change	13/21 (61.9%): side effects during treatment; 3/21 (14.3%): dropped out because of severity of side effects	*Maintenance:* 200 mL
2007	Buchanan et al[18] Pilot study 1. Rush 2. Buildup 3. Maintenance 24 mo	Egg (n = 7)	1–7 y (mean, 4 y)	7/7 (100%)	4/7 (57%) 3 mo after treatment: 2/7 (29%)	After 24 mo: ↑ IgG$_4$ ↓ IgE (71%)	7/7 (100%): mild side effects during rush phase 1/7 (14%): significant side effects at start of buildup phase	*Maintenance:* 300 mg

Year	Study	Intervention	Age				Side effects	Maximum dose
2007	Staden et al[19] Randomized clinical trial 1. Induction 2. Maintenance 21 mo (median), 2 mo elimination before food challenge	Milk (n = 14) Egg (n = 11) Control: elimination (n = 20)	0.6–12.9 y (median: 2.5)	16/25 (64%)	9/16 (56%; 36% of total) Note: 3 (19%; 12% of total) tolerant with regular intake, 4 (25%; 16% of total) experienced partial response	OIT patients: ↓ IgE Control patients with spontaneous allergy resolution (7/20, 35%): ↓ IgE	OIT patients: 16/25 (64%): mild side effects 9/25 (36%): dropped out because of severity of side effects during induction Control patients: 5/20 (25%): accidental ingestion	Maximum (end point of induction): Milk: 250 mL Egg: 2800 mg Maintenance: Milk: 100 mL Egg: 1600 mg
2008	Longo et al[20] Randomized clinical trial 1. Rush 2. Slow increase over 1 y	Milk (n = 30) Control: elimination (n = 30)	5–17 y (mean, 7.9 y)	27/30 (90%)	11/27 (41%; 37% of total) Note: 16 (59%; 53% of total) had increased tolerance, did not reach maintenance dose	OIT patients: ↓ IgE (50%)	OIT: 17/30 (57%): side effects at home 17/30: oral steroids 6/30: nebulized epinephrine 1/30: intramuscular epinephrine 3/30 (10%): dropped out because of severity of side effects Control: 6/30 (20%): accidental exposure	Maintenance: 150 mL

(continued on next page)

Table 1
(continued)

Year	Study	Allergen(s)	Age	Completed Study	Completed Food Challenge	Immunologic Changes	Side Effects	Doses
2008	Skripak et al[21] Randomized, double-blind, placebo-controlled trial 1. Build-up day 2. Home dose, weekly dose increases 3. Daily maintenance	Milk (n = 13) Control: placebo (n = 7) (active/placebo ratio, 2:1)	6–17 y (median OIT, 9 y, median placebo, 11 y)	12/13 (92%)	4/12 (8%)	OIT patients: ↑ IgG (predominantly IgG₄) No IgE change Control: No change in IgE or IgG	OIT patients: 35% median side effect frequency, side effects in 45% of daily doses, epinephrine = 0.2% total doses; 1/20 patients: Dropped out because of severe eczema Control: 1% median side effect frequency, side effects in 11% of daily doses	*Initial dose:* 40 mg *Maximum after OIT:* 5140 mg (median) 2540–8140 mg (range) *Minimum home dose:* 295 mg
2009	Clark et al[22] Case series 1. Increasing daily doses 2. 6 weeks maintenance	Peanut (n = 4)	9–13 y	4/4 (100%)	3/4 (75%)	n/a	Mild side effects common, no epinephrine	*Maintenance:* 800 mg

Year / Study	Food	Age					
2009 Jones et al[7] Open-label study 1. Initial day escalation 2. Build-up 3. Maintenance	Peanut (n = 39)	12–111 mo (median at enrollment: 57.5 mo)	29/39 (74%)	27/29 (93%; 69% of total) Note: 2/29 (7%) showed increased tolerance	After 6 mo: ↓ SPT response ↓ Basophil activation ↓ mast cells 6–12 mo: in vitro PBMCs: ↑ IL-10, IL-5, IFN-γ, TNF-α 12–18 mo: ↓ IgE ↑ IgG$_4$ 0–12 mo: ↑ FoxP3⁺ Tregs (↓ after 12 mo) Downregulation of apoptosis genes in T cells	Build-up: mild-to-moderate adverse reactions, oropharyngeal, skin, nausea/abdominal pain, diarrhea/emesis, mild wheezing (18%–69% of total doses) Maintenance: 0.7% of home doses, 2 epinephrine doses (2 subjects)	Maximum: 3.9 mg (16 peanuts)
2010 Blumchen et al[23] 1. Rush w/roasted peanut 2. Maintenance (8 wk) 3. Elimination (2 wk)	Peanut (n = 23)	3.2–14.3 y	14/23 (61%)	3/14 (21%; 13% of total) Note: median tolerance of peanut increased after OIT	↑ IgG$_4$ in vitro PBMCs: ↓ IL-5, IL-4, IL-2	2.6% of daily doses (mild-to-moderate), pulmonary obstruction symptoms in 1.3% 1/23 (4%): Dropped out of initial rush phase because of adverse effects 4/22 (18%): discontinued OIT because of adverse effects	After Rush: 0.15 g (median tolerated dose) Final dose: 0.5 g Final tolerance: 1 g (median)

(continued on next page)

Table 1
(continued)

Year	Study	Allergen(s)	Age	Completed Study	Completed Food Challenge	Immunologic Changes	Side Effects	Doses
2011	Varshney et al[24] Randomized, double-blind, placebo-controlled trial 1. Initial escalation (1 day) 2. Build-up + home dosing (~44 wk) 3. Maintenance (1 month)	Peanut (n = 19) Control: Placebo (n = 9) (active/placebo ratio, 2:1)	28–126 mo (median, 69 mo)	16/19 (84.2%)	16/16 (100%)	*OIT patients:* ↓ SPT response ↓ Il-5 ↓ IL-13 ↑ IgG ↑ IgG_4 ↑ FoxP3[hi]:FoxP3[int] Tregs 2–9 mo: ↑ IgE (no significant change at OFC) 9 mo: ↑ TGF-β (no significant change at OFC) *Placebo patients:* No significant changes	Initial escalation: 9/19 (47%) of OIT patients, 2 epinephrine doses (2 subjects) Build-up: 1.2% of OIT doses Home: 1 epinephrine dose (1 subject) in placebo group 2/19 (10.5%): Dropped out of initial escalation because of adverse effects 1/19 (5.3%): discontinued OIT because of adverse effects	*Initial rush:* End point: ≥1.5 mg, 6 mg maximum Cumulative: 12 mg *Maintenance:* Dose: 4000 mg OFC: Cumulative: 5000 mg

Abbreviations: n/a, not applicable; OFC, oral food challenge; SPT, skin prick test.

Data from Land M, Kim EH, Kim D, Burks W. Oral desensitization for food hypersensitivity. Immunol Allergy Clin North Am 2011;31:367–76; and Nowak-Wegrzyn A, Sampson HA. Future therapies for food allergies. J Allergy Clin Immunol 2011;127(3):558–73.

patients treated with OIT, 14 completed the induction phase within a year, and 2 completed the induction phase more slowly because of infections or pollen allergies. The remaining 9 patients (36%) did not complete the induction phase because of side effects. After completing OIT, oral tolerance was evaluated through having patients follow a strict elimination diet for 2 months before a follow-up oral food challenge. Of the 16 patients who completed OIT, 9 (36% of the original 25 patients) showed tolerance in the follow-up challenge (OIT tolerance group). In the elimination group, 7 of the 20 (35%) developed spontaneous tolerance. The rate of tolerance between the oral (36%) and spontaneous (35%) groups was therefore similar.[19]

Levels of allergen-specific IgE decreased significantly in the children who experienced response to OIT (geometric mean, pre–milk-specific IgE, ~10 kU/L and post–milk-specific IgE, ~2 kU/L; $P<.001$) and in those who developed spontaneous tolerance (geometric mean, pre–milk-specific IgE, ~4 kU/L and post–milk-specific IgE, ~0.5 kU/L; $P<.05$), but not in the children who remained allergic. Children with continued food allergy (ie, nonresponders) showed no change in their allergen-specific IgE levels. These results therefore supported the idea that OIT contributes to immunologic suppression of specific IgE responses, but the ability of OIT to induce tolerance was not conclusive.[1]

Longo and colleagues, 2008

Initial OIT trials excluded patients with severe allergic disease. To tackle this subgroup, Longo and colleagues[20] performed a randomized clinical trial to evaluate the use of OIT versus a strict elimination diet for children with severe cow's milk–induced allergic reactions. Additionally, because the children were older (mean age, 7.9 years) and because of the presence of high cow's milk–specific IgE levels, they were less likely to develop spontaneous tolerance.[1] Before desensitization, the milk-specific IgE levels in 47 of the 60 subjects were greater than 100 kU/L, and all were greater than 85 kU/L. The OIT protocol consisted of an in-hospital rush phase over 10 days, followed by a slow increasing phase performed at home, in which dairy products such as yogurt and cheese were added to patients' diets after they reached a daily dose of 150 mL. Thirty patients were randomly assigned to follow the OIT protocol, and another 30 were assigned to an elimination diet as control.[20] After 1 year, 11 (36%) of the patients treated with OIT tolerated a daily intake of at least 150 mL of cow's milk, with several following an unrestricted diet. Another 16 (54%) were able to consume 5 to 150 mL (criterion for partial tolerance) of milk daily. None of the children in the elimination group showed any desensitization on undergoing a follow-up DBPCFC, and none was able to tolerate even 5 mL of milk, representing a statistically significant difference ($P<.001$) between the groups.

Of the 30 patients in the OIT group, 15 exhibited a significant decrease in cow's milk–specific IgE, although most levels remained greater than 100 kU/L. No statistically significant IgE decrease was evident in the control group. Because of the severity of the allergies of the patients, the frequency of side effects in the OIT group was high, with 4 patients receiving intramuscular epinephrine once each during the rush phase and 2 treated in the emergency department during home dosing. Nebulized epinephrine was administered to 24 children: 22 doses to 18 children during the rush phase, and 9 doses to 6 children during the home phase. Three (10%) of the patients treated with OIT were unable to complete the study because of the severity of side effects experienced, and 6 patients in the comparison group experienced mild reactions because of accidental exposure to milk.[20] Most significantly, this study showed that OIT could be administered even to patients with very severe food allergies.

Skripak and colleagues, 2008

Skripak and colleagues[21] performed the first double-blind, placebo-controlled OIT clinical trial. Before their study, all OIT studies had compared OIT with elimination diets, the current standard of care.[1] Twenty children with cow's milk allergy (age range, 6–17) were randomly assigned to an OIT or a placebo group (13 active patients, 7 placebo patients). The OIT protocol consisted of three phases: build-up day, then daily doses at home with weekly in-office dose increases, followed by daily maintenance doses for 3 to 4 months.[21] Of the 20 patients, 19 completed the treatment. Children in the OIT group showed a marked increase in the amount of milk they were able to tolerate without a reaction (40 mg at baseline to a median of 5140 mg after OIT). This result differed significantly from that of the placebo group, in which all children reacted at 40 mg (P = .0003). No significant change in milk-specific IgE levels was observed in either group, but milk IgG levels, particularly IgG_4 levels, increased significantly in patients in the active treatment group. Side effects were considerably higher in the active group than in the placebo group, with patients reporting that 45% of daily doses resulted in symptoms in the active group, compared with 11% in the placebo group. Four patients received one dose of epinephrine each during the trial (0.2% of doses): 2 during build-up and 2 during home maintenance. Overall, the use of milk OIT was found to be effective in increasing the amount of milk tolerated in the subjects ingesting milk versus those ingesting placebo.[12,21]

Clark and colleagues, 2009

Despite the prevalence of peanut allergies and the dangers they pose, peanuts were not a major focus of OIT before 2009. Previous OIT studies primarily focused on cow's milk and egg allergies.[1] In 2009, Clark and colleagues[22] reported four cases of children with peanut allergy (age range, 9–13 years) who underwent OIT. The OIT protocol consisted of daily doses of peanut flour, increasing from 5 to 800 mg, with increases occurring twice weekly; this was followed by 6 weeks of maintenance treatment. All four children showed an increased threshold tolerance for peanut during the post-OIT food challenge. No immunologic changes were recorded. Mild side effects occurred commonly during dosing, but despite the severe nature of peanut allergy, no epinephrine was needed to treat any adverse reactions.[1,12,22]

Jones and colleagues, 2009

Jones and colleagues[7] reported a larger peanut OIT study in 2009. They enrolled 39 patients (median age, 57.5 months) in an open-label study. The OIT protocol consisted of three phases: initial day escalation, build-up, and maintenance. Of the 39 patients, 29 (74%) completed the trial in 8 to 18 months, During the final food challenge, 27 of these patients were able to safely consume 16 peanuts (3.9 mg peanut protein) and the other 2 consumed 9 peanuts. These amounts are significantly higher than would be expected to occur in accidental ingestion. Four (10%) patients withdrew from the trial because of side effects, and 6 withdrew for personal reasons. Mild adverse reactions were common during the build-up phase, and some adverse reactions were observed during the maintenance phase. Two subjects received one dose each of epinephrine during the maintenance phase.[7]

Several immunologic changes were noted in the patients who had successfully completed OIT, implicating many of the cells and molecules known to be involved in the allergic response. SPT responses decreased significantly by the 6-month mark, as did activation of basophils. By 12 to 18 months, peanut-specific IgE levels had decreased significantly and IgG_4 levels had increased significantly. IgE-peanut complex formation was inhibited by serum factors in an IgE-facilitated allergen binding assay. In vitro secretion of interleukin (IL)-10, IL-5, interferon (IFN)-γ, and tumor necrosis factor (TNF)-α from peripheral blood mononuclear cells (PBMCs) in response to peanut stimulation increased over 6 to 12 months. Additionally, numbers of peanut-specific FoxP3$^+$ T regulatory cells (Tregs) increased for 12 months, after which they decreased. Microarray analysis of T cells showed downregulation of genes related to apoptosis.[1,7,12]

Blumchen and colleagues, 2010

Blumchen and colleagues[23] published a subsequent peanut OIT study in 2010 in which 23 subjects (age range, 3.2–14.3 years) were enrolled in a protocol involving a rush phase with roasted peanut OIT followed by an 8-week maintenance phase. This was then followed by 2 weeks of a peanut elimination diet, after which a final DBPCFC was performed. A median of 0.15 g peanut was tolerated during the rush phase. Of the 23 patients, 22 continued with the long-term protocol and 14 (60%) reached a protective dose of 0.5 g of peanut after 7 to 18 months of OIT. The final DBPCFC showed an increase in the threshold of the amount of peanut tolerated by the subjects, with a median tolerance of 1000 mg compared with a median tolerated dose of 190 mg at baseline.[23] This finding showed that the threshold increase persisted beyond the discontinuation of OIT for at least 2 weeks, suggesting that tolerance may be achievable. In the patients treated with OIT, peanut-specific serum IgG$_4$ increased significantly, and in vitro production of IL-5, IL-4, and IL-2 through peanut-stimulated PBMCs decreased.[12,23] No change in T$_H$1 cytokines was observed, suggesting that OIT may act via clonal anergy or deletion.[1] Four of the 22 patients (18%) discontinued OIT because of adverse effects. Mild to moderate side effects were observed in 2.6% of the OIT doses.

Varshney and colleagues, 2011

In 2011, Varshney and colleagues[24] published the results of the first randomized double-blind, placebo-controlled study of OIT for peanut allergy. Of 28 subjects enrolled (median age, 69 months; range, 28–126 months), 19 were assigned to the OIT group and 9 to the placebo group. The median base peanut-specific IgE level was 106 kU$_A$/L. During initial escalation phase, 2 patients required epinephrine. Of the 19 patients treated with OIT, 16 (84%) completed the OIT protocol, reaching the maintenance dose of 4000 mg peanut by 40 weeks. All patients treated with OIT were able to tolerate a cumulative final dose of 5000 mg of peanut versus a median cumulative dose of 280 mg in the placebo patients, and only 1 OIT patient reacted with clinically significant symptoms to the food challenge, compared with 8 of the 9 patients treated with placebo.[24] This study showed that OIT induced desensitization among patients with peanut allergy, greatly increasing the subjects' levels of tolerance of peanut protein after 1 year of therapy. Long-term tolerance was not assessed, but the trial is continuing, with the goal of evaluating whether tolerance is induced.[24] Among patients treated with OIT, SPT wheal sizes decreased significantly between baseline and the oral food challenge (OFC; $P<.001$). Peanut-specific levels of IgE increased initially, but were unchanged at 12 months compared with initial levels. Peanut-specific IgG and IgG$_4$ increased significantly at all time points ($P<.05$ and $P\leq.001$, respectively). The ratio of FoxP3^{hi}:FoxP3^{int}CD4$^+$CD25$^+$ Tregs increased significantly between baseline and 12 months.[24] The study indicated that OIT is reasonably safe in a monitored clinical setting, and showed that OIT can decrease the severity of reactions to accidentally ingested doses of peanut.

TRENDS IN OIT

From examining these OIT trials, certain patterns emerge (**Box 1**). First, although many patients can be successfully desensitized, allergic reactions occurred in most participants during the desensitization in all the studies. Although most of these reactions were mild, many were severe, thus presenting a significant safety concern, especially if patients need to continue taking doses at home to maintain desensitization. The severity of these reactions resulted in the withdrawal of 10% to 25% of patients during the initial rush phase in most of the OIT studies. Of those who had significant allergic reactions but remained in the study, the rate of allergen dose escalation was slowed or halted prematurely.[12] This finding suggests that some patients may be more difficult than others to desensitize. For example, in the study reported by Longo and colleagues[20] of patients with severe milk allergy, only 36% of the subjects could tolerate 150 mL of cow's milk after 12 months of desensitization. The difficulty in desensitizing these patients required an unshakable commitment from patients and their entire families and medical teams to the OIT protocol. The simple availability of 24-hour telephone contact turned out to be crucial for supporting and counseling the parents who followed the home schedule. Therefore, OIT is not a universal solution, and significant safety risks exists, particularly in the subgroup of desensitization-resistant subjects.

The specific features that might identify this difficult-to-treat population, which includes those who withdraw or require slower advancement, are not yet clear. In the study reported by Longo and colleagues,[20] subjects with milk-specific IgE greater than 100 IU/mL had no detected reduction in their specific IgE levels at 12 months, suggesting that patients with very high levels of food-specific IgE might be a feature of this group. This finding might correlate with studies of the natural history of milk allergy, indicating that milk-specific IgE levels greater than 50 kU/L are associated with the failure of milk allergy to resolve spontaneously.[25] Conversely, patients who are successfully desensitized display decreased levels of IgE and increased levels of IgG_4, suggesting that the failure to significantly decrease food-specific IgE or significantly increase food-specific IgG_4 might also identify this difficult-to-treat group.[1,12] Additional specific biomarkers, component- or epitope-specific IgE and IgG_4 levels, profiles of food-induced cytokine production, or immune profiling of phosphoepitopes might also be useful in identifying this group of patients, which may require more

---

Box 1
Key features of OIT

1. OIT provides an effective intervention for food allergy that reduces the severity of accidental food ingestion in most patients, and may provide a potential cure for food allergy in some patients.

2. The specific, most effective protocol for OIT, in terms of dosing and timing, has not yet been established.

3. The safety of OIT is still problematic, with allergic reactions, including mild and severe reactions, developing in most patients undergoing OIT.

4. Although many patients successfully complete OIT, a sizable fraction of patients are difficult to desensitize because of severe allergic reactions.

5. Long-term tolerance has not yet been adequately assessed.

6. The mechanisms of OIT are not fully understood.

aggressive therapy, with agents such as anti-IgE mAb (see below) or other adjunctive immunomodulatory therapy to improve the safety and efficacy of OIT.

Another common feature in most studies of OIT was that, on average, 50% to 75% of patients were desensitized and could tolerate very large quantities of the food, whereas 10% to 20% of patients achieved only partial desensitization, tolerating larger quantities of the food than before the study but not reaching the maintenance dose.[12] Increasing the duration of OIT trials may lead to greater desensitization, but this has not been proven. In patients treated with aeroallergen immunotherapy, longer duration of therapy has been found to correlate with persistence of the beneficial effects even after discontinuation of therapy.[26] Although partial desensitization can have profound benefits for patients with food allergy, whether this limited desensitization can be maintained after discontinuation of daily allergen administration is not yet clear. Almost all OIT studies showed the generation of some degree of desensitization in patients, but assessment for the induction of permanent tolerance was not usually performed.

IGE IN PATIENTS WITH FOOD ALLERGY

In children with IgE-mediated food allergy, food-specific IgE plays a prominent role. First, the presence of food-specific IgE indicates the absence of oral tolerance to that food. Second, immediate skin tests are usually positive for the offending food, and reactions to food often include anaphylaxis occurring rapidly after food allergen exposure.[27] Food-specific IgE binds to high-affinity FcεRI receptors on basophils and mast cells and to low-affinity FcεRII receptors on lymphocytes, eosinophils, monocytes, macrophages, and platelets. Reexposure to the allergen triggers the production of molecules and mediators involved in the inflammatory response, such as histamine and prostaglandins, and also stimulates the production of cytokines that trigger the so-called late-phase response.[28] These observations suggest neutralization of IgE might be effective as treatment for food allergy.

Although the precise level of food-specific IgE in serum does not directly correlate with the severity of the disease, high concentrations of food-specific IgE antibodies in the serum are related to lowered probability of spontaneous allergy resolution.[25] In addition, a high food-specific IgE may identify a desensitization-resistant population. However, significant reduction in levels of food-specific IgE may indicate successful completion of OIT.[1,12] The precise mechanisms through which OIT might influence IgE concentrations are unclear, but could be related to deletion, anergy, or development of food-specific Treg cells.

ANTI-IGE MONOCLONAL ANTIBODIES
Omalizumab

Currently, the most widely used anti-IgE mAb is omalizumab (Xolair; Genentech, South San Francisco, CA, USA). Omalizumab is a recombinant humanized antibody (molecular weight, 150 kD) composed of a human IgG$_1$ skeleton (95%) and murine complementarity-determining regions (5%).[29] It selectively binds to the CHε3 domain of IgE with high affinity. Omalizumab is FDA-approved for treating children and adults ($\geq$12 years of age in the United States, $\geq$6 years in Europe) who have moderate-to-severe persistent asthma with evidence of aeroallergen sensitivity and who are inadequately controlled with inhaled corticosteroids.[30,31] Dosing is based on the patient's pretreatment serum IgE level and weight, with a minimal dosage of 0.016 mg/kg (IU/mL) IgE per 4 weeks in divided subcutaneous doses. Several clinical trials have shown its safety and efficacy in treating patients with severe steroid-requiring asthma, resulting in decreased hospitalization and reduction in the use of oral and inhaled corticosteroids.[32–35] In addition, omalizumab has been shown to be clinically efficacious in the treatment of seasonal and perennial allergic rhinitis, with significant improvements in nasal symptom severity scores, use of rescue antihistamines, and specific quality-of-life scores, although the FDA has not approved it for this indication.[36–38]

Several large clinical trials have also examined the efficacy and safety of adding omalizumab treatment to specific immunotherapy, and have shown that combination therapy significantly reduced symptom load during the pollen season.[39–41] Moreover, pretreatment of patients with omalizumab showed added safety to the rush phase of allergen immunotherapy, with prevention of acute allergic reactions,[39,41] suggesting that anti-IgE mAb might also reduce the side effects associated with food-specific OIT (see later discussion).

Talizumab

Talizumab (TNX-901; Tanox, Houston, TX, USA) is a humanized IgG$_1$ mAb administered subcutaneously. Similar to omalizumab, it recognizes and masks an epitope in the CHε3 region of IgE responsible for binding to both FcεRI receptors on mast cells, basophils, and dendritic cells (DCs). In addition to markedly down-regulating the expression of these receptors on basophils, it is also to believed to inhibit allergen-specific T-cell activation through interfering with antigen processing and presentation activities mediated by these receptors.[42] Because of multiple legal battles surrounding patent infringement, talizumab is currently not commercially available. However, in several peanut-allergic populations, talizumab was found to be effective in reducing peanut-induced allergic reactions (discussed later).

MECHANISMS OF ANTI-IGE MAB

Each IgE molecule has two CHε3 sites, and therefore can bind two molecules of omalizumab or talizumab simultaneously (**Fig. 1**). These small, soluble, biologically inert IgE/anti-IgE complexes develop when anti-IgE mAb is administered to patients, and are cleared from the circulation so as not to cause immune complex–related conditions. Anti-IgE mAb does not bind receptor-bound IgE and is therefore unable to stimulate the IgE receptor and mast cell degranulation.[42] Many of the important biologic effects of anti-IgE mAb center around the reduction of both circulating free IgE (by 96%–99%) and IgE binding to its cell surface receptors, FcεRI and FcεRII.[43]

The FcεRI is expressed mainly on mast cell and basophils. Blocking IgE binding not only prevents degranulation of these cells (therefore affecting histamine and lipid mediator release) but also dramatically reduces expression of the receptor itself by approximately 97%.[44] This action interrupts a positive feedback loop in which circulating IgE induces the synthesis of its own high-affinity receptor. This function thereby decreases the responsiveness of mast cells and basophils to antigen challenge and inhibits the allergic cascade.[45]

The FcεRII receptor is expressed on multiple antigen-presenting cells, including DCs and IgE-switched B cells. Inhibition of its interaction with IgE potentially interferes with total IgE production by B cells and decreases the synthesis of IgE-stimulating cytokines, such as IL-4 and IL-13. Because IgE/anti-IgE complexes cannot bind to IgE receptors, additional effects of therapy include the neutralization of allergens through the binding of circulating allergen to IgE/anti-IgE complexes.[46]

Through blocking IgE binding to its receptors and decreasing DC FcεRI receptor expression, omalizumab may also reduce antigen presentation to T cells and the

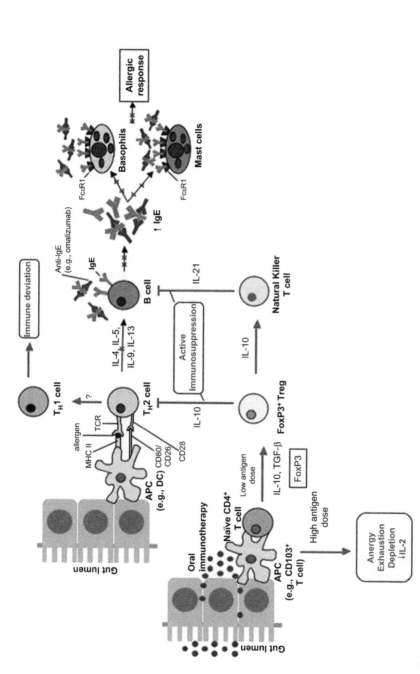

Fig. 1. Possible mechanisms of OIT and anti-IgE therapy. Oral immunotherapy, in combination with anti-IgE mAb therapy, allows desensitization to allergens through various mechanisms that interfere with the allergic response. Red indicates effects of oral immunotherapy. Magenta indicates effects of anti-IgE mAb therapy. APC, antigen-presenting cell; FoxP3, forkhead box P3; IFN, interferon; Ig, immunoglobulin; IL, interleukin; MHC II, major histo-compatibility complex protein class II; TCR, T-cell receptor; T_H, T-helper cell.

production of T_H2 cytokines. In correlate, studies have shown attenuation in the production of several T_H2 cytokines (eg, IL-4, IL-5, and IL-13) with anti-IgE mAb therapy.[47] Anti-IgE mAb has also been shown to reduce peripheral, sputum, and bronchial eosinophilia in patients with moderate-to-severe persistent IgE-mediated asthma after 16 weeks.[48] Studies of cutaneous responses to allergens have also provided evidence of the anti-inflammatory effects of omalizumab. One study showed a significant reduction of the late-phase skin reaction and cellular infiltration in skin biopsies after intradermal allergen challenges were performed in 24 atopic allergic volunteers who had been treated with omalizumab for 12 weeks. Skin biopsy results showed decreased levels of $CD3^+$ T cells and eosinophils in the omalizumab-treated group compared with the placebo group, suggesting that omalizumab prevented eosinophil influx and T-cell priming responses.[49]

When considering the above-mentioned biologic effects of anti-IgE mAb, several potential biomarkers can be measured to monitor its therapeutic effects. Because anti-IgE mAb only binds free circulating IgE, serial measurements of free IgE and not total IgE (which includes anti-IgE/IgE complexes) in serum are important in determining the timing of the potential inhibitory effects of anti-IgE.[50]

ANTI-IGE MAB IN RUSH SUBCUTANEOUS IMMUNOTHERAPY FOR RAGWEED

Omalizumab pretreatment before immunotherapy was first examined in a four-arm, double-blind, placebo-controlled study with rush immunotherapy for ragweed-induced allergic rhinitis. Patients with ragweed-induced allergic rhinitis received 9 weeks of omalizumab or placebo, followed by a 1-day rush or placebo immunotherapy (up to a 2-μg dose), then weekly increases to a 12-μg dose along with omalizumab or placebo. The total omalizumab period was 21 weeks. The combination of anti-IgE (omalizumab) with rush ragweed injection immunotherapy for seasonal allergic rhinitis resulted in a greater reduction in systemic allergic side effects versus immunotherapy alone.[51] These results showed a protective effect against acute allergic reactions that occur during rush ragweed-specific immunotherapy. Although other studies showed that the combination of chronic treatment with omalizumab with allergen-specific immunotherapy was more effective than immunotherapy alone in reducing clinical symptoms,[39] the results of this study are consistent with the possibility that omalizumab treatment might reduce acute allergic reactions associated with rapid OIT for food allergy.

ANTI-IGE IN FOOD ALLERGY

To date, clinical studies investigating the effect of anti-IgE mAb in food allergy have been limited. In 2003, Leung and colleagues[42] published a landmark study supporting its beneficial role, using talizumab to prevent or reduce the severity of allergic symptoms that might develop on accidental ingestion. This randomized, double-blind, placebo-controlled, dose-ranging study evaluated, 84 patients aged 12 to 60 years with a history of immediate hypersensitivity to peanuts and total IgE levels between 30 and 1000 IU/mL and a positive SPT to peanut. Before enrollment, a randomized, double-blind, placebo-controlled food challenge to peanut confirmed reactivity, and patients were randomly assigned to receive varying doses of talizumab (150, 300, or 450 mg) or placebo every 4 weeks. The mean amount of peanut flour that elicited objective symptoms and resulted in stopping of the food challenge (the sensitivity threshold) increased in all groups, with an apparent dose-response, but it was statistically significant only in the group receiving the highest anti-IgE dose (450 mg). In this group, the sensitivity threshold increased from approximately one-half of a peanut

(178 mg) to almost 9 peanuts (2805 mg), as evidenced by a final oral food challenge performed 2 to 4 weeks after the last dose (week 20). This study showed the safety and efficacy of anti-IgE mAb treatment as an important therapeutic option for patients with peanut allergy, specifically for increasing the threshold of reactivity in situations of accidental ingestion.[42]

To confirm these results, Sampson and colleagues[52] studied children aged 6 years and older with peanut allergy using a different anti-IgE mAb preparation (omalizumab). Similar to the study with talizumab, this study was designed to determine whether omalizumab (given at a dose of 0.016 mg/kg/IgE) was effective in preventing allergic reactions that might occur on accidental ingestion of peanut. Although the trial was terminated prematurely and most subjects did not reach the study end point, omalizumab seemed to be able to increase tolerance to peanut: 44.4% of omalizumab-treated subjects versus 20% of subjects receiving placebo could tolerate a peanut challenge of greater than 1000 mg.[52]

The third study of anti-IgE mAb in a food allergy examined the use of omalizumab in patients with severe food allergy with severe atopic dermatitis.[53] This phase I, randomized, double-blind, placebo-controlled study of omalizumab in eight patients aged 4 to 22 years (mean, 11.6 years) with food allergy and severe refractory atopic dermatitis examined the safety and efficacy trends of omalizumab using a higher dosing frequency of omalizumab to neutralize the higher levels of IgE (up to 3000 IU/mL; mean, 1068 IU/mL). Because both treatment and placebo groups had marked clinical improvement, no difference was noted between the treatment and placebo groups. However, several important inflammatory markers were markedly reduced with omalizumab treatment, including thymus and activation-regulated chemokine (by 60%–80% in three of four patients), thymic stromal lymphopoietin (by 50%–75% in four of four patients), and OX40 ligand (by 70%–80% in four of four patients). In addition, IL-10 levels were increased between 80% and 100% in patients treated with omalizumab compared with those treated with placebo. These results suggest that omalizumab might prevent IgE-mediated activation and reduce allergic inflammation.[53]

COMBINING ANTI-IGE MAB WITH OIT

Given the recent success of food allergen OIT in multiple previous studies for egg, milk, and peanut allergy, and the observations that anti-IgE mAb can reduce allergic reactions to food allergen challenges,[42,52,53] recent studies have been initiated to examine the efficacy of anti-IgE mAb in combination with OIT. Combined treatment with anti-IgE mAb and specific food-allergen OIT is attractive because of not only the potential ability of anti-IgE mAb to decrease immediate side effects from OIT but also the possibility to enhance the development of tolerance. Although OIT protocols for desensitization vary, all involve an allergen-specific approach with an incremental dose escalation, or buildup phase, of the implicated food.

In the first study of omalizumab in combination with OIT, Nadeau and colleagues[54] showed that pretreatment with omalizumab was safe and allowed for rapid oral desensitization in most subjects with significant IgE-mediated cow's milk allergy. This pilot study included 11 subjects (mean age, 10.2 years) with significant milk allergy (mean milk-specific IgE, 98 kU/L; median milk-specific IgE, 50 kU/L[54]). After treatment with omalizumab for 9 weeks, the children underwent rush desensitization to milk, increasing the dose of oral milk from 0.1 to 1000 mg over a 6-hour period, and to 2000 mg over 7 to 11 weeks. Throughout the dose-escalation period, subjects remained on omalizumab. One withdrawal occurred after the initial rapid desensitization phase because of abdominal symptoms that were not deemed to be allergic in origin, particularly because the subject was later diagnosed with abdominal migraines. Nine of the 10 patients who remained in the study later passed a DBPCFC, with a cumulative dose of 7250 mg of milk (equivalent to 220 mL of milk) and an additional open challenge of greater than 4000 mg (120 mL) of milk without symptoms. The tenth patient tolerated the 500-mg dose in the DBPCFC (total cumulative dose, 1000 mg). The 9 patients who passed the DBPCFC, and who are currently taking daily oral milk, are now able to tolerate essentially normal amounts of milk ($\geq$240 mL (8000 mg) per day) in their diet.[54]

Compared with previous studies of oral milk desensitization, this study suggests that omalizumab pretreatment could substantially improve the rapidity and likelihood of success of oral desensitization in patients with significant milk allergy. Oral desensitization without omalizumab pretreatment as previously described required many months to complete, and was successful (as shown by the ability of subjects to take a dose of milk greater than 8000 mg [>240 mL] per day without symptoms at study conclusion) in fewer than half of the subjects (36% and 42%, respectively, in two studies).[20,21] In contrast, in this small pilot study with omalizumab pretreatment, full desensitization occurred rapidly over a 7- to 11-week period in most patients, including those with very high milk-specific IgE. On the first day of rush desensitization, 9 of the 11 patients tolerated a dose of 250 mg, and 7 tolerated the full dose of 1000 mg. At study conclusion, 82% of the subjects (9/11) attained full desensitization and were able to safely take a dose of milk greater than 8000 mg/d without symptoms.[54] These results suggest that the goal of desensitization should not merely to be able tolerate accidental ingestion of the food, but rather to be able to tolerate normal daily dietary quantities of the food.

Although the frequency of allergic reactions during the desensitization process was low in this study using omalizumab pretreatment given the rapidity of the desensitization, the allergic reactions that were observed occurred primarily during the rush phase of the desensitization. Epinephrine was required in one of these patients. In contrast, fewer allergic reactions, which were mostly mild to moderate, were observed during the dose-escalation phase. Epinephrine was also administered in two patients with mild to moderate reactions at week 23 and 31, which the investigators believed to be related partly to compliance issues and viral infection, the latter of which may reduce tolerance to milk.[54] Other groups have also observed an association between viral infection and increased rates of reactions to previously tolerated doses in food desensitization protocols (without omalizumab).[13]

This first study of omalizumab and OIT by Nadeau and colleagues has several limitations.[54] First, the study sample size was small, because it was a pilot safety study. However, most of the patients were successfully and rapidly desensitized, suggesting that the observations may be reproduced in future studies with larger sample sizes. Second, the study did not include a placebo group. Nevertheless, because the results greatly exceeded those of previous studies of oral milk desensitization with regard to the rapidity and success of desensitization and the ability to tolerate milk at study conclusion,[20,21] this study provides proof-of-concept that omalizumab enables more-rapid and safe OIT even in patients with significant food allergy. However, additional confirmatory studies of omalizumab in OIT are clearly required before any strong conclusions can be made.

Although this study was restricted to cow's milk desensitization, it is possible that pretreatment with omalizumab, which neutralizes IgE of all specificities, could greatly reduce allergic reactions and be useful for desensitization to virtually any food allergen. In this regard, additional studies are currently being conducted to extend and confirm the idea that anti-IgE mAb can improve the success and effectiveness of OIT. For example, Dr Hugh Sampson is conducting a double-blind, placebo-controlled study of omalizumab as pretreatment for milk OIT in subjects aged 7 to 35 years (ClinicalTrials.gov). The subjects must first fail a DBPCFC with milk at a dose of less than 2 g of milk powder, and have an SPT wheal of 3 mm or greater or milk-specific IgE of 0.35 kU$_A$/L or greater. Dr Wes Burks is conducting another study using omalizumab with peanut OIT in subjects aged 12 years or older with an SPT wheal of 3 mm or greater or peanut-specific IgE of 5 kU$_A$/L or greater, and a history of significant clinical symptoms occurring within 60 minutes after ingesting peanuts.[55] A third study is being conducted at Children's Hospital Boston using omalizumab with peanut OIT in subjects aged 7 to 25 years with an SPT wheal greater than 10 mm, peanut-specific IgE greater than 20 kU$_A$/L, and who fail a DBPCFC with peanut at a dose 100 mg or less of peanut flour (ClinicalTrials.gov). These studies should help elucidate the role that anti-IgE mAb might play in the conduct of OIT, and whether anti-IgE mAb may allow all patients with food allergy, including those who are desensitization-resistant, to safely and rapidly benefit from OIT.

OTHER IMMUNOTHERAPEUTIC APPROACHES IN FOOD ALLERGY

In addition to anti-IgE mAb as adjunctive therapy for food-allergy OIT, several other studies of promising immunotherapeutic approaches for food allergy are underway. These include the modification of the protein used in the immunotherapy (eg, the use of heat-denatured protein or engineered major protein to improve tolerability to the allergen), sublingual administration of the food allergen in immunotherapy, and Chinese herbal medicine to decrease allergic reactions during immunotherapy.[1,10,12] In addition, the use of probiotics and modified probiotic agents to modulate the micro-environment of the gastrointestinal system is currently under examination (eg, lactobacillus transfected with IL-12 or modified parasite components).[56] These approaches have been recently reviewed elsewhere.[1,10,12]

SUMMARY AND FUTURE DIRECTIONS IN FOOD OIT

Many studies have shown the efficacy of OIT protocols in desensitizing patients with food allergy, suggesting that a clinical desensitization therapy may be available for patients with food allergy in the near future. However, many issues still need to be resolved. For example, the OIT studies performed thus far have focused almost exclusively on IgE-mediated food allergy (immediate sensitivity), and whether food-related problems, such as atopic dermatitis or eosinophilic esophagitis, may benefit from OIT is currently unclear. Second, safety remains an important issue, because allergic side effects, including anaphylaxis, are extremely common during OIT protocols, particularly during initial rush phases. These reactions might be less common with anti-IgE mAb pretreatment and sublingual methods of desensitization.[10,12,54] Because the maximum dose of antigen is somewhat limited in sublingual protocols, opportunities may exist to combine sublingual immunotherapy and OIT through administering lower oral doses safely and quickly sublingually and then proceeding to higher oral doses in an accelerated fashion. Furthermore, additional studies of anti-IgE mAb as pretreatment for OIT are needed to fine-tune this regimen, because this combination could result in a greatly reduced incidence of allergic reactions. In any case, because most OIT doses in any protocol are administered at home, patients must be vigilant for unexpected reactions, which may be aggravated by asthma exacerbations, fever, menses, exercise, or taking doses on an empty stomach.[13] Finally, because the development of eosinophilic esophagitis may occur without warning while on oral allergen treatment, long-term safety monitoring must continue in patients undergoing OIT, particularly for symptoms of persistent vomiting.[57]

Although most allergic reactions can be controlled and most patients with food allergy can be successfully desensitized, a subpopulation of patients may exist who are considered difficult-to-treat or desensitization-resistant, who develop significant allergic reactions during desensitization, require slower dose advancement, and often drop out of desensitization studies. These patients pose significant safety risks, and are difficult to identify based on their past clinical histories. Anti-IgE mAb may be able to help reduce the risk of allergic reactions that occur during OIT in these patients, or allow more rapid desensitization, although further studies must be performed to confirm this impression. Given that anti-IgE mAb decreases inflammatory cytokines and increases tolerogenic cytokines in patients with food allergy, and the promising preliminary results in patients with high levels of food-specific IgE, further studies of this adjunctive therapy are clearly warranted.

A third issue that could delay the introduction of OIT for general clinical use is long-term safety. Although desensitization is the first step toward a cure for food allergy, the precise dietary instructions for the years after desensitization completion are unclear. In some OIT studies, the goal has been to reduce allergic reactions occurring with accidental ingestions; in other studies, many patients are able to fully introduce the food into their diets in normal quantities. Until the issue of long-term tolerance is addressed, patients who complete OIT may need frequent, possibly daily, oral dosing to maintain desensitization, and may therefore require long-term monitoring. Based on studies of subcutaneous immunotherapy for aeroallergen sensitivity and bee venom sensitivity,[26,58] true tolerance may require a period of maintenance oral exposure for 2 to 5 years before tolerance (or cure) is established. Furthermore, examination of the immunologic mechanisms through which OIT produces its beneficial effects may help to better monitor the evolution from desensitization to tolerance. This research may in turn help develop better protocols for OIT; for example, with adjunctive methods such as anti-IgE mAb or Chinese herbal medicines, modified allergens, or different methods of allergen exposure (epicutaneous or sublingual).

Finally, before OIT can be promoted for general public use, some degree of standardization must be developed. For example, standardization of antigens, similar to what has been done for dust mite, cat, and grass allergens for subcutaneous immunotherapy, would be of great benefit, as might be standardization of food allergen preparation, measurement, and administration. Moreover, a phase III study using a consensus food OIT protocol (with or without anti-IgE mAb) to formalize a specific protocol would best serve patients, ensuring that a safe and effective therapy is available for the treatment and possible cure of food allergy.

REFERENCES

1. Land M, Kim EH, Burks W. Oral desensitization for food hypersensitivity. Immunol Allergy Clin North Am 2011;31:367–76.
2. Bock SA, Sampson HA. Food allergy in infancy. Pediatr Clin North Am 1994;41: 1047–67.
3. Chafen JJ, Newberry SJ, Riedl MA, et al. Diagnosing and managing common food allergies: a systematic review. JAMA 2010;303:1848–56.
4. Mills C, van Ree R, Breteneder H. Food allergy and intolerance in Europe—future directions within the ERA. Allergen Bureau Web site. Available at: http://www.allergenbureau.net/downloads/projects-and-resources/Food_Allergy_in_Europe.pdf. Accessed September 19 2011.

5. Food allergy and food intolerance. European Food Information Council Web site. Available at: http://www.eufic.org/article/en/expid/basics-food-allergy-intolerance/. Accessed September 19 2011.
6. Shek LP, Lee BW. Food allergy in Asia. Curr Opin Allergy Clin Immunol 2006;6(3): 197–201.
7. Jones SM, Pons L, Roberts JL, et al. Clinical efficacy and immune regulation with peanut oral immunotherapy. J Allergy Clin Immunol 2009;124(2):292–300, 300.e1–97.
8. Sampson HA, Rosen JP, Selcow JE, et al. Intradermal skin tests in the diagnostic evaluation of food allergy. J Allergy Clin Immunol 1996;98:714–5.
9. Sampson HA, Munoz-Furlong A, Campbell RL, et al. Second symposium on the definition and management of anaphylaxis: summary report—second National Institute of Allergy and Infectious Disease/Food Allergy and Anaphylaxis Network symposium. Ann Emerg Med 2006;47:373–80.
10. Nowak-Wegrzyn A, Muraro A. Food allergy therapy: is a cure within reach? Pediatr Clin North Am 2011;58:511–30.
11. Scurlock AM, Burks AW, Jones SM. Oral immunotherapy for food allergy. Curr Allergy Asthma Rep 2009;9:186–93.
12. Nowak-Wegrzyn A, Sampson HA. Future therapies for food allergies. J Allergy Clin Immunol 2011;127(3):558–73.
13. Scurlock AM, Vickery BP, Hourihane JO, et al. Pediatric food allergy and mucosal tolerance. Mucosal Immunol 2010;3(4):345–54.
14. Patriarca C, Romano A, Venuti A, et al. Oral specific hyposensitization in the management of patients allergic to food. Allergol Immunopathol (Madr) 1984; 12(4):275–81.
15. Bauer A, Ekanayake Mudiyanselage S, Wigger-Alberti W, et al. Oral rush desensitization to milk. Allergy 1999;54(8):894–5.
16. Patriarca G, Nucera E, Roncallo C, et al. Oral desensitizing treatment in food allergy: clinical and immunological results. Aliment Pharmacol Ther 2003;17: 459–65.
17. Meglio P, Bartone E, Plantamura M, et al. A protocol for oral desensitization in children with IgE-mediated cow's milk allergy. Allergy 2004;59:980–7.
18. Buchanan AD, Green TD, Jones SM, et al. Egg oral immunotherapy in nonanaphylactic children with egg allergy. J Allergy Clin Immunol 2007;119(1):199–205.
19. Staden U, Rolinck-Werninghaus C, Brewe F, et al. Specific oral tolerance induction in food allergy in children: efficacy and clinical patterns of reaction. Allergy 2007;62:1261–9.
20. Longo G, Barbi E, Berti I, et al. Specific oral tolerance induction in children with very severe cow's milk-induced reactions. J Allergy Clin Immunol 2008;121(2):343–7.
21. Skripak JM, Nash SD, Rowley H, et al. A randomized, double-blind, placebo-controlled study of milk oral immunotherapy for cow's milk allergy. J Allergy Clin Immunol 2008;122(6):1154–60.
22. Clark AT, Islam S, King Y, et al. Successful oral tolerance induction in severe peanut allergy. Allergy 2009;64(8):1218–20.
23. Blumchen K, Ulbricht H, Staden U, et al. Oral peanut immunotherapy in children with peanut anaphylaxis. J Allergy Clin Immunol 2010;126(1):83.e1–91.e1.
24. Varshney P, Jones SM, Scurlock AM, et al. A randomized controlled study of peanut oral immunotherapy: clinical desensitization and modulation of the allergic response. J Allergy Clin Immunol 2011;127(3):654–60.
25. Skripak JM, Matsui EC, Mudd K, et al. The natural history of IgE-mediated cow's milk allergy. J Allergy Clin Immunol 2007;120(5):1172–7.

26. Durham SR, Walker SM, Varga E-M, et al. Long-Term Clinical Efficacy of Grass-Pollen Immunotherapy. N Engl J Med 1999;341(7):468–75.
27. Sicherer SH. Food allergy. Mt Sinai J Med 2011;78(5):683–96.
28. Burks W, Ballmer-Weber BK. Food allergy. Mol Nutr Food Res 2006;50(7): 595–603.
29. Pelaia G, Renda T, Romeo P, et al. Omalizumab in the treatment of severe asthma: efficacy and current problems. Ther Adv Respir Dis 2008;2(6):409–21.
30. Xolair: Omalizumab. United States Food and Drug Administration Web site. Available at: http://www.accessdata.fda.gov/drugsatfda_docs/label/2007/103976s5102lbl.pdf. Accessed October 12, 2011.
31. Xolair (omalizumab). European Medicines Agency Web site. Available at: http://www.ema.europa.eu/ema/index.jsp?curl=pages/medicines/human/medicines/000606/human_med_001162.jsp&mid=WC0b01ac058001d124&jsenabled=true. Accessed October 12, 2011.
32. Humbert M, Beasley R, Ayres J, et al. Benefits of omalizumab as add-on therapy in patients with severe persistent asthma who are inadequately controlled despite best available therapy (GINA 2002 step 4 treatment): INNOVATE. Allergy 2005; 60:309–16.
33. Corren J, Casale T, Deniz Y, et al. Omalizumab, a recombinant humanized anti-IgE antibody, reduces asthma- related emergency room visits and hospitalizations in patients with allergic asthma. J Allergy Clin Immunol 2003;111: 87–90.
34. Lanier B, Bridges T, Kulus M, et al. Omalizumab for the treatment of exacerbations in children with inadequately controlled allergic (IgE-mediated) asthma. J Allergy Clin Immunol 2009;124:1210–6.
35. Rodrigo GJ, Neffen H, Castro-Rodriguez JA. Efficacy and safety of subcutaneous omalizumab versus placebo as add on therapy to corticosteroids for children and adults with asthma: a systematic review. Chest 2011;139(1):28–35.
36. Casale TB, Condemi J, LaForce C, et al. Omalizumab Seasonal Allergic Rhinitis Trail Group. Effect of omalizumab on symptoms of seasonal allergic rhinitis: a randomized controlled trial. JAMA 2001;286:2956–67.
37. Chervinsky P, Casale T, Townley R, et al. Omalizumab, an anti- IgE antibody, in the treatment of adults and adolescents with perennial allergic rhinitis. Ann Allergy Asthma Immunol 2003;91:160–7.
38. Okubo K, Ogino S, Nagakura T, et al. Omalizumab is effective and safe in the treatment of Japanese cedar pollen- induced seasonal allergic rhinitis. Allergol Int 2006;55:379–86.
39. Kuehr J, Brauburger J, Zielen S, et al. Efficacy of combination treatment with anti-IgE plus specific immunotherapy in poly- sensitized children and adolescents with seasonal allergic rhinitis. J Allergy Clin Immunol 2002;109(2):274–80.
40. Kopp MV, Brauburger J, Riedinger F, et al. The effect of anti-IgE treatment on in vitro leukotriene release in children with seasonal allergic rhinitis. J Allergy Clin Immunol 2002;110:728–35.
41. Kopp MV, Stenglein S, Kamin W, et al. Omalizumab (Xolair) in children with seasonal allergic rhinitis: leukotriene release as a potential in vitro parameter to monitor therapeutic effects. Pediatr Allergy Immunol 2007;18:523–7.
42. Leung DY, Sampson HA, Yunginger JW, et al. Effect of anti-IgE therapy in patients with peanut allergy. N Engl J Med 2008;348(11):986–93.
43. Corren J, Shapiro G, Reimann J, et al. Allergen skin tests and free IgE levels during reduction and cessation of omalizumab therapy. J Allergy Clin Immunol 2008;121(2):506–11.

44. MacGlashan DW Jr, Bochner BS, Adelman DC, et al. Downregulation of FcεRI expression on human basophils during in vivo treatment of atopic patients with anti-IgE antibody. J Immunol 1997;158:1438–45.
45. Stone KD, Prussin C, Metalfe DD. IgE, mast cells, basophils, and eosinophils. J Allergy Clin Immunol 2010;125(2):S73–80.
46. Belliveau PP. Omalizumab: a monoclonal anti-IgE antibody. MedGenMed 2005; 7(1):27.
47. Noga O, Hanf G, Kunkel G. Immunological changes in allergic asthmatics following treatment with omalizumab. Int Arch Allergy Immunol 2003;131:46–52.
48. Djukanovic R, Wilson SJ, Kraft M. Effects of treatment with anti-immunoglobulin E antibody omalizumab on airway inflammation in allergic asthma. Am J Respir Crit Care Med 2004;170(6):583–93.
49. Ong YE, Menzies-Gow A, Barkans J, et al. Anti-IgE (omalizumab) inhibits late-phase reactions and inflammatory cells after repeat skin allergen challenge. J Allergy Clin Immunol 2005;116(3):558–64.
50. Lowe PJ, Tannenbaum S, Gautier A, et al. Relationship between omalizumab pharmacokinetics, IgE pharmacodynamics and symptoms in patients with severe persistent allergic (IgE-mediated) asthma. Br J Clin Pharmacol 2009;68(1):61–76.
51. Casale TB, Busse WW, Kline JN, et al. Omalizumab pretreatment decreases acute reactions after rush immunotherapy for ragweed-induced seasonal allergic rhinitis. J Allergy Clin Immunol 2006;117(1):134–40.
52. Sampson HA, Leung DY, Burks AW, et al. A phase II, randomized, double-blind, parallel-group, placebo-controlled oral food challenge trial of Xolair (omalizumab) in peanut allergy. J Allergy Clin Immunol 2011;127(5):1309.e1–10.e1.
53. Iyengar SR, Hoyte EG, Loza A, et al. Safety of omalizumab treatment in children (>4 years) with high serum IgE and severe atopic dermatitis and food allergy. J Allergy Clin Immunol 2008;121(2):S1–32.
54. Nadeau KC, Schneider LC, Hoyte L, et al. Rapid oral desensitization in combination with omalizumab therapy in patients with cow's milk allergy. J Allergy Clin Immunol 2011;127(6):1622–4.
55. Available at: http://www.clinicaltrials.gov/ct2/show/NCT00932282?term=burks%2C+peanut&rank=2. Accessed November 14, 2011.
56. Cross ML, Gill HS. Can immunoregulatory lactic acid bacteria be used as dietary supplements to limit allergies? Int Arch Allergy Immunol 2001;125(2):112–9.
57. Ridolo E, De Angelis GL, Dall'Aglio P. Eosinophilic esophagitis after specific oral tolerance induction for egg protein. Ann Allergy Asthma Immunol 2011;106(1): 73–4.
58. Golden DB. Insect sting allergy and venom immunotherapy: a model and a mystery. J Allergy Clin Immunol 2005;115(3):439–47.

Alternative and Complementary Treatment for Food Allergy

Julia Ann Wisniewski, MD[a],*, Xiu-Min Li, MD, MS[b]

KEYWORDS

- Food allergy • Complementary and alternative medicine
- Traditional Chinese medicine • Acupuncture
- Immunotherapy • Peanut

Despite increased consumer interest in complementary and alternative medicine (CAM) for the treatment of food allergy, there remains a relative paucity of knowledge regarding the clinical efficacy, mechanisms of action, and safety of most CAM treatments available to consumers. A comprehensive review of CAM for food allergy shows that Food Allergy Herbal Formulation-2 (FAHF-2), the only herbal formulation currently in phase II clinical trials, is safe and has promise to induce tolerance in food-allergic patients. Several mechanisms of action may underlie the therapeutic effect of FAHF-2 on food-induced immune responses. These include a systemic shift in T-helper 1 (Th1)/Th2 effector responses, as well as direct effects on mast cell and basophil reactivity. FAHF-2 seems to promote tolerance to food allergens without systemic immune suppression that is associated with steroids and other immune-modulating pharmaceuticals used in mainstream treatment of allergic diseases. Other novel approaches to diagnosis and treatment of food allergy are reviewed, but have not been formally validated for clinical use.

FOOD ALLERGY AND CAM

Food allergy research is receiving increased attention because of the high prevalence and severity of food-related conditions.[1] Recent efforts to develop effective treatments for food allergy have incorporated concepts from CAM and other novel avenues of immunotherapy to reduce the prevalence of food allergy and morbidity

---

[a] Department of Pediatrics, Division of Allergy and Immunology, University of Virginia, 409 Lane Road, Box 801355, Charlottesville, VA 22908, USA
[b] Department of Pediatrics, Jaffe Food Allergy Institute, Mount Sinai Hospital, One Gustave L Levy Place, New York, NY 10029, USA
* Corresponding author.
E-mail address: jaw4he@virginia.edu

Immunol Allergy Clin N Am 32 (2012) 135–150
doi:10.1016/j.iac.2011.11.001
0889-8561/12/$ – see front matter © 2012 Published by Elsevier Inc.

immunology.theclinics.com

caused by accidental food ingestions in sensitized individuals. Current trends in the availability of herbal supplements, acupuncture, and homeopathic remedies to Western health care consumers,[2,3] combined with new interest in the potential immune-modulating effects of these products among Western physicians,[4,5] have led to what has been referred to as a renaissance of complementary medicine.[6] Approximately 6 in 10 Americans report using some type of dietary supplement, and 1 in 6 Americans report using herbal remedies on a regular basis.[7] Patients who use CAM for their allergies are younger, more educated, motivated by the assumption of few side effects, and unsatisfied with conventional medicine.[8] In 2001, 4 procedures accounted for most of the CAM use in Europe: homeopathy (35%), autologous blood injection (28%), acupuncture (17%), and bioresonance (10%). European medical doctors provided 60% of CAM therapies and received reimbursement from insurance companies for 50% of services at a median cost of €41 (range €15–205) per treatment and €205 (range €15–1278) for a 4-treatment course.[8] The therapeutic mechanisms, safety, and clinical efficacy of these previously non-evidence-based therapies are being tested by standards of Western medicine.[9] Within the subspecialty of allergy, the clinical efficacy and potential mechanism of action of specific CAM components have been reported and reviewed for treatment of asthma,[10–13] atopic dermatitis,[14] and hay fever.[10,15–18] In 2002, remedies for the treatment of food allergy accounted for 11% of CAM use reported by CAM users with allergic conditions.[8] In 2005, 18% of patients seen in United States food allergy clinics reported using CAM for treatment of their food allergies.[19] This article focuses on recent advances in CAM for food allergy, including acupuncture, herbal medicine, probiotics, and alternative approaches to allergen immunotherapy. Whereas most patients who consult practitioners of alternative allergy seek alternative treatments for established allergic diseases, others seek alternative methods of allergy diagnosis to explain clinical symptoms when conventional allergy testing is negative.[20] This article therefore briefly discusses the evidence for alternative approaches to the diagnosis of food allergy, but focuses on alternative approaches to the treatment of food allergy. Other novel approaches to treatment, including anti-immunoglobulin E (IgE) therapy, have been reviewed recently.[21–23]

CURRENT CONCEPTS IN MECHANISMS OF ORAL TOLERANCE AND A ROLE FOR CAM

Food allergy results from the failure to establish oral tolerance or loss of preexisting tolerance-sustaining mechanisms. Factors central to the development of food allergy include those that promote and amplify Th2 responses in the gut, such as thymic stromal lymphopoietin (TSLP),[24] and factors that bypass normal gut mucosal tolerance, such as exposure to allergens through the skin or respiratory track.[25] Effector molecules and cellular pathways involved in oral tolerance remain areas of active investigation.[26,27] Scientists interested in CAM have begun to investigate how CAM therapies may interact with these complex pathways to either enhance tolerant responses or reduce Th2 responses to ingested food antigens.

THE SCOPE OF CAM

Complementary medicine encompasses treatments beyond the scope of conventional allopathic medicine, including acupuncture, homeopathy, Chinese herbal medicine, Ayurveda, and other ancient Eastern traditions, as well as household remedies such as probiotics and nonpharmaceutical supplements.[28] In 2005 chiropractors, homeopaths, and acupuncturists provided most of the therapies for food-allergic patients seeking alternative treatments.[19] CAM is currently not emphasized in the curriculum of Accreditation Council for Graduate Medical Education–accredited training programs in allergy and immunology, even though this is a field where patients often seek or use CAM for treatment of allergic disease.[4,5] The intrinsic barriers to measuring the efficacy of complementary medicine using evidence-based medicine include large placebo response rates, sampling error, and reduced within-group variation.[29] Central to understanding the medicinal benefit of many of these alternative treatments is acceptance of the relationship between the mind and body, which influence health and illness. Activation of neuroimmunomodulatory pathways has been reported to have dramatic effects on immunity, and has been suggested to explain the mechanism by which placebos exert their effects.[30] However, without extensive supporting data to support this mechanism, CAM treatments have been shown to improve quality-of-life scores in patients with allergic disease.[31] This article focuses on the best scientific evidence supporting the safety, therapeutic benefit, and other plausible mechanisms of action of alternative therapies.

ALTERNATIVE APPROACHES TO DIAGNOSIS OF FOOD ALLERGY

Complementary diagnostic techniques are used mainly in food-allergy intolerance.[32] At present, the only noninvestigational treatment for food allergy is strict food-allergen avoidance and prescription medicines to treat symptoms caused by accidental exposures.[33] Because strict avoidance is mandated, children with multiple food allergies can develop vitamin and other nutritional deficiencies.[34] These children also suffer from social isolation at school age, and psychological problems resulting in poorer overall health and limitations in social activities.[35] Given the known risk for social, psychological, and nutritional side effects of food avoidance, the use of unproven diagnostic tools for food allergy diagnosis is highly controversial[19,36–39] but, nonetheless, appealing to some families. Immunoglobulin G (IgG) antibodies to food allergens likely reflect normal and potentially protective immune responses to food intake. Moreover, the measurement of food-specific IgG levels in blood as a diagnostic tool for food allergy has been disproved by double-blind placebo-controlled food challenge (DBPCFC), where no correlation was found between symptoms resulting from ingestion of the food antigens and levels of food-specific IgG or IgG4 antibodies.[38] Similar unproven tests in allergy diagnosis include cytotoxic food-allergy testing, leukocytotoxic testing, the provocation/neutralization sublingual or subcutaneous test, the heart-ear reflex test, hair analysis, iridology, bioresonance, electrodermal testing (electroacupuncture), reflexology, and applied kinesiology.[32,36–38] Despite being costly to administer, these tests lack scientific rationale, are not reproducible, and do not correlate with clinical evidence of allergy.[38] The gold standard for food-allergy diagnosis remains positive skin-prick testing or detectable food-allergen–specific IgE antibodies in parallel with a positive food challenge or documented allergic symptoms within 2 hours of food ingestion.[33] The only evidenced exception to this is with regard to delayed IgE-mediated food allergies caused by sensitization to galactose-α-1,3-galactose (α-gal).[40] These food-allergic patients are diagnosed by positive intradermal skin tests (often negative skin-prick tests), IgE antibodies to α-gal, and clinical allergic symptoms within 3 to 6 hours of food ingestion.[40] Other established food-related conditions that cannot be tested by detection of IgE antibodies, but do improve with food-avoidance diets, include eosinophilic gastrointestinal disease, food protein-induced enterocolitis syndrome, and celiac disease.[41] Although the molecular basis of food intolerance remains poorly defined, existing alternative diagnostic tests such as those mentioned earlier are unlikely to lead patients and physicians in the right direction. Rather, they may cause additional confusion and place patients at an increased risk for the nutritional side effects associated with strict avoidance diets.

SAFETY OF CAM

Although the overall risk to public health seems to be low, certain groups of traditional remedies have been associated with potentially serious side effects.[42,43] The Food and Drug Administration (FDA) has only recently provided a plan to begin to address issues related to manufacturing processes and quality control of the dietary supplement industry, which includes herbs and probiotics.[7] Experience has shown that using herbal remedies without adequate thought about what the active drug components are, or their mechanism of action, may actually worsen rather than treat allergic disease.[20,44] For example, injection of specific Chinese herbs for treatment of upper airway symptoms was reported to cause anaphylaxis,[43] and the use of several topical herbal remedies was reported to cause allergic contact dermatitis and, more rarely, IgE-mediated sensitization.[44] Royal jelly and propolis are honeybee products used in traditional medicine for their reported antioxidant and anti-inflammatory effects.[45,46] Surveillance of toxicologic problems associated with the use of traditional and herbal remedies and herbal supplements between 1991 and 1997 at the Medical Toxicology Unit at Guy's Hospital, London, identified 785 adverse reactions attributed to herbal treatments among 1297 symptomatic enquiries.[42] These complaints included liver problems after the use of traditional Chinese medicine (TCM) for skin problems, allergic reactions from royal jelly and propolis, and heavy-metal poisoning caused by remedies from the Indian subcontinent.[42] Because of these past concerns, herbal remedies currently under investigation for the treatment of food allergy underwent extensive safety testing[47–49] before attaining FDA approval for use in human clinical trials.[50,51] Safety monitoring in murines and humans to date has shown no evidence of end-organ toxicity, heavy-metal contamination, or global immune suppression with FAHF-1 or FAHF-2 (**Tables 1** and **2**). Safety concerns regarding the health risks of acupuncture treatments in the United States, such as the potential for disease transmission through nonsterile needle use, were addressed in 1996, when the FDA removed the experimental status tag on acupuncture needles. The FDA reclassified acupuncture needles, regulating them as it does other medical devices such as surgical scalpels and hypodermic syringes. Acupuncture needles must now be manufactured according to single-use standards of sterility, and are regulated to be used by licensed practitioners. At least 40 states and the District of Columbia use an examination administered by the National Certification Commission for Acupuncture and Oriental Medicine. Studies of acupuncture for the treatment of asthma, atopic dermatitis, and allergic rhinitis remain conflicting with regard to efficacy; however, they have established the safety of acupuncture treatments by licensed practitioners, including safe use in children.[18,52–57] In the authors' experience several patients with food allergy have anecdotally reported satisfaction and subjective benefits from acupuncture treatments, but they have not identified any published studies that formally investigate the use of acupuncture for the treatment of food allergy, nor was any published evidence identified for the use of homeopathy for the treatment of food allergy.

HERBAL MEDICINE FOR THE TREATMENT OF FOOD ALLERGY

One in 6 Americans report using herbal remedies on a regular basis,[7] and remedies for food allergy account for 11% of CAM used for allergic conditions.[8] Despite high consumer interest, wider acceptance into mainstream medicine has been hindered until more recently by a relative paucity of knowledge regarding the active ingredients and mechanism of action of herbal formulations on food tolerance induction. Most of the herbal formulas studied include combinations of medical plants derived from TCM and, less often, ayurvedic medicine.[58] Food restriction for treatment of respiratory allergy has been a long-term practice in ayurvedic medicine,[59] and principles of ayurveda have been reported as beneficial for the treatment of food intolerance,[60] but the authors could not identify any study that evaluated the efficacy of ayurveda for the treatment of IgE-mediated food allergy. Based primarily on in vitro studies, numerous herbal formulations demonstrate the ability to modulate cytokine activity and alter both gene and protein expression, suggesting that their therapeutic efficacy may be related to such effects at a transcriptional level.[58] The most rigorous investigations of mechanism of action, identification of active compounds, and standardization of formula content for the treatment of food allergy have related to FAHF-1 and FAHF-2. Despite centuries of use of TCM for a variety of allergic conditions, modern definitions of food allergy are not described in the TCM literature.[47] Recent approaches to food-allergy treatment, which incorporate components of TCM, have shown promising results in preclinical trials in terms of both safety and efficacy. The first evidence-based report of TCM for food allergy tested in an animal model of peanut (PN) allergy was FAHF-1, developed in 2001 from a combination of herbs with anti-inflammatory and antiallergy properties.[47]

Food Allergy Herbal Formula

FAHF-1 was the first TCM formulation proved to protect against PN-induced anaphylaxis in mice.[47] FAFH-2 is a refined version of FAHF-1 which lacks 2 herbs thought to be non-key herbs and potentially toxic in humans, if they are not processed correctly.[48] FAHF-2 was shown to be equally protective against anaphylaxis in PN-allergic mice[48] and is safe for food-allergic patients who are older than 12 years in clinical trials.[50,51] The observed decrease in symptoms of anaphylaxis with FAHF-2 treatment is associated with suppression of Th2 cytokines, PN-specific IgE, histamine levels, numbers of peripheral blood basophils, and peritoneal mast cells, as well as diminished FcεRI expression on mast cells.[48,61,62] Establishment of tolerance in PN-allergic mice was further associated with increased numbers of Th1 and mesenteric interferon-γ (IFN-γ)-producing CD8$^+$ cells.[63] It was later shown that CD8$^+$ T cells are the major source of IFN-γ and that neutralization of IFN-γ or depletion CD8 T cells attenuated the efficacy of FAHF-2.[61] In vitro, FAHF-2 inhibits proliferation of IgE-producing B cells and mast cell activation. At the cellular level, 3 compounds in 1 of the herbs, berberine, palmatine, and jatrorrhizine, were shown to directly inhibit mast-cell degranulation by suppressing spleen tyrosine kinase phosphylation.[62] Because binding of monomeric IgE to FcεRI promotes mast-cell and basophil survival, the reduction in levels of PN-specific IgE associated with FAHF-2 treatment has been proposed as one explanation for the observed reduction in peripheral basophils and mast cells.[62] Enhanced levels of IgG2a, which interfere with mast-cell degranulation by blocking FcεRI cross-linking via antigen interception, may further contribute to the FAHF-2 effects on mast cell and basophil reactivity.[61] Because basophil numbers were reduced without effects on surface FcεRI expression, the potential effect of FAHF-2 on basophil survival has been proposed to be mediated through basophil survival factors, such as interleukin (IL)-3 and/or IL-33 signaling.[62] Despite the dramatic effect of FAHF-2 on several effector immune cells, treatment with no single FAHF-2 herb alone provided full protection against anaphylaxis, indicating that the medicinal benefit of FAHF-2 likely depends on synergistic effects of each of its 11 component herbs.[61,64] To reduce the size and dose of FAHF-2 pills for use in children, butanol extraction effectively decreased the dose by fivefold without altering its

Table 1
Preclinical trials in food-allergic mice treated with Chinese herbal medicine

Herbal Treatment	Evidence of Action	Duration of Action	Mechanism(s) of Action	Safety
FAHF-1[a] (21 mg) given twice daily for 7 wk before oral challenge[47]	Protected mice from anaphylaxis induced by 10 mg of crude PN challenge	Single challenge at end of 7 wk therapy Peanut-specific IgE remained reduced at least 4 wk after discontinuing treatment	Reduced mast cell (MC) degranulation and histamine release Reduced peanut-specific IgE Suppressed Th2 cytokines	Therapeutic dose given for double the treatment course (14 wk) showed no damage to kidney, liver, blood cell lines, or other organs. No global immune-suppressive effect on B or T cells
FAHF-2[b] (20 mg) given twice daily for 7 wk[48]	Protected mice from anaphylaxis induced by 200 mg of ground peanut	Protective response at 1 wk, persisted at 3 wk, and 5 wk post therapy	Blocked vascular leakage associated with anaphylaxis Suppressed Th2 responses to recall peanut stimulation	In a Lethal Dose 50 (LD50) protocol, mice were fed 12 times the daily therapeutic dose. LD50 was 24 times the therapeutic dose
FAHF-2[b] (32 mg) given twice daily for 7 wk[63]	Protected mice from anaphylaxis induced by 200 mg of ground peanut	Protective response at 24 h, persisted at 4 wk post therapy	Increased peanut-specific IgG2a Increased numbers of mesenteric interferon (IFN)-γ^+ CD8 T cells	
Dry herb extracts equivalent to dose of herb present in the FAHF-2[b] formula given twice daily for 7 wk[64]	FAHF-2, but none of the constituent herbs, protected 100% of mice from anaphylaxis *Huang bai* protected 25% of mice challenged	Full or partial protection was documented at 5 wk post therapy	*Huang bai*–treated mice showed reduced histamine release and Th2-cytokine production FAHF-2, but no constituent herb alone, induced a significant reduction in IgE and increase in IgG2a	

FAHF-2[c] (32 mg) given twice daily for 7 wk[61]	Protected mice from anaphylaxis induced by 200 mg of ground peanut	Full protection persisted up to 6 mo post therapy, including 6 separate oral challenges; partial protection lasted 9 mo post therapy	In vivo neutralization of IFN-γ abrogated protective effect of FAHF-2 on suppression of anaphylaxis, peanut-IgE, and Th2-cytokine production	No physical, histologic, or laboratory evidence of toxicity to mice at 16 mo post treatment
B-FAHF-2[d] (12.8 mg) given daily for 7 wk[49]	Protected mice from anaphylaxis induced by 200 mg of ground peanut	Full protection persisted up to 8 mo post therapy, including 6 separate oral challenges; partial protection lasted 12 mo post therapy. A second treatment course restored protection	In vitro suppression of peanut-induced Th2-cytokine secretion and enhanced peanut-induced Th1-cytokine secretion. Dose-dependent inhibition of IgE production by human B cells and inhibition of MCs	
FAHF-2[c] (32 mg) given twice daily for 7 wk[62]	Protected mice from anaphylaxis induced by 200 mg of ground peanut	Protective response at 24 h, persisted at 4 wk post therapy	Reduced numbers of peripheral basophils, peritoneal MCs, and cutaneous MC degranulation	MC/9 mast cells remained viable with FAHF-2 (20 μl/ml) in culture

[a] Food Allergy Herbal Formula-1 (FAHF-1) contains 11 traditional Chinese medicinal herbs (*Latin name*), including fruiting body of Ling Zhi (*Ganoderma lucidum*), root of Fu Zi (*Radix lateralis aconite carmichaeli praeparata*), fruits of Wu Mei (*Prunus mume*), seed of Chuan Jiao (*Zanthoxyli bungeani*), whole Xi Xin (*Herba cum radice asari*), root of Huang Lian (*Coptis chinensis* or *Rhizoma coptidis*), bark of Huang Bai (*Phellodendron chinense*), rhizome of Gan Jiang (*Zingiber officinalis*), twigs of Gui Zhi (*Cinnamomum cassia*), roots of Ren Shen (*Panax ginseng*), and roots of Dang Gui (*Angelica sinensis*).[47]

[b] Food Allergy Herbal Formula-2 (FAHF-2) is a simplified formulation of FAHF-1 that lacks 2 components of the original formula, Fu Zi (*Radix lateralis aconite carmichaeli praeparata*), and Xi Xin (*Herba cum radice asari*).[48]

[c] On the basis of organoleptic and microscopic examination, the raw herbs used in FAHF-2 were confirmed to be 9 herbs (*Latin names*): (1) *Zanthoxylum schinifolium*, (2) *Ganoderma lucidum*, (3) *Prunus mume*, (4) *Coptis chinensis*, (5) *Phellodendron chinense*, (6) *Zingiber officinalis*, (7) *Cinnamomum cassia*, (8) *Panax ginseng*, and (9) *Angelica sinensis*. Note: *Zanthoxylum schinifolium* replaced *Zanthoxyli bungeani*.[61]

[d] Butanol-extracted Food Allergy Herbal Formula-2 (B-FAHF-2) comprises the active ingredients in FAHF-2 concentrated to one-fifth of the effective daily dose of FAHF-2 (64 mg).[49]

Table 2
Clinical trials in food-allergic patients and healthy controls treated with Chinese herbal medicine

Clinical Trial	Clinical Outcome	Tolerability	Immunologic Outcomes	Overall Safety
Phase I clinical trial: food-allergic patients treated with FAHF-2[a] or placebo for 7 days[50]	18 food-allergic patients completed the therapy (12 received FAHF-2 and 6 received placebo)	1 FAHF-2–treated patient reported loose stools; 1 subject developed a flare of underlying eczema	No change in specific IgE or skin-prick tests; Reduced IL-5 in vitro allergen-stimulated PBMC cultures in FAHF-2 treated subjects	Levels of heavy metals, pesticides, and ethanol residues were below recommended limits; No serious adverse events occurred
Phase I clinical trial: 3.3 g (6 tablets) FAHF-2[a] taken three times a day for 6 mo[51]	18 food-allergic subjects enrolled; 14 subjects completed the study. Dropouts were related to noncompliance (3) and pregnancy (1)	1 subject temporarily stopped FAHF-2 because of a recurrence of eosinophilic esophagitis	Significant reduction in basophil activation markers in response to ex vivo stimulation at 6 mo	No toxicity in kidney, liver, lungs, or heart in any subjects
Phase II clinical trial: 10 tablets FAHF-2[a] taken three times a day for 6 mo (ClinicalTrials.gov identifier: NCT00602160)	FAHF-2 and placebo-treated groups will undergo DBPC food challenges and the beginning and after 6 mo of treatment	NA	NA	Ongoing study of 68 subjects aged 12–45 years expected to end by June 2012

Abbreviations: DBPC, double-blind placebo-controlled; NA, not available; PBMC, peripheral blood mononuclear cell.

[a] FAHF-2 (0.55 g per tablet), produced by Xiyuan Chinese Medicine Research and Pharmaceutical Manufacturer (Beijing, China) and was approved by the FDA. The product is composed of 9 herbal extracts (*Latin names*): (1) fruits of Wu Mei [*Prunus mume*] or Japanese apricot, 20.0%], (2) seed of Chuan Jiao [*Zanthoxyli bungeani*] or Pricklyash peel, 2.0%], (3) roots of Dang Gui [*Angelica sinensis*] or Angelica root, 6.0%], (4) rhizome of Gan Jiang [*Zingiber officinalis*] or ginger, 6.0%], (5) twigs of Gui Zhi [(*Cinnamomum cassia*) or cassia cinnamon, 4.0%], (6) roots of Ren Shen [(*Panax ginseng*) or ginseng, 4.0%], (7) bark of Huang Bai [*Phellodendron chinense*) or Phellodendron, 4.0%], (8) root of Huang Lian [*Rhizoma coptidis*) or Goldthread, 6.0%], and (9) Ling Zhi [(*Ganoderma lucidum*) or Reishi mushroom, 46.0%].

protective benefit.[49] At present, the immune-modulatory capacity of FAFH-2 in PN-allergic mice seems temporary, lasting 6 to 12 months post treatment, but can be restored by a second treatment course.[49] In addition to providing safety information for treatment in humans, results of phase I clinical trials support evidence of an FAHF-2–mediated immune-modulatory effect similar to the effect seen in animal models. In phase I clinical trials, patients who received 3.3 g (6 tablets) of FAHF-2 3 times a day demonstrated a significant reduction in basophil activation markers in response to ex vivo stimulation, and a downward trend in total numbers of blood eosinophils and basophils at the end of a 6-month treatment course.[51] Current evidence, summarized in **Tables 1** and **2**, suggests that several mechanisms may underlie the therapeutic effect of FAHF-2 on PN-induced immune responses. These include a systemic shift in Th1/Th2 effector responses, as well as direct effects on mast cell and basophil reactivity. FAHF-2 seems to promote tolerance to PN allergen without systemic immune suppression that is associated with steroids and other immune-modulating pharmaceuticals used in the mainstream treatment of allergic diseases.

Herbal Formulations Implicated for Possible Treatment of Food Allergy

The safety of herbal agents other than FAHF-2 for the treatment of food allergy has not been tested in humans, but several reports have identified alternative formulations with potentially beneficial immune-modulatory benefits. Investigation of more than 210 crude herbal compounds used in traditional Japanese medicines (Kampo medicine) revealed only 2 functionally immune-suppressive herbs, Notopterygii Rhizoma and Saussureae Radix. Isolation of the active components of Saussureae Radix proved this herb to be cytotoxic; however, in an epicutaneous sensitization model, topical treatment with Notopterygii Rhizoma suppressed delayed-type hypersensitivity to ovalbumin (OVA). The anti-inflammatory effect of Notopterygii Rhizoma seems to occur via suppression of expression of inducible nitric oxide synthase and inhibition of lipopolysaccharide (LPS)-induced dendritic-cell (DC) maturation by its active component falcarindiol.[65] Kakkonto is one of the most common traditional Japanese herbal medicines, comprising seven constituents and widely used for the treatment of cold, headaches, and myalgia[66] and, more recently, proposed to be beneficial for the treatment of food allergy.[67] Pretreatment with Kakkonto of OVA-sensitized mice suppressed development of allergic diarrhea when mice were challenged with OVA. Decreased symptoms were associated with reduced mucosal mast-cell numbers and reduced Th1 and Th2 cytokines in the colon, suggesting that Kakkonto has the potential to interfere with infiltration of mast cells in the colon of food-allergic mice.[67] Quercetin, a flavonoid polyphonic compound, was also recently proposed to have immune-modulatory effects similar to FAHF, and is being investigated as another novel therapeutic for food allergy.[68] Pentagalloylglucose (PGG) is a natural polyphenolic compound and major constituent of plant-derived tannins from *Phyllanthus emblica* L, a subtropical tree located in China, India, and Indonesia. The fruit and juice that contain PGG are reported to have anti-inflammatory properties, and have been used by local people for treatment of eczema and diarrhea.[69] In another mouse model of food allergy, PGG was shown to reduce allergic symptoms on challenge via suppression of FcεRI on mast cells in the gut.[70] Although most studies have focused on identifying the effects of herbal formulations on global Th1/Th2-cytokine-mediated effects or directly on mast cells and basophils, evidence also suggests that certain herbal formulations may exert direct effects on airway smooth muscle cells and attenuate airway constriction that accompanies food-induced anaphylaxis, a mechanism most relevant to food-allergic patients with underlying asthma.[71] Herbal formulations developed specifically for the treatment of asthma have entered clinical trials,[72] but are beyond the scope of this article.

ALTERNATIVE IMMUNOTHERAPY

Conventional immunotherapy with food allergens has a significantly higher rate of adverse events compared with those associated with aeroallergen and insect venom, thus making the injection of crude allergen extract unsafe for the treatment of food allergy.[73] Current investigational approaches to food-allergen immunotherapy have begun to address this problem by creating formulations of food allergens that induce cellular mechanisms of tolerance without cross-linking IgE on the surfaces of effector cells. Suggested alternatives to the classic subcutaneous injection of whole allergen extracts include oral[74] or sublingual administration of whole allergen,[75] engineered food-allergen proteins,[76] synthetic allergen peptides,[77] and adjuvant therapy.[78]

Central to understanding the mechanism of oral immunotherapy is the notion that administration of crude extracts of raw[74] or cooked[79] food allergens somehow engages the natural mechanisms of oral tolerance via the gut mucosa. The enhanced safety and efficacy of cooked food allergens for the treatment of food allergy are thought to occur because the process of heating alters allergen epitopes, making the cross-linking of IgE less efficient than in the raw form. A more refined way to reduce food-allergen reactivity is to engineer food-allergen proteins, which contain altered amino acid residues within epitope regions and thereby reduce the efficiency of the food allergen to cross-link IgE. These engineered proteins have been shown to lack the capacity to bind to IgE and, when injected subcutaneously, partially desensitize PN-allergic mice.[80] Despite the inability to cross-link IgE, these engineered proteins maintained their ability to interact with T cells and to promote tolerance via suppression of Th2 cytokines and induction of IFN-γ and transforming growth factor β.[80]

Adjuvants have long been used in vaccination to promote long-term immunity against infectious diseases. More recently, their immune-activating properties have been explored for enhancing tolerant immune responses to food allergens. In the first approach, PN-sensitized mice treated with modified PN allergens in the presence of *Listeria monocytogenes* or *Escherichia coli* showed enhanced protection against anaphylaxis compared with treatment with modified PN allergen alone.[80] In the second approach, when heat-killed *E coli* (HKE) overexpressing modified PN allergens were administered to PN-allergic mice before oral food challenge, the mice showed reduced anaphylaxis symptoms and reduced plasma histamine levels that were associated with a reduction of PN-specific IgE and Th2 cytokines.[76]

The mechanism by which these bacterial adjuvants enhance tolerogenic responses to food allergens likely involves activation of innate signaling pathways via toll-like receptors (TLRs) expressed on the surface of professional antigen-presenting cells. Recent work suggests that the induction of tolerance to PN using a bacterial adjuvant system depends on the ability of HKE to engage TLR signaling pathways, and that blocking TLR signaling abrogates the effect of HKE.[78]

NUTRITION

The most marked change in paradigm with regard to dietary intake and food allergy is that avoidance of food allergens during pregnancy, lactation, or infancy is no longer believed to prevent allergic disease.[81] Although rigorous studies of the role of nutrition and allergic disease are lacking, specific nutrients, including antioxidants, oligosaccharides, polyunsaturated fatty acids, folic acid, retinoic acid, probiotics, and other vitamins, have documented effects on immune function.[82] A recent systematic review of evidence-related nutritional supplements and allergic disease found epidemiologic evidence to support intake of vitamins A, D, E, and zinc; fruits and vegetables; and the Mediterranean diet for prevention of asthma.[83] A birth cohort of 2423 Swedish children, who started taking multivitamins before age 4 years, had a decreased risk for sensitization to food allergens, measured in blood at the age of 8 years.[84] Similarly, adults who reported higher levels of vitamin E intake had lower levels of food sensitization.[85] No prospective studies have evaluated these nutritional components for the prevention or treatment of food allergy.

PROBIOTICS AND SOY ISOFLAVONES

An extension of the use of nutrition and bacterial adjuvants for the treatment of food allergy is the use of probiotics to enhance the gut's natural microflora and engage innate signaling pathways that promote tolerance. The therapeutic benefit of soy products to protect against food-induced anaphylaxis was first demonstrated in a PN-allergic mouse model, in which oral administration of a fermented soy product (processed by a koji fungus Aspergillus oryzae) called ImmuneBalance reduced anaphylaxis scores in parallel with reduced plasma histamine and PN-specific IgE levels.[86] The major active isoflavones present in soybean (genistein, daidzein, and glycitein) are examples of naturally derived immunologically active compounds alleged to combat a wide variety of diseases. The role of soy in the treatment of PN allergy poses interesting questions because, in addition to the known immune-regulatory effects of isoflavones, soybean proteins share significant amino acid sequence homology to PN allergens. Nonetheless, the incidence and severity of soy allergy are far less compared with PN, and the active components of soy may prevent initiation of PN allergy or otherwise diminish responsiveness of effector cells in models of PN anaphylaxis. Dietary intake of high levels of soy has been associated with improved lung function in asthmatics.[87] In mice, genistein and daidzein supplementation before oral sensitization reduced symptoms of anaphylaxis caused by PN oral challenge by 35% to 40%.[88] In this model, the reduction in symptoms was associated with significantly reduced skin mast-cell degranulation, β-chymase release by intestinal mucosal mast cells, and allergen-specific IgE production. Furthermore, soy isoflavones were shown to inhibit human DC maturation in vitro.[88] The immune-regulatory effects of soy may include both a primary regulatory response to PN allergen and a secondary suppression of responsiveness to PN allergen exposure in sensitized patients, by attenuating the responsiveness of effector cells.

SUMMARY

Historically most of the medicines we use originate from natural products and their synthetic derivatives.[15] It is not surprising, therefore, that traditional herbal formulations would contain immune-modulating characteristics and the ability to alter or suppress allergic disease at a cellular level. Compared with the long history of ancient traditions, such as TCM for a variety of other illnesses, alternative herbal therapy and immunotherapy for food allergy remains in its infancy. As evidence favoring CAM strengthens, the distinction between CAM and other novel approaches to the treatment of food allergy becomes clouded. This gray area is likely to transform into a modern era of truly integrative medicine. It is insufficient to investigate the clinical efficacy of CAM without giving priority to elucidating the mechanistic actions of these therapies. In food-allergy research, as we struggle to define the roles of specific immune cells, portals for allergen sensitization, and the role of food allergy in setting the stage for more severe allergic diseases later in life, it is important to incorporate what we learn from CAM into this paradigm.

The scope of CAM for the treatment of food allergy is slowly increasing. In addition, the scope of potential use for agents that promote oral tolerance extends beyond treatment of food allergy.[89] Similarly, health care expenditures have increased in this sector. As health care practitioners we have an obligation to our patients to understand their reasoning and interest in complementary treatments and to help them to make educated decisions about the potential risks and benefits of each. For patients with severe disease and limited conventional therapeutic options, or for those who have suffered from unwanted side effects of conventional therapies, we should break the cultural and social barriers to accessing complementary therapies that have been proved to be safe and beneficial.

REFERENCES

1. Sicherer SH. Epidemiology of food allergy. J Allergy Clin Immunol 2011;127: 594–602.
2. Barnes PM, Bloom B, Nahin RL. Complementary and alternative medicine use among adults and children: United States, 2007. Natl Health Stat Report 2008;(12):1–23.
3. Eisenberg DM, Kessler RC, Foster C, et al. Unconventional medicine in the United States. Prevalence, costs, and patterns of use. N Engl J Med 1993;328:246–52.
4. Engler RJ, Silvers WS, Bielory L. Complementary and alternative medicine education: need for expanded educational resources for American Academy of Allergy, Asthma & Immunology members. J Allergy Clin Immunol 2009;123: 511–2.
5. Engler RJ, With CM, Gregory PJ, et al. Complementary and alternative medicine for the allergist-immunologist: where do I start? J Allergy Clin Immunol 2009;123: 309–16.
6. Vozeh S. Is the increasing use of evidence-based pharmacotherapy causing the renaissance of complementary medicine? Br J Clin Pharmacol 2003;56:292–6.
7. Gershwin ME, Borchers AT, Keen CL, et al. Public safety and dietary supplementation. Ann N Y Acad Sci 2010;1190:104–17.
8. Schafer T, Riehle A, Wichmann HE, et al. Alternative medicine in allergies—prevalence, patterns of use, and costs. Allergy 2002;57:694–700.
9. Staud R. Effectiveness of CAM therapy: understanding the evidence. Rheum Dis Clin North Am 2011;37:9–17.
10. Li XM. Complementary and alternative medicine in pediatric allergic disorders. Curr Opin Allergy Clin Immunol 2009;9:161–7.
11. Li XM, Brown L. Efficacy and mechanisms of action of traditional Chinese medicines for treating asthma and allergy. J Allergy Clin Immunol 2009;123:297–306 [quiz: 7–8].
12. Sorkness RL. CAM and respiratory disease. Nutr Clin Pract 2009;24:609–15.
13. Lewith GT, Watkins AD. Unconventional therapies in asthma: an overview. Allergy 1996;51:761–9.
14. Boneberger S, Rupec RA, Ruzicka T. Complementary therapy for atopic dermatitis and other allergic skin diseases: facts and controversies. Clin Dermatol 2010; 28:57–61.
15. Kulka M. The potential of natural products as effective treatments for allergic inflammation: implications for allergic rhinitis. Curr Top Med Chem 2009;9: 1611–24.

16. Matkovic Z, Zivkovic V, Korica M, et al. Efficacy and safety of *Astragalus membranaceus* in the treatment of patients with seasonal allergic rhinitis. Phytother Res 2010;24:175–81.
17. Witt CM, Brinkhaus B. Efficacy, effectiveness and cost-effectiveness of acupuncture for allergic rhinitis—an overview about previous and ongoing studies. Auton Neurosci 2010;157:42–5.
18. Brinkhaus B, Witt CM, Ortiz M, et al. Acupuncture in seasonal allergic rhinitis (ACUSAR)—design and protocol of a randomised controlled multi-centre trial. Forsch Komplementmed 2010;17:95–102.
19. Ko J, Lee JI, Munoz-Furlong A, et al. Use of complementary and alternative medicine by food-allergic patients. Ann Allergy Asthma Immunol 2006;97:365–9.
20. Kay AB, Lessof MH. Allergy. Conventional and alternative concepts. A report of the Royal College of Physicians Committee on Clinical Immunology and Allergy. Clin Exp Allergy 1992;22(Suppl 3):1–44.
21. Burks W, Kulis M, Pons L. Food allergies and hypersensitivity: a review of pharmacotherapy and therapeutic strategies. Expert Opin Pharmacother 2008;9:1145–52.
22. Nowak-Wegrzyn A, Muraro A. Food allergy therapy: is a cure within reach? Pediatr Clin North Am 2011;58:511–30, xii.
23. Nowak-Wegrzyn A, Sampson HA. Future therapies for food allergies. J Allergy Clin Immunol 2011;127:558–73 [quiz: 74–5].
24. Blazquez AB, Mayer L, Berin MC. Thymic stromal lymphopoietin is required for gastrointestinal allergy but not oral tolerance. Gastroenterology 2010;139:1301–9.
25. Lack G, Fox D, Northstone K, et al. Factors associated with the development of peanut allergy in childhood. N Engl J Med 2003;348:977–85.
26. DePaolo RW, Abadie V, Tang F, et al. Co-adjuvant effects of retinoic acid and IL-15 induce inflammatory immunity to dietary antigens. Nature 2011;471:220–4.
27. Weiner HL, da Cunha AP, Quintana F, et al. Oral tolerance. Immunol Rev 2011;241:241–59.
28. Wieland LS, Manheimer E, Berman BM. Development and classification of an operational definition of complementary and alternative medicine for the Cochrane collaboration. Altern Ther Health Med 2011;17:50–9.
29. Bausell RB, Lee WL, Soeken KL, et al. Larger effect sizes were associated with higher quality ratings in complementary and alternative medicine randomized controlled trials. J Clin Epidemiol 2004;57:438–46.
30. Watkins AD. The role of alternative therapies in the treatment of allergic disease. Clin Exp Allergy 1994;24:813–25.
31. Brinkhaus B, Witt CM, Jena S, et al. Acupuncture in patients with allergic rhinitis: a pragmatic randomized trial. Ann Allergy Asthma Immunol 2008;101:535–43.
32. Passalacqua G, Compalati E, Schiappoli M, et al. Complementary and alternative medicine for the treatment and diagnosis of asthma and allergic diseases. Monaldi Arch Chest Dis 2005;63:47–54.
33. Boyce JA, Assa'ad A, Burks AW, et al. Guidelines for the diagnosis and management of food allergy in the United States: report of the NIAID-sponsored expert panel. J Allergy Clin Immunol 2010;126:S1–58.
34. Noimark L, Cox HE. Nutritional problems related to food allergy in childhood. Pediatr Allergy Immunol 2008;19:188–95.
35. Flokstra-de Blok BM, Dubois AE, Vlieg-Boerstra BJ, et al. Health-related quality of life of food allergic patients: comparison with the general population and other diseases. Allergy 2010;65:238–44.

36. Senna G, Gani F, Leo G, et al. Alternative tests in the diagnosis of food allergies. Recenti Prog Med 2002;93:327–34 [in Italian].
37. Beyer K, Teuber SS. Food allergy diagnostics: scientific and unproven procedures. Curr Opin Allergy Clin Immunol 2005;5:261–6.
38. Wuthrich B. Unproven techniques in allergy diagnosis. J Investig Allergol Clin Immunol 2005;15:86–90.
39. Weiss J. IgG food allergies—a subject of controversy. Dtsch Med Wochenschr 2011;136:p3 [in German].
40. Commins SP, Satinover SM, Hosen J, et al. Delayed anaphylaxis, angioedema, or urticaria after consumption of red meat in patients with IgE antibodies specific for galactose-alpha-1,3-galactose. J Allergy Clin Immunol 2009;123:426–33.
41. Nomura I, Morita H, Hosokawa S, et al. Four distinct subtypes of non-IgE-mediated gastrointestinal food allergies in neonates and infants, distinguished by their initial symptoms. J Allergy Clin Immunol 2011;127:685–8.e1–8.
42. Shaw D, Leon C, Kolev S, et al. Traditional remedies and food supplements. A 5-year toxicological study (1991-1995). Drug Saf 1997;17:342–56.
43. Ji K, Chen J, Li M, et al. Comments on serious anaphylaxis caused by nine Chinese herbal injections used to treat common colds and upper respiratory tract infections. Regul Toxicol Pharmacol 2009;55:134–8.
44. Niggemann B, Gruber C. Side-effects of complementary and alternative medicine. Allergy 2003;58:707–16.
45. Watanabe MA, Amarante MK, Conti BJ, et al. Cytotoxic constituents of propolis inducing anticancer effects: a review. J Pharm Pharmacol 2011;63:1378–86.
46. Yanagita M, Kojima Y, Mori K, et al. Osteoinductive and anti-inflammatory effect of royal jelly on periodontal ligament cells. Biomed Res 2011;32:285–91.
47. Li XM, Zhang TF, Huang CK, et al. Food Allergy Herbal Formula-1 (FAHF-1) blocks peanut-induced anaphylaxis in a murine model. J Allergy Clin Immunol 2001;108:639–46.
48. Srivastava KD, Kattan JD, Zou ZM, et al. The Chinese herbal medicine formula FAHF-2 completely blocks anaphylactic reactions in a murine model of peanut allergy. J Allergy Clin Immunol 2005;115:171–8.
49. Srivastava K, Yang N, Chen Y, et al. Efficacy, safety and immunological actions of butanol-extracted food allergy herbal formula-2 on peanut anaphylaxis. Clin Exp Allergy 2011;41:582–91.
50. Wang J, Patil SP, Yang N, et al. Safety, tolerability, and immunologic effects of a food allergy herbal formula in food allergic individuals: a randomized, double-blinded, placebo-controlled, dose escalation, phase 1 study. Ann Allergy Asthma Immunol 2010;105:75–84.
51. Patil SP, Wang J, Song Y, et al. Clinical safety of food allergy herbal formula-2 (FAHF-2) and inhibitory effect on basophils from patients with food allergy: extended phase I study. J Allergy Clin Immunol 2011;128:1259–65.
52. Lin CH, Wang MH, Chung HY, et al. Effects of acupuncture-like transcutaneous electrical nerve stimulation on children with asthma. J Asthma 2010;47:1116–22.
53. Choi JY, Jung HJ, Kim JI, et al. A randomized pilot study of acupuncture as an adjunct therapy in adult asthmatic patients. J Asthma 2010;47:774–80.
54. Wechsler ME, Kelley JM, Boyd IO, et al. Active albuterol or placebo, sham acupuncture, or no intervention in asthma. N Engl J Med 2011;365:119–26.
55. Witt CM, Reinhold T, Jena S, et al. Cost-effectiveness of acupuncture in women and men with allergic rhinitis: a randomized controlled study in usual care. Am J Epidemiol 2009;169:562–71.

56. Witt CM, Pach D, Brinkhaus B, et al. Safety of acupuncture: results of a prospective observational study with 229,230 patients and introduction of a medical information and consent form. Forsch Komplementmed 2009;16:91–7.

57. Pfab F, Huss-Marp J, Gatti A, et al. Influence of acupuncture on type I hypersensitivity itch and the wheal and flare response in adults with atopic eczema—a blinded, randomized, placebo-controlled, crossover trial. Allergy 2010;65:903–10.

58. Burns JJ, Zhao L, Taylor EW, et al. The influence of traditional herbal formulas on cytokine activity. Toxicology 2010;278:140–59.

59. Sharman J, Kumar L, Singh S. Allergenicity of common foods restricted in respiratory allergy. Indian J Pediatr 2000;67:713–20.

60. Arora D, Kumar M. Food allergies—leads from Ayurveda. Indian J Med Sci 2003; 57:57–63.

61. Srivastava KD, Qu C, Zhang T, et al. Food allergy herbal formula-2 silences peanut-induced anaphylaxis for a prolonged posttreatment period via IFN-gamma-producing CD8+ T cells. J Allergy Clin Immunol 2009;123:443–51.

62. Song Y, Qu C, Srivastava K, et al. Food allergy herbal formula 2 protection against peanut anaphylactic reaction is via inhibition of mast cells and basophils. J Allergy Clin Immunol 2010;126:1208–17.e3.

63. Qu C, Srivastava K, Ko J, et al. Induction of tolerance after establishment of peanut allergy by the food allergy herbal formula-2 is associated with up-regulation of interferon-gamma. Clin Exp Allergy 2007;37:846–55.

64. Kattan JD, Srivastava KD, Zou ZM, et al. Pharmacological and immunological effects of individual herbs in the food allergy herbal formula-2 (FAHF-2) on peanut allergy. Phytother Res 2008;22:651–9.

65. Mitsui S, Torii K, Fukui H, et al. The herbal medicine compound falcarindiol from Notopterygii Rhizoma suppresses dendritic cell maturation. J Pharmacol Exp Ther 2010;333:954–60.

66. Furuichi M, Hara H, Asano Y, et al. Letter: Fixed drug eruption caused by the Japanese herbal drug kakkonto. Dermatol Online J 2010;16:13.

67. Yamamoto T, Fujiwara K, Yoshida M, et al. Therapeutic effect of kakkonto in a mouse model of food allergy with gastrointestinal symptoms. Int Arch Allergy Immunol 2009;148:175–85.

68. Chirumbolo S. Quercetin as a potential anti-allergic drug: which perspectives? Iran J Allergy Asthma Immunol 2011;10:139–40.

69. Zhang YJ, Abe T, Tanaka T, et al. Phyllanemblinins A-F, new ellagitannins from *Phyllanthus emblica*. J Nat Prod 2001;64:1527–32.

70. Kageyama-Yahara N, Suehiro Y, Maeda F, et al. Pentagalloylglucose down-regulates mast cell surface FcepsilonRI expression in vitro and in vivo. FEBS Lett 2010;584:111–8.

71. Ghayur MN, Gilani AH, Janssen LJ. Ginger attenuates acetylcholine-induced contraction and Ca2+ signalling in murine airway smooth muscle cells. Can J Physiol Pharmacol 2008;86:264–71.

72. Zhang T, Srivastava K, Wen MC, et al. Pharmacology and immunological actions of a herbal medicine ASHMI on allergic asthma. Phytother Res 2010;24:1047–55.

73. Oppenheimer JJ, Nelson HS, Bock SA, et al. Treatment of peanut allergy with rush immunotherapy. J Allergy Clin Immunol 1992;90:256–62.

74. Thyagarajan A, Varshney P, Jones SM, et al. Peanut oral immunotherapy is not ready for clinical use. J Allergy Clin Immunol 2010;126:31–2.

75. Kim ST, Han DH, Moon IJ, et al. Clinical and immunologic effects of sublingual immunotherapy on patients with allergic rhinitis to house-dust mites: 1-year follow-up results. Am J Rhinol Allergy 2010;24:271–5.

76. Li XM, Srivastava K, Grishin A, et al. Persistent protective effect of heat-killed *Escherichia coli* producing "engineered," recombinant peanut proteins in a murine model of peanut allergy. J Allergy Clin Immunol 2003;112:159–67.

77. Rupa P, Mine Y. Oral immunotherapy with immunodominant T-cell epitope peptides alleviates allergic reactions in a Balb/c mouse model of egg allergy. Allergy 2011 Sep 27. [Epub ahead of print]. DOI: 10.1111/j.1398–9995.2011.02724.x.

78. Pochard P, Vickery B, Berin MC, et al. Targeting Toll-like receptors on dendritic cells modifies the T(H)2 response to peanut allergens in vitro. J Allergy Clin Immunol 2010;126:92–7 e5.

79. Lemon-Mule H, Sampson HA, Sicherer SH, et al. Immunologic changes in children with egg allergy ingesting extensively heated egg. J Allergy Clin Immunol 2008;122:977–83.e1.

80. Li XM, Srivastava K, Huleatt JW, et al. Engineered recombinant peanut protein and heat-killed *Listeria monocytogenes* coadministration protects against peanut-induced anaphylaxis in a murine model. J Immunol 2003;170:3289–95.

81. Prescott SL, Bouygue GR, Videky D, et al. Avoidance or exposure to foods in prevention and treatment of food allergy? Curr Opin Allergy Clin Immunol 2010; 10:258–66.

82. West CE, Videky DJ, Prescott SL. Role of diet in the development of immune tolerance in the context of allergic disease. Curr Opin Pediatr 2010;22:635–41.

83. Nurmatov U, Devereux G, Sheikh A. Nutrients and foods for the primary prevention of asthma and allergy: systematic review and meta-analysis. J Allergy Clin Immunol 2011;127:724–33.e1–30.

84. Marmsjo K, Rosenlund H, Kull I, et al. Use of multivitamin supplements in relation to allergic disease in 8-y-old children. Am J Clin Nutr 2009;90:1693–8.

85. Sausenthaler S, Loebel T, Linseisen J, et al. Vitamin E intake in relation to allergic sensitization and IgE serum concentration. Cent Eur J Public Health 2009;17: 79–85.

86. Zhang T, Pan W, Takebe M, et al. Therapeutic effects of a fermented soy product on peanut hypersensitivity is associated with modulation of T-helper type 1 and T-helper type 2 responses. Clin Exp Allergy 2008;38:1808–18.

87. Smith LJ, Holbrook JT, Wise R, et al. Dietary intake of soy genistein is associated with lung function in patients with asthma. J Asthma 2004;41:833–43.

88. Masilamani M, Wei J, Bhatt S, et al. Soybean isoflavones regulate dendritic cell function and suppress allergic sensitization to peanut. J Allergy Clin Immunol 2011;128:1242–50.

89. Mayer L, Shao L. Therapeutic potential of oral tolerance. Nat Rev Immunol 2004; 4:407–19.

Paradigm Shift in the Management of Milk and Egg Allergy: Baked Milk and Egg Diet

George N. Konstantinou, MD, PhD, MSc[a,b], Jennifer S. Kim, MD[a,*]

KEYWORDS

- Food allergy • Egg allergy • Milk allergy • Baked milk diet
- Baked egg diet • Thermal processing • Heat treatment
- Allergenicity

Cooking can make food more palatable, change flavor, texture, or even color, and improve digestibility. In addition to flavor and texture enhancement, thermal processing, such as pasteurization or sterilization, is used to eliminate microorganisms and thus ensure microbiological safety. These alterations in sensory, nutritional, and physical properties are the result of protein denaturation during thermal processing. The effect of heat on allergenicity is variable and food dependent. For peanut (dry roasting)[1] and shrimp (boiling),[2] high temperatures seem to increase allergenicity. However, for cow's milk and hen's egg, allergenicity is attenuated. These recent findings, in both the laboratory setting (mouse) and clinical setting (man), have set the stage for a paradigm shift in food allergy management. Strict avoidance has been the standard of care for food allergy for decades, but more recent studies have supported the safety and potential benefits of inclusion of extensively heated products containing milk and/or egg into the diet of those who are nonreactive.

EFFECT OF THERMAL PROCESSING ON ANTIGENICITY AND ALLERGENICITY

Epitopes are defined as the portions of the antigenic molecules, typically proteins, that can bind with the complementary site of an antibody. There are 2 types of epitopes: (1) sequential or continuous or linear (based on the primary structure of the molecule), in which the antibody binds to a contiguous stretch of amino acid residues within the

[a] Division of Allergy and Immunology, Department of Pediatrics, Jaffe Food Allergy Institute, Mount Sinai School of Medicine, 1 Gustave L. Levy Place, Box 1198, New York, NY 10029, USA
[b] Department of Allergy, 424 General Military Training Hospital, Periferiaki Odos, Nea Efkarpia, Thessaloniki 56429, Greece
* Corresponding author.
E-mail address: jennifer.kim@mssm.edu

Immunol Allergy Clin N Am 32 (2012) 151–164
doi:10.1016/j.iac.2011.11.003
0889-8561/12/$ – see front matter © 2012 Elsevier Inc. All rights reserved.

peptide, and (2) conformational or discontinuous (based on the secondary or tertiary structure of the molecule), in which the antibody binds to noncontiguous amino acid segments that are distantly separated within the protein and are brought into proximity by the folding of the molecule (**Fig. 1**).[3] The structure of an epitope and the physico-chemical properties of the component amino acids define the antigenic specificity of this epitope. Any change in the structure, including a single amino acid substitution or destruction, may influence antigenicity.

When food allergens are exposed to heat, allergenic activity may be unchanged, decreased (perhaps abolished), or even increased.[4] These phenomena can be explained by inactivation, denaturation, or destruction of epitope structure; formation of new epitopes (neotopes); or exposure of hidden epitopes after unfolding (cryptotopes).[5,6]

The clinical (symptomatic) expression of food allergy, specifically to milk and egg, has been attributed to individual epitopes in case-control, cross-sectional,[7–12] and longitudinal cohort studies.[13] Transient and persistent allergy have been attributed to recognition of primarily conformational and sequential epitopes, respectively. Greater IgE epitope diversity recognition and higher binding affinity are also associated with increased severity and persistence of disease.[13]

Thus, the aforementioned heat-induced changes on the physical and biological properties of cow's milk and hen's egg are expected to affect predominantly conformational epitopes, existing only when the tertiary and secondary molecular structure remains intact, whereas more limited effects are expected on sequential epitopes.

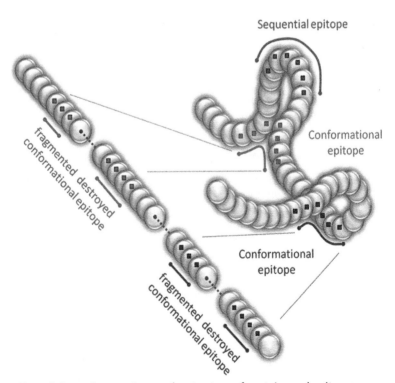

Fig. 1. Effect of thermal processing on the structure of proteins and epitopes.

Cow's Milk

Strict avoidance has been the standard of care for decades, but since as early as 1966 thermal processing was proposed to have a potential preventative role in cow's milk allergy.[14] Evidence published in the ensuing 45 years has elucidated many of the effects of heat on allergenicity of cow's milk proteins and its immunologic consequences (**Table 1**). Cow's milk contains 3.3% total protein. There are 2 major categories: casein and whey, which differ in their chemical composition and physical properties (**Table 2**).[15]

Pasteurization and homogenization

Cow's milk is consumed in homogenized and pasteurized forms by humans living in industrialized countries. Homogenization is a process by which the fat particles of the milk are broken up and dispersed uniformly so as to prevent or delay the natural separation of cream from the rest of the emulsion; this occurs at 60°C to 72°C. Pasteurization minimizes the number of viable microbes so that they are unlikely to become pathogenic, destroys undesirable enzymes to improve the keeping quality of milk, and extends shelf life. Pasteurization temperatures vary depending on the method utilized (72°C–150°C) but are generally higher than homogenization temperatures.[16] These processes occur within 1 to 15 seconds.

Although the purpose of such processing is to enhance safety as well as improve digestibility and texture, it is of great interest to understand their effects on antigenicity

Table 1
Sensitivity of cow's milk and hen's egg proteins and allergens to thermal processing

		Protein	Allergen	Thermal Process	
				Effect on Molecule	Effect on Allergenicity
Cow's milk	Caseins	β-Casein	Bos d 8 beta	Heat resistant	Partially heat labile
		α$_{s1}$-Casein	Bos d 8 alpha-s1		
		α$_{s2}$-Casein	Bos d 8 alpha-s2		
		κ-Casein	Bos d 8 kappa		
	Whey	α-Lactalbumin	Bos d 4	Heat labile[73,74]	Heat labile
		β-Lactoglobulin	Bos d 5	Heat labile	Heat labile
		Lactoferrin	Bos d Lactoferrin	Heat labile	Heat labile
Hen's egg	Egg white	Ovalbumin	Gal d 2	Heat labile	Heat labile
		Ovomucoid	Gal d 1	Relatively heat resistant	Partially heat labile
		Ovotransferrin (conalbumin)	Gal d 3	Heat labile	Heat labile
		Lysozyme	Gal d 4	Relatively heat resistant	Heat labile
		Ovoinhibitor	—	N/A	N/A
		Ovomucin	—	Heat labile	Heat labile
	Egg yolk	Phosvitin[75,76]	—	Partially heat labile	Partially heat labile
		α-Livetin[77]	Gal d 5	Partially heat labile	Partially heat labile
		β-Livetin[76,78,79]	—	Contradictory evidence	Unknown
		γ-Livetin	—	Unknown	Unknown
		Glycoprotein 42[80]	Gal d 6	Heat resistant	Heat resistant

Abbreviation: N/A: not available.

Table 2
Cow's milk proteins

	Casein	Whey (Serum Proteins)
Percentage of milk protein (%)	82	18
Components	β-Casein (approximately 45%) (Bos d 8 beta) α_{s1}-Casein (approximately 40%) (Bos d 8 alpha-s1) α_{s2}-Casein (approximately 10%), (Bos d 8 alpha-s2) κ-Casein (approximately 5%) (Bos d 8 kappa)	β-Lactoglobulin (approximately 55%) (Bos d 5) α-Lactalbumin (approximately 24%) (Bos d 4) Immunoglobulins (approximately 15%) (Bos d 7) Bovine serum albumin (approximately 5%) (Bos d 6) Lactoferrin (Bos d Lactoferrin), transferrin, and other minor proteins and enzymes
Characteristics	Contains phosphorus Coagulates/precipitates at pH 4.6	Does not contain phosphorus Soluble at pH 4.6

and allergenicity in mouse and man. Heat has a significant effect on milk protein stability, particularly the whey fraction.

A recent mouse model[17] elegantly demonstrated that pasteurization (62°C for 33 minutes or 72°C for 2 minutes) affected allergenicity but not antigenicity of whey proteins. Pasteurization significantly reduced the ability of both α-lactalbumin and β-lactoglobulin to induce anaphylaxis when administered orally to sensitized mice. Casein, however, retained its allergenicity after pasteurization. The explanation for this discrepancy was attributed to redirected intestinal epithelial uptake of whey proteins, particularly β-lactoglobulin. Pasteurization, by inducing aggregation, inhibited uptake of whey proteins by enterocytes (whereby native whey proteins transcytose). Bypassing intestinal epithelial cells, antigens enter into Peyer patches, thereby enhancing sensitization and promoting food allergy induction. In contrast, casein exists in an aggregated form (micelles), which hinders its crossing of the epithelial barrier, and is thus taken up by Peyer patches, characteristics that do not change with heat treatment. The importance of the route of sensitization in addition to allergen structure in anaphylaxis induction was also demonstrated by this study.[17] Allergic responses in these mice could not be triggered by aggregates of milk proteins when administered orally. Only soluble milk allergens could interact with the intestinal mast cells after they were transcytosed from the intestinal epithelium. Systemically introduced aggregates could, however, cause clinical anaphylaxis. Similar enhancements in allergenicity because of homogenization have been shown in other mouse models as well.[18–20] However, it was not clear if these increases were because of thermal or emulsifying effects.

The impact of pasteurization clinically (in man) has not been well characterized, although casein is generally considered the major allergen in milk-allergic patients, followed by the whey proteins α-lactalbumin and β-lactoglobulin. Antibodies to casein, but not consistently to α-lactalbumin and β-lactoglobulin, are readily detected in nearly all milk-allergic individuals.[21,22]

There is only one study to the authors' knowledge in which the effects of pasteurization and homogenization on milk allergenicity were examined in a double-blind placebo-controlled manner. Five toddlers with milk allergy were challenged to raw untreated milk, pasteurized milk (at 75°C for 15 sec), and homogenized/pasteurized milk.

Extensively hydrolyzed casein formula was used as a placebo. No significant differences were found in challenge outcomes or skin prick test (SPT) responses.[23] However, the small number of subjects examined does not allow for definitive conclusions.

Cooking

Cooking is defined as food preparation by use of heat, such as baking, broiling, roasting, boiling, stewing, and frying, generally for periods significantly longer than in pasteurization. In animal models, heat-treated cow's milk preparations have been shown to considerably decrease anaphylactic sensitizing capacity.[17,24–27] As indicated earlier, the casein and whey fractions have different responses to heat treatment. Casein has been shown to be unaffected after cooking at 95°C for longer than 30 minutes. However, bovine serum protein has been found to be heat labile in milk at 85°C for 120 minutes[28] and even when heated at 100°C for 5 minutes.[29] In another study, boiling skimmed milk at 100°C for 10 minutes resulted in decreased IgE binding for caseins and α-lactalbumin and abolished it for β-lactoglobulin and bovine serum albumin.[30]

The heat-labile nature of β-lactoglobulin, the major whey protein, has been extensively studied.[31–35] Inhibition enzyme-linked immunosorbent assay results for β-lactoglobulin showed no IgE binding effect when milk was heated at 72°C for 30 seconds (pasteurization). However, heating at 90°C for 4 minutes had a clear effect, reducing IgE binding and increasing half maximal inhibitory concentration (IC_{50}) from 0.20 (for fresh untreated milk) to 4.96 µg/ml in one study.[36] Similar results were shown in another study, in which heating at 90°C for 60 minutes increased IC_{50} from 2.03 to 8.45 µg/ml.[37] When low-fat milk was boiled at 100°C for 15 minutes, the IC_{50} for IgE binding to β-lactoglobulin increased from 2.03 to 109 µg/ml. This change was magnified with extended heat exposure (60 minutes), even at a lower temperature (90°C); IC_{50} increased to 245 µg/ml.[37] Thus, the presence of fat may hinder heat-induced changes to milk protein.

From these studies it is evident that β-lactoglobulin is heat labile as a whole, although some sequential epitopes remain extremely heat stable even after extensive heat treatement.[38] It cannot be ruled out, nevertheless, that neotopes are created or cryptotopes are revealed via the heating process. This was suggested by experiments in which heat-induced conformational changes of the β-lactoglobulin molecule were shown to affect the binding of anti-β-lactoglobulin monoclonal antibodies to different epitopes[39] and also that showed there was an anti-β-lactoglobulin monoclonal antibody specific only for the heat-denatured form.[40]

Clinical heterogeneity with immunologic specificities between children tolerant to heated milk and those reactive to unheated milk has also been demonstrated. In a study by Nowak-Wegrzyn and colleagues,[41] it has been shown that most (approximately 75%) children with milk allergy can tolerate baked milk (heated to 350°F/177°C for 30 minutes). Subjects having undetectable serum milk-specific IgE levels or skin prick test wheal size less than 5 mm were shown to be nonreactive to foods containing baked-in milk (eg, muffins or waffles). In contrast, 85% of those with milk-specific IgE levels greater than 35 kU/L were reactive to baked milk products, some with anaphylaxis.

Thus, stability and IgE-binding capacity of cow's milk proteins is partially dependent on temperature and time but has great interpatient variation.[42] In addition, fatty acids can also affect IgE binding,[37] underscoring the potentially significant impact of the food matrix on allergenicity.

Hen's Egg

Like cow's milk, sensitivity of hen's egg proteins and allergens to thermal processing varies (see **Table 1**). The dominant antigens in hen's egg are distinguished according to their location: white and yolk (**Table 3**). Egg proteins are sensitive not only to

Table 3 Hen's egg proteins		
	White	**Yolk**
Components	Ovalbumin (or Gal d 2) (~54%)[a]	Serum albumin protein or α-livetin
	Ovomucoid (or Gal d 1) (~11%)[a]	(Gal d 5)
	Ovotransferrin (or Gal d 3) (~12%)[a]	β-Livetin (α2 glycoprotein,)
	Ovomucin (~3.5%)[a]	γ-Livetin (IgY)
	Lysozyme (or Gal d 4) (~3.4%)[a]	Yolk glycoprotein 42 (Gal d 6)
	Ovoglobulin G2 (~4%)[a]	Vitellins
	Ovoglobulin G3 (~4%)[a]	Phosvitins
	Ovoinhibitor (~1.5%)[a]	Protease and protease inhibitors
	Ovoglycoprotein	Other enzymes
	Plavoprotein	
	Ovomacroglobulin	
	Avidin cystatin	

[a] Of total egg white proteins.

temperature and time but also to pH (unlike cow's milk). In general, the biological activity of ovomucoid decreases with increased heating times, an effect that is more dramatic at alkaline (higher pH) rather than acidic environments.

Pasteurization and proteolysis

The effects of heat and enzymatic activity on whole egg with regard to antigenicity and allergenicity have been examined in a carefully performed study. The technological processes utilized included (1) pasteurization of liquid eggs (at 67°C for 6 minutes), (2) first stirring at 250 rpm (at 65°C for 10 minutes), (3) first proteolysis (at 55°C for 2 hours), (4) second stir-heating (at 75°C for 10 minutes), (5) second proteolysis (at 55°C for 2 hours), and (6) third stir-heating (at 90°C for 30 minutes). Pasteurization seemed to affect only lysozyme. The second stir-heating was the only step that changed protein composition considerably. It is not clear if this was a direct heat effect or if the first enzyme became more active at a higher temperature before becoming inactivated. In the last step, nearly all proteins were undetectable. Regarding IgE binding, very low immunoreactivity was observed at the end of the process. Here, technologically altered egg showed substantially diminished allergenicity below 1% of the initial raw material without, according to the authors, significantly affecting texture and flavor. This suggests that even those egg proteins typically characterized as heat resistant can lose their antigenicity and allergenicity after an extended thermal and proteolytic process.[43]

Clinically it seems that children who can tolerate pasteurized egg can also tolerate raw egg white based on a study that challenged 32 children with egg allergy to both pasteurized and fresh raw egg white. In addition, results from immunoblotting, immunoblotting inhibition, and ImmunoCAP (Thermo Fisher Scientific Inc., Waltham, MA, USA) inhibition (with fresh and pasteurized raw egg white) were identical.[44] However, the same cannot be said of boiling.[45]

Cooking

Similar to cow's milk, heat treatment for different periods affect egg allergenicity. Boiling (100°C) for 5 minutes was sufficient in a mouse model to reduce allergenicity (>93%) of egg white proteins significantly.[46] The binding activities of IgE antibodies in individuals allergic to egg were evaluated in 1985 using Western blot in one of the first relevant studies that implemented this technique for this purpose. A significant decrease in allergenicity (after heating egg white at 90°C for 15 minutes) was observed in more than half of the 36 patients tested positive for egg allergy. Three patients showed a slight increase in IgE binding.[47]

Binding of IgG (antigenicity) and IgE (allergenicity) antibodies from individuals allergic to egg to native and heat-treated egg white was examined and compared with that of rabbit anti–egg white IgG antibodies.[48] After careful protein purification to avoid overestimation of antigenicity and allergenicity due to contamination,[49,50] heat treatment of purified egg white proteins at 95°C for 15 minutes decreased antigenicity in all components: ovalbumin (from 21.1% to 17%), ovomucoid (from 77.5% to 19.2%), ovotransferrin (from 45.6% to 16.8%), lysozyme (from 79.4% to 47.7%), and ovomucin (from 7.3% to 0.9%) (values are expressed as percentage binding activity of IgG antibodies to native whole egg white). Binding affinities of ovalbumin-specific IgE antibodies from patients allergic to egg in other studies were variable. One study showed 90.6% less binding with heat-treated ovalbumin (100°C for 3 minutes) compared with native ovalbumin.[51] However, in another study, both antigenic and allergenic activities of thermally treated ovalbumin at 80°C for 10 minutes were similar to untreated protein.[52] It is not clear if this discrepancy can be attributed to the difference in temperature applied or to patient variability in IgE specificities.

According to human IgE binding specificities, ovomucoid is the most dominant allergen followed by ovotransferrin, ovalbumin, and lysozyme. Heating significantly affected IgE binding with ovomucoid (from 85.5% to 17.8%), ovotransferrin (from 48.3% to 11.4%), and ovalbumin (from 46.8% to 18.2%) but not lysozyme (from 43.1% to 42.5%). In the same study, it was shown that heating affected the secondary structure of ovotransferrin and ovalbumin but had less of an effect on ovomucoid and lysozyme. The differences in binding affinities between human and rabbit anti–egg white protein antibodies in these studies may be species specific or secondary to route of allergen sensitization, underscoring the importance of interpreting antigenicity and allergenicity according to the reagents used. Overall, antiovalbumin IgE recognizes more sequential epitopes than antiovomucoid IgE. On the other hand, antiovomucoid IgE and antilysozyme IgE may recognize not only sequential but also conformational epitopes of the corresponding proteins that may remain partially intact after heating process.[48]

In addition, pH plays an important role in egg allergenicity because the pH of a fresh egg gradually increases from 7.6 (fresh egg) to 9.7 during storage, that is, the fresher the egg is, the more allergenic it is expected to be.[53–57] The effects of pH on pepsin digestibility of raw and boiled (for 10 minutes) egg white at different acidic pH values were assessed in vitro using Western blot. Binding to heated ovalbumin was abolished at pH 1.5 to 2.5 after a 30-minute incubation period, whereas raw ovalbumin allergenic epitopes were found to be only partially labile to enzymatic digestion at all pH values up to 4. On the other hand, ovomucoid allergenic epitopes were found to be susceptible after 30- to 60-minute pepsin incubation independently of heat treatment.[58]

Digestibility of heat-treated ovalbumin (boiled for 15 minutes) was also assessed in a mouse model. Sensitized mice consuming heat-treated ovalbumin did not experience any clinical reactions in contrast with mice fed with unheated ovalbumin that did react. This finding strongly indicates that heat-treated ovalbumin does not retain its allergenicity.[59]

Using serum from children reactive to heated egg, it was demonstrated that heat did not destroy IgE-binding capacity of ovalbumin and ovomucoid. However, digestibility in vitro was enhanced for heated ovalbumin but not heated ovomucoid. Both heated ovalbumin and heated ovomucoid demonstrated diminished basophil activation.[60] These findings suggest the important synergistic role that digestion (gut permeability) has with heat treatment in minimizing allergenicity of egg protein, ovalbumin in particular.

Furthermore, wheat/gluten has been proposed to have a matrix effect on egg protein specifically. Baking egg whites with wheat flour induces irreversible denaturation of ovomucoid leading to loss of antigenic properties. Gluten has been proposed to be responsible for this through disulfide exchange reactions. Antigenicity of heated (180°C for 10 minutes) and unheated wheat–egg white mixtures was assessed using rabbit antiovomucoid antibodies. Almost no ovomucoid was detected in the heated mixture, whereas it was readily identifiable in the unheated mixture and found to be slightly reduced when egg white was heated alone. These findings indicate that the coexistence of wheat accelerated antigenic inactivation or insolubilization when exposed to a thermal process. This matrix effect was evident only for gluten and not for soy protein or milk casein.[61,62]

In the clinical setting, Urisu and colleagues[63] demonstrated that 21 of 38 subjects with positive double-blind placebo-controlled food challenges to freeze-dried egg white showed negative responses to egg white heated at 90°C for 60 minutes. Subjects with positive challenges had significantly higher ovomucoid-specific IgE levels than those with negative challenges. In addition, among the 17 subjects reactive to heated egg, 16 had negative responses when challenged to heated ovomucoid-depleted egg white. These results implicate a significant clinical role of ovomucoid as a heat-resistant allergen in egg allergy compared with more heat-susceptible allergens such as ovalbumin, ovotransferrin, and lysozyme.

In another study of 60 children, 73% of children allergic to egg who were older than 5 years tolerated baked egg in a cake, although the amount of egg protein per serving and degree of heat applied were not reported. Children tolerant to baked egg had significantly smaller SPT responses to total egg, egg white, and egg yolk.[64]

The immunologic background of children tolerant to heated egg (muffin/waffle) but allergic to regular egg (scrambled/French toast) was described by Lemon-Mule and colleagues[65] in a cohort with a mean age of 7 years. These patients had lower egg white–specific, ovomucoid-specific, and ovalbumin-specific IgE levels and smaller SPT wheal responses than patients reactive to heated egg. However, none of these parameters could accurately predict the outcome. The investigators of this study indicated that performing challenges with baked egg remains the only conclusive test to determine tolerance to baked egg products in patients allergic to egg. This cohort was challenged to a serving size of baked egg (muffin/waffle) approximately equivalent to one-third of an egg.

In contrast, another study by Ando and colleagues[66] showed that an ovomucoid-specific IgE antibody level less than 1.2 kU/L had a negative predictive value of 97% and a value more than 11.8 kU/L had a positive predictive value of 88% in predicting challenge outcomes to heated egg. In this study, among 67 children allergic to raw egg white, only 29 (43%) passed their heated egg white challenge. However, challenges were performed with heated egg white prepared by heating liquid egg white at 90°C for 60 minutes. After freeze-drying, the preparation was milled into a powder. Oral provocations were conducted by administering up to the equivalent of approximately 1 egg mixed in 50 mL of assorted fruit juices.[66] The differences demonstrated in these 2 studies may be attributable to the differences in study methodology, specifically with regard to allergen dose and preparation. It is likely that baking egg within a wheat matrix is a confounding factor.

Most children challenged in the clinical setting who tolerate boiled or scrambled egg are subsequently able to introduce egg ad lib into their diets. However, there are at least 2 examples of children tolerating hard-boiled eggs who later developed anaphylaxis to less-cooked or raw versions of egg-containing products. Skin testing revealed smaller wheal sizes to hard-boiled egg, boiled ovomucoid, and boiled ovalbumin compared with raw egg and native ovomucoid and ovalbumin.[45]

THE ROLE OF THERMAL PROCESSING IN THE NATURAL HISTORY OF EGG AND MILK ALLERGY
Cow's Milk

The standard of care for treatment of milk allergy has consistently been strict avoidance.[67,68] However, as previously noted,[41] most (approximately 75%) children with cow's milk allergy tolerate extensively heated (baked) milk products. A follow-up study regarding outcomes was recently published by the same group.[69] Children evaluated for tolerance to baked milk (muffin containing 1.3 g of milk protein cooked at 350°F/177°C for 30 minutes) underwent sequential food challenges to baked cheese (pizza, 4.6 g of milk protein cooked at 425°F/218°C for 13 minutes) followed by unheated milk (8–10 g of milk protein) over a median of 37 months (range, 8–75 months). Among 65 subjects initially tolerant to baked milk, 39 (60%) tolerated unheated milk by the end of the study compared with only 2 of 23 (9%) among the group reactive to baked milk. Subjects who were initially tolerant to baked milk were 28 times more likely to become tolerant to unheated milk than those reactive to baked milk (P value <.001). Median casein IgG4 levels in the group tolerant to baked milk increased significantly (P value <.001). Median milk-specific IgE values did not change significantly. In addition, among the 172 challenges performed, only 10% were completed in subjects who were initially reactive to baked milk. Epinephrine was administered during challenges at a higher rate among the group reactive to baked milk than among the group tolerant to baked milk (17% vs 3%, P value = 0.04). Thus, tolerance of baked milk was deemed a marker of transient IgE-mediated cow's milk allergy, whereas reactivity to baked milk predicted a more persistent phenotype. The addition of baked milk to the diet of children tolerating such foods seemed to be associated with more rapid development of unheated milk tolerance compared with strict avoidance.[69] Children who were tolerant to baked milk but reactive to unheated milk were also found to have higher frequencies of casein-specific $CD4^+$ $CD25^+$ $CD27^+$ T-regulatory cells in their circulation, which supports their tendency toward a tolerizing phenotype.[70] Further prospective trials are necessary to confirm these findings.

Hen's Egg

The possibility that baked egg might alter the natural history of egg allergy was proposed for the first time in humans by Konstantinou and colleagues.[71] In this study, 12- to 48-month-old children who were allergic to egg (n = 55) plus those sensitized to egg white (N = 39, no prior ingestion) were challenged to increasing quantities of a cake baked with 1 egg. Of these 94 children, 87 (93%) could tolerate baked egg. Serum egg white–specific IgE levels were not predictive of outcomes. All children who passed baked egg challenges were advised to eat a piece of cake daily. The amount of egg protein was gradually increased from approximately 100 μg (approximately one-tenth of a teaspoon) up to a total of 1.5 g (approximately one-sixth of an egg) per piece of cake. After a period of 6 months, 83 of 87 (95%) children passed open challenges to boiled egg white, suggesting an immunomodulatory effect leading toward egg white tolerance. The immunologic changes in these patients occurred predominantly during the first trimester of baked egg introduction. These changes included decreases in egg white SPT wheal sizes and ovalbumin-specific IgE levels

> **Key Clinical Concepts**
>
> There are 2 different phenotypes of IgE-mediated milk allergy in children. Tolerance of baked milk is a marker of transient IgE-mediated cow's milk allergy, whereas reactivity to baked milk prognosticates a more persistent phenotype. Given the risk of anaphylaxis in children reactive to baked milk products, addition of such foods should be performed under the supervision of a physician with expertise in food allergy.
>
> Most children with egg allergy are likely to tolerate heated or baked egg, but only an oral food challenge provides a definitive diagnosis. It has been suggested that ovomucoid-specific IgE levels may be helpful as a distinguishing factor, but further studies are needed to confirm these findings.
>
> The addition of baked milk or heated egg to the diet of children tolerating such foods may hasten the development of unheated milk or egg tolerance compared with strict avoidance.
>
> Allergenicity of foods is affected not only by heat and time but also by other factors such as preparation (baked in wheat matrix) and digestibility (pH).

as well as increases in ovalbumin- and ovomucoid-specific IgG_4 levels, changes suggestive of tolerance development to unheated egg.[65]

In another study, children allergic to egg were challenged, annually, to well-cooked egg (sponge cake baked at 180°C for 20 minutes) or uncooked egg (commercially available uncooked pasteurized whole egg "nuggets"). Tolerance to well-cooked egg developed approximately twice as fast as to that of uncooked egg. Median ages at which tolerance to cooked and uncooked egg occurred were 5 and 10 years, respectively.[72]

SUMMARY

The past 5 decades have brought about a plethora of studies elucidating the effect that thermal processing has on food protein structure and subsequent effects on allergenicity. It is a complex interplay involving acid and enzymatic degradation as well as the associated matrix (fat, gluten) in which the food is presented. It seems that tolerance to baked goods containing milk and egg is a positive prognostic indicator for tolerance to raw forms of these foods. It is yet unconfirmed as to whether and how ingestion of extensively heated forms of these foods accelerates tolerance development. Nevertheless, application of the knowledge gleaned thus far has provided leads in the development of personalized medicine, honing the ability to minimize disease effects and produce positive effects on childhood nutrition and familial quality of life.

REFERENCES

1. Beyer K, Morrow E, Li XM, et al. Effects of cooking methods on peanut allergenicity. J Allergy Clin Immunol 2001;107(6):1077–81.
2. Carnes J, Ferrer A, Huertas AJ, et al. The use of raw or boiled crustacean extracts for the diagnosis of seafood allergic individuals. Ann Allergy Asthma Immunol 2007;98(4):349–54.
3. Barlow DJ, Edwards MS, Thornton JM. Continuous and discontinuous protein antigenic determinants. Nature 1986;322(6081):747–8.
4. Thomas K, Herouet-Guicheney C, Ladics G, et al. Evaluating the effect of food processing on the potential human allergenicity of novel proteins: international workshop report. Food Chem Toxicol 2007;45(7):1116–22.
5. Besler M, Steinhart H, Paschke A. Stability of food allergens and allergenicity of processed foods. J Chromatogr 2001;756(1–2):207–28.

6. Van Regenmortel MH. What is a B-cell epitope? Methods Mol Biol 2009;524:3–20.
7. Jarvinen KM, Beyer K, Vila L, et al. B-cell epitopes as a screening instrument for persistent cow's milk allergy. J Allergy Clin Immunol 2002;110(2):293–7.
8. Jarvinen KM, Beyer K, Vila L, et al. Specificity of IgE antibodies to sequential epitopes of hen's egg ovomucoid as a marker for persistence of egg allergy. Allergy 2007;62(7):758–65.
9. Chatchatee P, Jarvinen KM, Bardina L, et al. Identification of IgE- and IgG-binding epitopes on alpha(s1)-casein: differences in patients with persistent and transient cow's milk allergy. J Allergy Clin Immunol 2001;107(2):379–83.
10. Chatchatee P, Jarvinen KM, Bardina L, et al. Identification of IgE and IgG binding epitopes on beta- and kappa-casein in cow's milk allergic patients. Clin Exp Allergy 2001;31(8):1256–62.
11. Vila L, Beyer K, Jarvinen KM, et al. Role of conformational and linear epitopes in the achievement of tolerance in cow's milk allergy. Clin Exp Allergy 2001;31(10):1599–606.
12. Cooke SK, Sampson HA. Allergenic properties of ovomucoid in man. J Immunol 1997;159(4):2026–32.
13. Wang J, Lin J, Bardina L, et al. Correlation of IgE/IgG4 milk epitopes and affinity of milk-specific IgE antibodies with different phenotypes of clinical milk allergy. J Allergy Clin Immunol 2010;125(3):695–702, 702 e691–6.
14. Kocho K. Milk allergy with special reference to a histopathologico-anatomic study of its prevention. II. Prevention of intestinal hypersensitivity by means of digestive ferments and heating of milk. Nihon Shonika Gakkai Zasshi 1966;70(7):606–14 [in Japanese].
15. Farrell HM Jr, Jimenez-Flores R, Bleck GT, et al. Nomenclature of the proteins of cows' milk—sixth revision. J Dairy Sci 2004;87(6):1641–74.
16. Lewis MJ, Heppell NJ. Continuous thermal processing of foods: pasteurization and UHT sterilization. MD: Aspen Publishers, Inc; 2000.
17. Roth-Walter F, Berin MC, Arnaboldi P, et al. Pasteurization of milk proteins promotes allergic sensitization by enhancing uptake through Peyer's patches. Allergy 2008;63(7):882–90.
18. Poulsen OM, Hau J, Kollerup J. Effect of homogenization and pasteurization on the allergenicity of bovine milk analysed by a murine anaphylactic shock model. Clin Allergy 1987;17(5):449–58.
19. Poulsen OM, Nielsen BR, Basse A, et al. Comparison of intestinal anaphylactic reactions in sensitized mice challenged with untreated bovine milk and homogenized bovine milk. Allergy 1990;45(5):321–6.
20. Nielsen BR, Poulsen OM, Hau J. Reagin production in mice: effect of subcutaneous and oral sensitization with untreated bovine milk and homogenized bovine milk. In Vivo 1989;3(4):271–4.
21. Docena GH, Fernandez R, Chirdo FG, et al. Identification of casein as the major allergenic and antigenic protein of cow's milk. Allergy 1996;51(6):412–6.
22. Shek LP, Bardina L, Castro R, et al. Humoral and cellular responses to cow milk proteins in patients with milk-induced IgE-mediated and non-IgE-mediated disorders. Allergy 2005;60(7):912–9.
23. Host A, Samuelsson EG. Allergic reactions to raw, pasteurized, and homogenized/pasteurized cow milk: a comparison. A double-blind placebo-controlled study in milk allergic children. Allergy 1988;43(2):113–8.
24. Kilshaw PJ, Heppell LM, Ford JE. Effects of heat treatment of cow's milk and whey on the nutritional quality and antigenic properties. Arch Dis Child 1982;57(11):842–7.

25. Anderson KJ, McLaughlan P, Devey ME, et al. Anaphylactic sensitivity of guinea-pigs drinking different preparations of cows' milk and infant formulae. Clin Exp Immunol 1979;35(3):454–61.
26. McLaughlan P, Anderson KJ, Widdowson EM, et al. Effect of heat on the anaphylactic-sensitising capacity of cows' milk, goats' milk, and various infant formulae fed to guinea-pigs. Arch Dis Child 1981;56(3):165–71.
27. Heppell LM, Cant AJ, Kilshaw PJ. Reduction in the antigenicity of whey proteins by heat treatment: a possible strategy for producing a hypoallergenic infant milk formula. Br J Nutr 1984;51(1):29–36.
28. Werfel SJ, Cooke SK, Sampson HA. Clinical reactivity to beef in children allergic to cow's milk. J Allergy Clin Immunol 1997;99(3):293–300.
29. Fiocchi A, Restani P, Riva E, et al. Heat treatment modifies the allergenicity of beef and bovine serum albumin. Allergy 1998;53(8):798–802.
30. Gjesing B, Osterballe O, Schwartz B, et al. Allergen-specific IgE antibodies against antigenic components in cow milk and milk substitutes. Allergy 1986;41(1):51–6.
31. Boye JI, Ismail AA, Alli I. Effects of physicochemical factors on the secondary structure of beta-lactoglobulin. J Dairy Res 1996;63(1):97–109.
32. Chen WL, Hwang MT, Liau CY, et al. Beta-lactoglobulin is a thermal marker in processed milk as studied by electrophoresis and circular dichroic spectra. J Dairy Sci 2005;88(5):1618–30.
33. Garcia-Hernandez E, Hernandez-Arana A, Zubillaga RA, et al. Spectroscopic and thermodynamic evidence for a complex denaturation mechanism of bovine beta-lactoglobulin A. Biochem Mol Biol Int 1998;45(4):761–8.
34. Iametti S, De Gregori B, Vecchio G, et al. Modifications occur at different structural levels during the heat denaturation of beta-lactoglobulin. Eur J Biochem 1996;237(1):106–12.
35. Sava N, Van der Plancken I, Claeys W, et al. The kinetics of heat-induced structural changes of beta-lactoglobulin. J Dairy Sci 2005;88(5):1646–53.
36. Ehn BM, Allmere T, Telemo E, et al. Modification of IgE binding to beta-lactoglobulin by fermentation and proteolysis of cow's milk. J Agric Food Chem 2005;53(9):3743–8.
37. Ehn BM, Ekstrand B, Bengtsson U, et al. Modification of IgE binding during heat processing of the cow's milk allergen beta-lactoglobulin. J Agric Food Chem 2004;52(5):1398–403.
38. Jarvinen KM, Chatchatee P, Bardina L, et al. IgE and IgG binding epitopes on alpha-lactalbumin and beta-lactoglobulin in cow's milk allergy. Int Arch Allergy Immunol 2001;126(2):111–8.
39. Kaminogawa S, Shimizu M, Ametani A, et al. Monoclonal antibodies as probes for monitoring the denaturation process of bovine beta-lactoglobulin. Biochim Biophys Acta 1989;998(1):50–6.
40. Negroni L, Bernard H, Clement G, et al. Two-site enzyme immunometric assays for determination of native and denatured beta-lactoglobulin. J Immunol Methods 1998;220(1–2):25–37.
41. Nowak-Wegrzyn A, Bloom KA, Sicherer SH, et al. Tolerance to extensively heated milk in children with cow's milk allergy. J Allergy Clin Immunol 2008;122(2):342–7, 347 e341–2.
42. Jost R, Monti JC, Pahud JJ. Reduction of whey protein allergenicity by processing. Adv Exp Med Biol 1991;289:309–20.
43. Hildebrandt S, Kratzin HD, Schaller R, et al. In vitro determination of the allergenic potential of technologically altered hen's egg. J Agric Food Chem 2008;56(5):1727–33.

44. Jurado-Palomo J, Fiandor-Roman AM, Bobolea ID, et al. Oral challenge with pasteurized egg white from Gallus domesticus. Int Arch Allergy Immunol 2010; 151(4):331–5.

45. Eigenmann PA. Anaphylactic reactions to raw eggs after negative challenges with cooked eggs. J Allergy Clin Immunol 2000;105(3):587–8.

46. Peng HJ, Chang ZN, Tsai LC, et al. Heat denaturation of egg-white proteins abrogates the induction of oral tolerance of specific Th2 immune responses in mice. Scand J Immunol 1998;48(5):491–6.

47. Anet J, Back JF, Baker RS, et al. Allergens in the white and yolk of hen's egg. A study of IgE binding by egg proteins. Int Arch Allergy Appl Immunol 1985;77(3): 364–71.

48. Mine Y, Zhang JW. Comparative studies on antigenicity and allergenicity of native and denatured egg white proteins. J Agric Food Chem 2002;50(9):2679–83.

49. Bernhisel-Broadbent J, Dintzis HM, Dintzis RZ, et al. Allergenicity and antigenicity of chicken egg ovomucoid (Gal d III) compared with ovalbumin (Gal d I) in children with egg allergy and in mice. J Allergy Clin Immunol 1994;93(6):1047–59.

50. Mine Y, Zhang J. The allergenicity of ovomucoid and its elimination from hen's egg white. J Sci Food Agric 2001;81:1540–6.

51. Honma K, Kohno Y, Saito K, et al. Specificities of IgE, IgG and IgA antibodies to ovalbumin. Comparison of binding activities to denatured ovalbumin or ovalbumin fragments of IgE antibodies with those of IgG or IgA antibodies. Int Arch Allergy Immunol 1994;103(1):28–35.

52. Elsayed S, Hammer AS, Kalvenes MB, et al. Antigenic and allergenic determinants of ovalbumin. I. Peptide mapping, cleavage at the methionyl peptide bonds and enzymic hydrolysis of native and carboxymethyl OA. Int Arch Allergy Appl Immunol 1986;79(1):101–7.

53. Gu JX, Matsuda T, Nakamura R. Antigenicity of ovomucoid remaining in boiled shell eggs. J Food Sci 1996;51:1448–50.

54. Gu JX, Matsuda T, Nakamura R, et al. Chemical deglycosylation of hen ovomucoid: protective effect of carbohydrate moiety on tryptic hydrolysis and heat denaturation. J Biochem 1989;106(1):66–70.

55. Van der Plancken I, Van Remoortere M, Van Loey A, et al. Trypsin inhibition activity of heat-denatured ovomucoid: a kinetic study. Biotechnol Prog 2004;20(1):82–6.

56. Baker C, Balch D. Molecular genetics of avian proteins, I. The egg proteins of the domestic fowl. Br Poult Sci 1962;3:161–74.

57. Lee JW, Lee KY, Yook HS, et al. Allergenicity of hen's egg ovomucoid gamma irradiated and heated under different pH conditions. J Food Prot 2002;65(7):1196–9.

58. Yoshino K, Sakai K, Mizuha Y, et al. Peptic digestibility of raw and heat-coagulated hen's egg white proteins at acidic pH range. Int J Food Sci Nutr 2004;55(8):635–40.

59. Joo K, Kato Y. Assessment of allergenic activity of a heat-coagulated ovalbumin after in vivo digestion. Biosci Biotechnol Biochem 2006;70(3):591–7.

60. Martos G, Lopez-Exposito I, Bencharitiwong R, et al. Mechanisms underlying differential food allergy response to heated egg. J Allergy Clin Immunol 2011; 127(4):990–7 e991–2.

61. Kato Y, Watanabe K, Matsuda T. Decrease in ovomucoid antigenicity in the processes of breadmaking supplemented with egg white. Food Sci Technol Int Tokyo 1997;3:362–5.

62. Kato Y, Watanabe H, Matsuda T. Ovomucoid rendered insoluble by heating with wheat gluten but not with milk casein. Biosci Biotechnol Biochem 2000;64(1): 198–201.

63. Urisu A, Ando H, Morita Y, et al. Allergenic activity of heated and ovomucoid-depleted egg white. J Allergy Clin Immunol 1997;100(2):171–6.
64. Des Roches A, Nguyen M, Paradis L, et al. Tolerance to cooked egg in an egg allergic population. Allergy 2006;61(7):900–1.
65. Lemon-Mule H, Sampson HA, Sicherer SH, et al. Immunologic changes in children with egg allergy ingesting extensively heated egg. J Allergy Clin Immunol 2008;122(5):977–83 e971.
66. Ando H, Moverare R, Kondo Y, et al. Utility of ovomucoid-specific IgE concentrations in predicting symptomatic egg allergy. J Allergy Clin Immunol 2008;122(3):583–8.
67. Fiocchi A, Brozek J, Schunemann H, et al. World Allergy Organization (WAO) Diagnosis and Rationale for Action against Cow's Milk Allergy (DRACMA) guidelines. Pediatr Allergy Immunol 2010;21(Suppl 21):1–125.
68. Fiocchi A, Schunemann HJ, Brozek J, et al. Diagnosis and Rationale for Action Against Cow's Milk Allergy (DRACMA): a summary report. J Allergy Clin Immunol 2010;126(6):1119–28 e1112.
69. Kim JS, Nowak-Wegrzyn A, Sicherer SH, et al. Dietary baked milk accelerates the resolution of cow's milk allergy in children. J Allergy Clin Immunol 2011;128(1):125–31 e122.
70. Shreffler WG, Wanich N, Moloney M, et al. Association of allergen-specific regulatory T cells with the onset of clinical tolerance to milk protein. J Allergy Clin Immunol 2009;123(1):43–52 e47.
71. Konstantinou GN, Giavi S, Kalobatsou A, et al. Consumption of heat-treated egg by children allergic or sensitized to egg can affect the natural course of egg allergy: hypothesis-generating observations. J Allergy Clin Immunol 2008;122(2):414–5.
72. Clark A, Islam S, King Y, et al. A longitudinal study of resolution of allergy to well-cooked and uncooked egg. Clin Exp Allergy 2011;41(5):706–12.
73. McGuffey MK, Epting KL, Kelly RM, et al. Denaturation and aggregation of three alpha-lactalbumin preparations at neutral pH. J Agric Food Chem 2005;53(8):3182–90.
74. Wang Q, Tolkach A, Kulozik U. Quantitative assessment of thermal denaturation of bovine alpha-lactalbumin via low-intensity ultrasound, HPLC, and DSC. J Agric Food Chem 2006;54(18):6501–6.
75. Chung SL, Ferrier LK. Heat Denaturation and Emulsifying Properties of Egg Yolk Phosvitin. J Food Sci 1995;60:906–8.
76. Dixon DK, Cotterill OJ. Electrophoretic and chromatographic changes in egg yolk proteins due to heat. J Food Sci 1981;46:981–3.
77. Quirce S, Maranon F, Umpierrez A, et al. Chicken serum albumin (Gal d 5*) is a partially heat-labile inhalant and food allergen implicated in the bird-egg syndrome. Allergy 2001;56(8):754–62.
78. Chang P, Powrie WD, Fennema O. Disc gel electrophoresis of protein in native and heat treatment albumen, yolk and centrifuged whole egg. J Food Sci 1970;35:774–8.
79. Le Denmat M, Anton M, Gandemer G. Protein denaturation and emulsifying properties of plasma and granules of egg yolk as related to heat treatment. J Food Sci 1999;64:194–7.
80. Amo A, Rodriguez-Perez R, Blanco J, et al. Gal d 6 is the second allergen characterized from egg yolk. J Agric Food Chem 2010;58(12):7453–7.

Food-Induced Anaphylaxis

Antonella Cianferoni, MD, PhD[a],*, Antonella Muraro, MD, PhD[b]

KEYWORDS

• Anaphylaxis • Food • Allergy

DEFINITION

Food-induced anaphylaxis (FIA) is a serious allergic reaction that may cause death rapidly in otherwise healthy individuals. There is no universal agreement on its definition or criteria for diagnosis.[1] In 2006 an international task force on anaphylaxis recommended a new working clinical definition of anaphylaxis, which tried to address such issues (**Box 1**).[2]

Based on this latest recommendation,[1,3] FIA is diagnosed when

1. Two or more of the following symptoms occur rapidly and acutely after exposure to a likely allergen and:
    • Involvement of the skin or mucosal tissue, respiratory compromise, cardiovascular compromise, persistent gastrointestinal symptoms
2. Hypotension after exposure to known allergen for that patient.

EPIDEMIOLOGY

The epidemiology of FIA has been difficult to quantify, with estimates varying widely[2]; however, there is general agreement that hospital admissions for FIA have more than doubled in the last decade.[4]

Epidemiologic challenges in determining the burden of FIA has been reviewed[5] and are listed in **Box 2**.

Bearing in mind the limitation cited in **Box 2**, it is estimated that the incidence of:

• *Fatal reaction due to FIA* is 1 in 800,000 per year in children and 1 in 4 million for adults

---

Funding sources: NIH K08 AI089982-01A1.

The content is solely the responsibility of the authors and does not necessarily represent the official views of the National Center for Research Resources or the National Institutes of Health.

Conflict of interest: The authors have no financial conflicts of interest to disclose.

[a] Allergy and Immunology Division, The Children's Hospital of Philadelphia, University of Pennsylvania, ARC 1216H, 3615 Civic Center Boulevard, Philadelphia, PA 19104, USA

[b] Department of Pediatrics, Food Allergy Referral Center, Padua General University Hospital, Via Giustiniani 3, 35128 Padua, Italy

* Corresponding author.

E-mail address: cianferonia@email.chop.edu

Immunol Allergy Clin N Am 32 (2012) 165–195

doi:10.1016/j.iac.2011.10.002

immunology.theclinics.com

Box 1
Clinical criteria for the diagnosis of anaphylaxis

Anaphylaxis is highly likely when any one of the following 3 criteria are fulfilled:

1. Acute onset of an illness (minutes to several hours) with involvement of the skin, mucosal tissue, or both (eg, generalized hives, itch or flushing, swollen lips, tongue, or uvula, rhinorrhea, conjunctivitis). And at least one of the following:

    a. Respiratory compromise (eg, dyspnea, bronchospasm, stridor, hypoxia)

    b. Cardiovascular compromise (eg, hypotension, collapse)

2. Two or more of the following that occur rapidly after exposure to a likely allergen for that patient (minutes to several hours):

    a. Involvement of the skin or mucosal tissue (eg, generalized hives, itch, flushing, swelling)

    b. Respiratory compromise (eg, dyspnea, bronchospasm, stridor, hypoxia)

    c. Cardiovascular compromise (eg, hypotension, collapse)

    d. Persistent gastrointestinal symptoms (eg, crampy abdominal pain, vomiting)

3. Hypotension after exposure to known allergen for that patient (minutes to several hours)

Hypotension for children is defined as systolic blood pressure <70 mm Hg from 1 month to 1 year [<70 mm Hg + (2 × age)] from 1 to 10 years, and <90 mm Hg from 11 to 17 years.

Data from Muraro A, Roberts G, Clark A, et al. The management of anaphylaxis in childhood: position paper of the European Academy of Allergology and Clinical Immunology. Allergy 2007;62(8):857–71.

- *Nonfatal reaction due to FIA* is reported to be between 0.5 and 16 cases per 100,000 person-years.[6–9]

These numbers may underestimate the actual burden of anaphylaxis or risk of anaphylaxis in the general population. Indeed it is estimated that 0.1% to 5% of children have a prescription for epinephrine,[10,11] and that in the United States the direct and indirect cost of hospitalization, emergency room visits, epinephrine prescription, and ambulance transport related to FIA is more than $40 million per year, with about 75% of these costs attributable to pediatric patients.[12]

Box 2
Epidemiologic challenges in determining the burden of food-induced anaphylaxis

1. Lack of universal consensus on consistent definition to identify anaphylaxis (especially for studies published before the new 2006 guidelines[2])

2. Difficulty in distinguishing anaphylaxis from other disorders

3. Selection bias based on hospital presentation

4. Use of different measures of disease occurrence to estimate disease burden (such as prevalence and incidence)

5. Limited ability of International Classification of Diseases (ICD) 995.6 code ("anaphylactic shock due to adverse food reaction") to identify specific allergic reactions in the emergency department, as it is not realistic to expect physicians (or health statistics) to code anaphylactic reactions defined as multisystem organ involvement, but not shock, with codes specifically including shock

Peanut/tree nuts anaphylaxis is estimated to have a prevalence of 0.25% to 0.95% in the United Kingdom and United States pediatric populations, and appears to be on the increase in the last decade.[13–15] This statistic mirrors the increased prevalence of peanut and tree nut allergy reported in United States children. Peanut allergy recently has been found to be 2.6% in the general population and 22.6% among children sensitized to peanut.[16] In general, the prevalence of adverse reactions to foods is higher in children than in adults; however, allergy to nuts is an important problem in adulthood, the prevalence of allergy to nuts being higher in adults (1.6%) than in children (0.6%).[14] As allergy to nuts persists over the years, these data could reflect a cumulative effect in adults because peanut and tree nut allergy seems to develop early in life, with most affected children in the United States and the United Kingdom developing symptoms before the age of 2 years.[17,18]

Shellfish anaphylaxis has a prevalence of 0.44% in the United States.[19] The consumption of seafood has risen by approximately 50% over the last 40 years, both in the United States and elsewhere,[20] corresponding to an increase in the incidence of seafood allergy over the same period, with significantly lower rates in children compared with adults[19,21] as happens for tree nut and peanut allergy.

TRIGGERS OF FIA

Food is one of the most common causes of anaphylaxis, with most surveys indicating that food-induced reactions account for 30% to 50% of anaphylaxis cases in North America, Europe, Asia, and Australia,[4,6,7,9,12,22] and for up to 81% of anaphylaxis cases in children.[23,24]

Although a wide range of foods has been reported as the cause of FIA, the most commonly implicated foods worldwide are peanut, tree nuts, milk, egg, sesame seeds, fish, and shellfish[2,3,5,6,9,25,26] in both adults and children (**Table 1**). However, the individual food allergy varies by culture and population. For example, peanut allergy is one of the most common causes of FIA in the United States, United Kingdom, and Australia, but is rare in Italy and Spain (where consumption of peanut is significantly lower than in the United States) or China (where peanut consumption is similar to that in the United States).[5,6,25,27–30]

Even if prior exposure is necessary for the development of sensitization, 72% patients with peanut and/or tree nut allergy reported symptoms during their first known exposure.[31] These patients may have had previous unknown exposures through breast milk, contamination with other foods, or use of topical products containing food oils (eg, peanut).[32]

Reports of anaphylaxis in exclusively breast-fed babies due to passage of food allergens from the mother to the infant are extremely rare,[33,34] and there are no reports in the literature of fatal FIA in exclusively breast-fed infants.

The spectrum of foods responsible for causing anaphylaxis appears to be broadening, to include fruits and other foods not previously commonly associated with anaphylaxis.

- Asero and colleagues[29] recently reported on a series of 1110 adolescent and adult Italian patients (mean age 31 years, range 12–79 years) diagnosed with food allergy based on history of reaction in the presence of positive skin prick test (SPT) or elevated food-specific serum IgE. Anaphylaxis was reported by 5% of food-allergic individuals, with the most common cause being lipid transfer protein (LTP). LTP is a widely cross-reacting plant pan-allergen. Offending food for LTP-allergic patients was most often peach, but included also other members

Table 1
Most common cause of FIA

Food	Type of Anaphylaxis	%	Country	Refs.	Age	Food	Type of Anaphylaxis	%	Country	Refs.	Age
Peanut	Fatal	42	Australia	38	Peds and adults	Egg	Fatal	2	UK	68	Peds and adults
		62	USA	69	Peds and adults		ED/Hospital	9	Australia	38	Peds and adults
		53	USA	67	Peds and adults			9	Israel	70	Peds
		19	UK	68	Peds and adults			2	USA	48	Peds
	ED/Hospital	23	Australia	38	Peds and adults		Registry	7	Germany	47	Peds
		0	Israel	70	Peds		Allergy office	11	Italy	71	Peds
		10	Italy	23	Adults			7	Spain	28	Peds
		22	USA	48	Peds			0	Italy	29	Adults
	Registry	22	Germany	47	Peds	Vegetables	Fatal	2	UK	68	Peds and adults
	Allergy office	0	Italy	71	Peds		ED/Hospital	10	Italy	47	Peds
		0	Spain	28	Peds		Allergy office	4	Italy	71	Peds
		3	Italy	29	Adults			3	Italy	29	Adults
Tree nuts	Fatal	28	USA	69	Peds and adults	Fruit	Fatal/near fatal	13	Israel	70	Peds
		25	USA	67	Peds and adults		ED/Hospital	8	USA	48	Peds
	ED/Hospital	19	UK	68	Peds and adults		Registry	4	Germany	47	Peds
		16	Australia	38	Peds and adults		Allergy office	11	Italy	71	Peds
		23	Israel	70	Peds			8	Spain	28	Peds
		18	USA	48	Peds						
	Registry	25	Germany	47	Peds	Cereal	Fatal/near fatal	31	Italy	29	Adults
	Allergy office	13	Italy	71	Peds		ED/Hospital				
		16	Spain	28	Peds						
		19	Italy	29	Adults						

Food	Setting	%	Country	Ref	Population	Setting	%	Country	Ref	Population
Fish	Fatal	14	Australia	[38]	Peds and adults	Registry	2	Germany	[47]	Peds
Shellfish		3	USA	[69]	Peds and adults	Allergy office	5	Italy	[71]	Peds
		6	USA	[67]	Peds and adults		5	Italy	[29]	Adults
		4	UK	[68]	Peds and adults	Soy	Fatal/near fatal			
	ED/Hospital	34	Australia	[38]	Peds and adults	ED/Hospital	4.5	Israel	[70]	Peds
		30	Italy	[23]	Adults		10	Italy	[23]	Adults
		5	USA	[48]	Peds	Registry	1	Germany	[47]	Peds
	Registry	5	Germany	[47]	Peds	Allergy office				
	Allergy office	30	Italy	[71]	Peds					
		22	Spain	[28]	Peds					
		18	Italy	[29]	Adults					
Milk	Fatal	3	USA	[69]	Peds and adults					
		12	USA	[67]	Peds and adults					
		12	UK	[68]	Peds and adults					
	ED/Hospital	8	Australia	[38]	Peds and adults					
		39	Israel	[70]	Peds					
		0	Italy	[23]	Adults					
		18	USA	[48]	Peds					
	Registry	9	Germany	[47]	Peds					
	Allergy office	22	Italy	[71]	Peds					
		47	Spain	[28]	Peds					
		0	Italy	[29]	Adults					

Abbreviations: ED, emergency department; Peds, pediatric patients.

of the *Rosaceae* family of fruits (apple, pear, cherry, plum, apricot, medlar, almond, strawberry), tree nuts, corn, rice, beer, tomato, spelt, pineapple, and grape.[35–37]

- Recently there have been several case reports of anaphylaxis resulting from ingestion of lupin flour, which is being increasingly used in bakery products in France and Mediterranean countries.[38,39]

- Moreover, some newly described food allergens appear to cause specific clinical subtypes of anaphylaxis.
  - Water-insoluble omega-5-gliadin (Tri a 19) has been identified as a major allergen in Finnish subjects with food-dependent exercise-induced anaphylaxis (FDEIA), with in vitro and in vivo cross-reactivity to rye allergens and barley allergens, but not oat allergens.[40,41]
  - A carbohydrate nonprotein food allergen, galactose-α-1,3-galactose (α-gal), is capable of eliciting delayed systemic symptoms of anaphylaxis, angioedema, or urticaria associated with eating beef, pork, or lamb 3 to 6 hours earlier, and appears to be more common in middle-aged men living in Virginia, North Carolina, Tennessee, Arkansas, and Missouri, as well as in Australia. Given the peculiar geographic distribution and the fact that more than 80% of the patients reported being bitten by ticks, researchers were able to provide evidence that tick (*Amblyomma americanum* or *Ixodes holocyclus*) bites are a (possibly singular) cause of IgE-mediated sensitization to α-gal in these areas of the United States and Australia.[42–44]

Peanut/Tree Nut Anaphylaxis

Peanut and tree nuts are overwhelmingly and disproportionately represented in case series of severe and fatal outcomes, severe allergic reaction, and visits to the emergency department for food anaphylaxis, particularly in United States, Germany, Australia, and the United Kingdom (see **Table 1**),[4,5,45–48] and allergy to peanut and tree nuts is becoming a significant health problem in many parts of the world.[49] Large surveys indicate that in comparison with other foods, allergic reactions to nuts seem to be particularly severe, with multisystemic or respiratory symptoms in up to 81% of the cases. Some studies indicate that severity of coexisting atopic diseases may be a risk factor in the development of life-threatening allergic reactions to peanut and tree nuts.[50]

Recent advances in allergy sequencing and the availability of platforms for IgE specific for single epitopes of the single allergens have increased our understanding of which epitopes are more important in the triggering of an allergic reaction. Major allergens described for peanut and tree nuts are listed in **Tables 2a** and **2b**. Serologic studies have shown that the diversity of IgE recognition of peanut proteins is associated more with clinical outcome than with recognition of individual allergens.[51] However, some studies suggest having IgE specific to Ara h 2 is associated with more severe (mostly respiratory) symptoms, whereas Ara h 8, a Bet v 1 cross-reactive allergen, more often causes less severe reaction such as oral syndrome.[52] Different food processing methods used in different countries may be responsible for increased or decreased peanut allergenicity, and consequently peanut allergy prevalence in countries with similar consumption such as China and the United States. Indeed the dry-roasting process (150°C) used in United States enhances the allergenicity of Ara h 1, 2, and 3, whereas boiling (100°C) or frying (120°C) used in China reduces the allergenic properties of these molecules.[30]

One of the most common reported tree nut allergies is that of the cashew. One-third of the patients reacting to cashew nuts are also allergic to pistachios, which belongs to the same botanic family (**Table 3**). Severe allergic reactions to hazelnuts, including systemic anaphylaxis, have also been described in patients sensitized to Cor a 8 (LTP) and Cor a 9 (11S globulin).[53] In United States children the most common tree nut allergies are walnut, almond, and pecan.[31] Allergic reactions to other nuts such as Brazil nuts, pistachios, macadamia nuts, pine nuts, and coconuts are less common triggers of FIA and have been reported anecdotally.[49] Chestnut allergy is generally observed in the context of latex-fruit syndrome.[54]

Assessment of cross-reactivity among tree nuts is complicated by shared allergens among the nuts and between nuts and other plant-derived foods and pollens. If skin test reactivity is a result of cross-reactivity to pollens, food reactions are typically absent or mild (ie, oral allergy syndrome) (see **Tables 2a** and **2b**).[49] Some nut allergens may be homologous and cause reactions (eg, in pistachio and cashew), whereas others may be homologous but rarely elicit clinical cross-reactivity (eg, proteins in coconut and walnut). Clinical relevant cross-reactivity is estimated to be around 30% to 40%; however, fatal reactions have been described from a first exposure to a nut in patients allergic to other nuts.[55] Hence, considering the potential severity of the allergy and issues with accurate identification of specific nuts in prepared foods, very often a total elimination of the nut family (perhaps with the exception of previously tolerated nuts eaten in isolation) is suggested by most clinicians.[55] Cross-reactions to seeds, such as sesame, mustard, and poppy, have also been reported.[56–64]

Cosensitization to allergenic foods, such as peanut, tree nuts, and seeds (sesame, poppy, and mustard) is common, although clinically significant cross-reacting proteins have not yet been described. Coallergy to peanut and tree nut has been reported as between 23% and 50% in referral populations of atopic patients and 2.5% in unselected populations.[56]

Seafood

Seafood is a common cause of anaphylaxis, and fatal events have been reported (see **Table 1**), with a rate of anaphylaxis among sensitized patients of about 20%.[20] Shellfish are a nontaxonomic group that includes crustaceans and mollusks, which are invertebrates, unlike fish (see **Table 3**). The major shellfish allergen has been identified as tropomyosin, an essential protein in muscle contraction, which is a pan-allergen responsible for in vivo and in vitro cross-reactivity between crustaceans (shrimp, crab, crawfish, lobster), insects (cockroaches), arachnids (house dust mites), and different classes of mollusks (**Table 2c**).[65]

The situation with fish is less certain, with reports of both polysensitization to multiple species (50%–92% of individuals) and monosensitization to a single fish type. The major allergens responsible for cross-reactivity among noncrustacean fish are the muscular parvalbumins (see **Table 2c**), pan-allergens resistant to thermal and enzymatic degradation.[65] Canned fish, which is cooked for up to 7 hours under pressure, may be less allergenic; however, anaphylaxis related to canned fish has been reported, so this food is not safe for patients with fish-induced anaphylaxis.[20]

Cross-reactivity between crustaceans and fish has been not reported, so affected individuals are usually advised to avoid either fish or crustaceans; however, up to 50% of individuals may be sensitive to both shellfish and fish.[20]

Despite a generalized belief within the medical community, allergies to shellfish do not increase the risk of reaction to intravenous contrast.[66]

Milk, Egg, and Soy

In the pediatric population, milk and egg allergy are a frequent cause of anaphylactic reactions.[67,68]

Table 2a
Allergen described in egg, cow's milk, soy, peanut

Allergen Name	Allergen Common Name	Clinical Relevance	Allergen Name	Allergen Common Name	Clinical Relevance
Hen's egg (*Gallus domesticus*)			Peanut (*Arachis hypogea*)		
Gal d 1	Ovomucoid		Ara h 1	Seed storage proteins	Heat stable
Gal d 2	Ovalbumin	Major allergen	Ara h 2	Seed storage proteins	Heat stable, associated with anaphylaxis
Gal d 3	Ovotransferrin/ conalbumin		Ara h 3	Seed storage proteins	
Gal d 4	Lysozyme		Ara h 4	Seed storage proteins	
Gal d 5	α-Livetin	Bird-egg syndrome	Ara h 5	Profilin (Bet v 2 like)	Cross-reactive with other plants; little clinical relevance
Cow's milk			Ara h 6	Seed storage proteins	Homology with Ara h 2. Allergy persists
Bos d 8	α−, α.2-n, β-, γ1, γ2 γs K-casein	Major allergen, heat stable	Ara h 7	Seed storage proteins	

Bos d 4	α-Lactalbumin	Major allergen, heat sensitive	Ara h 8	Bet v 1 family (PR-1 O, Bet v 1 like)	Responsible for cross-reactivity with birch pollen analogues
Bos d 5	β-Lactoglobulin	Major allergen, heat sensitive	Ara h 9	LTP	Low prevalence of recognition in USA and north Europe; more common in south Europe
Bos d 7	Immunoglobulin		Ara h 10	Oleosin plant lipid storage bodies	
Bos d 6	BSA	Cross-reactivity with beef	Ara h 11	Oleosin plant lipid storage bodies	
Soybean (Glycine max)					
Gly m 1	LTP				
Gly m 2	Defensin				
Gly m 3	Profilin				
Gly m 4	Bet v 1 family (PR-1 O, Bet v 1 like)	Cross-reactive with birch/peanut, mild oropharyngeal reaction			
Gly m 5	Vicilin	Severe reaction			
Gly m 6	Legumin	Severe reaction			

Abbreviations: BSA, bovine serum albumin; LTP, lipid transfer protein.

Table 2b
Allergens described in legumes, tree nuts, and seeds

Allergen Name	Allergen Common Name	Clinical Relevance	Allergen Name	Allergen Common Name	Clinical Relevance
Pea (*Pisum sativum*)			Sesame		
Pis s 1	Vicilin		Ses i 1	S albumin	
Pis s 2	Convicilin		Ses i 2	S albumin	
Green bean (*Phaseolus vulgaris*)			Ses i 3	7S globulin	
Pha v 3	nsLTP type 1		Ses i 4	Oleosin	
Hazelnut (*Corylus avellana*)			Ses i 5	Oleosin	
Cor a 1	PR-10 (Bet v 1 homologous)		Ses i 6	Basic subunit of 11S globulins	
Cor a 2	Profilin		Ses i 7	Basic subunit of 11S globulins	
Cor a 8	PR-14 (LPT) 9		Lupine (*Lupinus angustifolius*)		
Cor a 9	Globulin (11S)		Lup an 1	β-Conglutin (vicilin)	
Cor a 11	Vicilin (7S)		Lentil (*Lens culinaris*)		
Chestnut (*Castanea sativa*)			Len c 1	γ-Vicilin subunit	
Cas s 5	Chitinase Ib		Len c 2	Seed specific	
Cas s 8	PR-14 (LPT)	Oral allergy syndrome	Len c 3	nsLTP type 1	
Brazil nut			Cashew (*Anacardium occidentale*)		
Ber e 1	Albumin (2S)	Anaphylaxis	Ana o 1	Vicilin (7S)	
Ber e 2	Legumin (11S)	Anaphylaxis	Ana o 2	Legumin (11S)	
			Walnut (*Juglans regia*)		
			Jug r 1	Albumin (2S)	
			Jug r 2	Vicilin (7S)	
			Jug r 3	PR-14 (LTP)	
			Jug r 4	Legumin (11S)	

Table 2c
Allergens in seafood

Allergen Name	Allergen Common Name	Clinical Relevance
Fish		
Baltic cod (*Gadus callarias*), Atlantic cod (*Gadus morhua*), Atlantic salmon (*Salmo salar*), edible frog (*Rana esculenta*)		
Gad c 1 Gad m 1 Sal s 1 Ran e 1	Parvalbumin	Anaphylaxis cross-reactivity among multiple fish
Shellfish		
Greasyback shrimp (*Metapenaeus ensis*), brown shrimp (*Penaeus aztecus*), black tiger shrimp (*Penaeus monodon*), shrimp (*Penaeus indicus*), Crab (*Charybdis feriatus*), lobster (*Homarus americanus, Panulirus stimpsoni*), squid (*Todarodes pacificus*), Snail (*Helix aspera*), abalone (*Haliotis midae*)		
Met e 1 Pen a 1 Pen m 1 Pen i 1 Cha f 1 Hom a 1 Pan s 1 Tod p 1 Hel as 1 Hal m 1	Tropomyosin	Anaphylaxis cross-reaction with multiple shellfish and with house dust mite
Shrimp (*Penaeus indicus*)		
	Myosin light chain	Anaphylaxis
Black tiger shrimp (*Penaeus monodon*), shrimp (*Penaeus indicus*)		
	Sarcoplasmic calcium-binding protein	
Black tiger shrimp (*Penaeus monodon*)		

Milk is also the third most common food responsible for fatal or near-fatal food-induced anaphylactic reactions (8%–15% cases),[67–69] and appears to be globally one of the most common causes of anaphylaxis in young children (see **Table 1**).[28,48,70,71] Acute (IgE-mediated) reactions to milk are caused by various milk allergens mainly belonging to the family of caseins and whey proteins (see **Table 2a**).[72,73] Cooking diminishes the allergenicity of whey proteins, presumably by denaturation of heat-labile proteins, resulting in loss of conformational epitopes. Children reactive to extensively heated milk (but not egg) are at higher risk for systemic reactions treated with epinephrine than those children tolerant to heated milk but

Table 3
Family of most common allergenic foods: peanut, tree nuts, and seafood

Family	Species	Common Name	Common Cause of Anaphylaxis	Uncommon Cause of Anaphylaxis
Leguminoseae	*Arachis hypogea*	Peanut	+	
Betulaceae	*Corylus avellana*	Hazelnut	+	
Anacardiaceae	*Anacardium occidentale*	Cashew	+	
	Pistacia vera	Pistachio	+	
Juglandaceae	*Juglans regia*	Walnut	+	
	Carya illinoinensis	Pecan nut		+
Rosaceae	*Prunus dulcis*	Almond		+
Lecythidaceae	*Bertholletia excelsa*	Brazil nut	+	
Fagaceae	*Castanea sativa*	Chestnut		+
Pinaceae	*Pinus pinea*	Pine nut		+
Proteaceae	*Macadamia intergrifolia*	Macadamia nut		+
Palmaceae	*Cocos nucifera*	Coconut		+
Arthropods	Crustaceans	Crab, rock lobster, prawn, shrimp Shellfish	+	
Mollusks	Gastropods	Abalone, snail, whelk		+
	Bivalves	Clam, oyster, scallop, mussel, cockles		+
	Cephalopods	Squid (cuttlefish), octopus		+
Chordate	Teleosts	Tuna, salmon, carp, trout	+	+

Data from Lopata AL, O'Hehir RE, Lehrer SB. Shellfish allergy. Clin Exp Allergy 2010;40(6):850–8; and Crespo JF, James JM, Fernandez-Rodriguez C, et al. Food allergy: nuts and tree nuts. British J Nutr 2006;96(Suppl 2):S95–102.

reactive to unheated milk, suggesting a possible correlation between sensitivity toward different epitopes in the allergens and severity of reaction.[74] Indeed the importance of sequential epitope recognition in the persistence of cow's milk allergy has been highlighted in several studies.[75–79] Cooking-induced allergen denaturation may explain why many patients allergic to cow's milk tolerate extensively heated milk.[74,80] Similarly, yogurt cultures, which ferment and acidify milk, contain less intact whey protein, therefore individuals with cow's milk allergy exclusively sensitized to whey proteins may tolerate yogurt-based dairy products.[81] However, in children with near-fatal anaphylaxis it is prudent to avoid all forms of milk even in minor quantities. Mammals that are phylogenetically related have quite similar milk protein expression, hence no mammalian milk (ie, goat, donkey, and so forth) is safe for children with anaphylaxis to milk.[81]

Fatal reactions to egg are rare, but have been reported.[22] Food-dependent, exercise-induced anaphylaxis with egg as the trigger has also been reported.[82] Five major allergenic proteins from the egg of the domestic chicken (*Gallus domesticus*) have been identified, and are designated Gal d 1 to Gal d 5. Most of the allergenic egg proteins are found in egg white. Although ovalbumin (OVA) is the most abundant protein in hen's egg white, ovomucoid (OVM) has been shown to be the dominant allergen in egg. Egg-specific IgE molecules that identify sequential or conformational epitopes of OVM and OVA can distinguish different clinical phenotypes of egg allergy. It has been shown that patients with egg allergy with IgE antibodies reacting against sequential epitopes tend to have persistent allergy, whereas those with IgE antibodies primarily to conformational epitopes tend to have transient allergy. Studies have shown that ingestion of raw or undercooked egg may trigger more severe clinical reactions than well-cooked egg.[83] Manufactured food products often contain trace amounts of egg lecithin as emulsifiers, but ingestion of trace amounts of egg lecithin is probably insufficient to elicit allergic reactions.[84]

Although severe soy allergy reactions have been reported, they are quite rare and far less common than milk allergy (see **Table 1**).[85,86] The specificity of soy allergens is variable and complex. As many as 28 different soy proteins have been recognized as being allergenic; however, only a few are considered major allergens. Gly m 5 and Gly m 6 account for about 30% and 40% of the total seed proteins, respectively, and have been shown to be a potential indicator for severe allergic reactions to soy (see **Table 2a**).[87] Most individuals with anaphylaxis induced by cow's milk allergy tolerate soy if such patients have no IgE to soy.[81] Clinical cross-reactivity between peanut and soy, both legumes, is extremely rare despite the high degree of cross-sensitization, and is estimated to be less than 7%.[37,88,89]

RISK FACTORS

The major risk factor for FIA appears to be food allergy. Indeed the majority of patients with fatal or near-fatal FIA are known to be allergic to the food that caused the anaphylactic reaction.[2,28,67,90] The severity of previous allergic reaction is not predictive of the severity of future allergic reaction, as the experience accumulated with food challenge and reports on fatal FIA seems to indicate.[68,91] Therefore it is not surprising that recent National Institutes of Health (NIH) guidelines for the management of food allergy encourage clinicians to consider prescribing an epinephrine autoinjector for all patients with documented IgE-mediated food allergy reactions, because it is impossible to predict the severity of any subsequent reactions with accuracy.[45] The group at highest risk of FIA are young male children, while among adults women are at higher risk. Overall the group at highest risk for fatal anaphylaxis is young adults.[23,28,29,67,71,92] Among patients with food allergy, those at highest risk[45,67,68,93] are those with a history positive anaphylaxis, those with asthma (risk increases with the severity of asthma),[46,92] those with allergy to peanut, tree nuts, and shellfish, and adolescents.

Several factors can contribute to lower the "threshold" for anaphylaxis, possibly by increasing the allergen uptake (ie, exercise, alcohol, drugs that increase gastric pH) or by enhancing the inflammatory response (ie, febrile illness, asthma exacerbation, or nonsteroidal anti-inflammatory drug use); hence the unpredictability of future reaction.[94]

Higher income, living in an area with low sun exposure, and possible low level of vitamin D may predispose individuals to develop anaphylaxis.[95,96]

PATHOGENESIS

FIA is a typical IgE-mediated allergic reaction, being immediate, reproducible, and readily diagnosed by detection of food-specific IgE. FIA is initiated by the engagement of allergen-specific IgE antibody with its high-affinity receptor (FcεRI) that is expressed on mast cells and basophils. When a specific antigen binds the IgE linked to the FcεRI it determines a receptor cross-link and consequent release of preformed mediators (histamine, tryptase, carboxypeptidase A, proteoglycans, and some cytokines) and newly synthesized ones (leukotrienes, bradykinins, cytokines including tumor necrosis factor α, and platelet-activating factor [PAF]).[97,98] Ultimately, these mediators cause the characteristic clinical features of anaphylaxis, including vasodilation, angioedema, bronchoconstriction, and increased mucus production (**Table 4**).[99–101]

Even if initially it was thought that mast cells were the principal effector cells in IgE-mediated acute reaction, further studies have shown that basophils also play a major role in acute food allergy symptoms. Indeed patients with food allergy have higher rates of spontaneous release of histamine from basophils, which normalizes after

Table 4
Mediators involved in anaphylaxis

Mediators	Effects	Clinical Manifestation
Histamine	Agonist of H1 and H2 receptors, which causes increase in the vascular permeability, vasodilation, contraction of smooth muscle cells, increase in exocrine gland secretion, and irritation of sensory nerves	Urticaria, angioedema, asthma, hypotension, abdominal cramps, diarrhea
Lipooxygenase pathway products LTB$_4$ LTC$_4$ LTD$_4$	Chemotaxis Contraction of smooth muscle cells, increase in vascular permeability, increase in exocrine gland secretion (goblet cells)	Biphasic reaction, asthma, hypotension
Cyclooxygenase PGD$_2$ PGF$_{2a}$ TXA$_2$	Vasodilation, contraction of smooth muscle cells, coronary vasoconstriction, increase in exocrine gland secretion (goblet cells)	Asthma, hypotension, heart ischemia
PAF	Induction of arachidonic acid metabolites	Asthma, hypotension
Chemotactic factors for eosinophils and neutrophils	Tissue infiltration and activation of eosinophils and neutrophils	Possible role in biphasic or prolonged reactions
Tryptase	Activates complement through C$_3$ Cut fibrinogen Activates kallikrein	No clear physiologic role
Kininogenase of mast cells and basophil kallikrein	Activation of contact system, release of kinins	No clear physiologic role
Chymase	Degrades neuropeptides Conversion of angiotensin I to II	Hypotension and inhibition of neuropeptides
Heparin	Inhibition of coagulation, plasmin, kallikrein and complement	Possible anti-inflammatory role

Abbreviations: LTB, leukotriene B; LTC, leukotriene C; LTD, leukotriene D; PAF, platelet-activating factor; PGD, prostaglandin D; PGF, prostaglandin F; TXA, thromboxane A.

the offending food has been removed from the diet. Furthermore, normal serum tryptase levels (a specific marker of mast cell activation) in patients with FIA have been reported, suggesting an involvement of histamine release from tryptase-negative cells such as basophils. Moreover, in a peanut anaphylaxis animal model the combined deficiency of mast cells and phagocytes, but not mast cells and basophils, averted nearly all clinical and physiologic signs of anaphylaxis, suggesting that other cells of the innate immune system may play a role in anaphylaxis.[102]

Histamine is one of the major preformed mediators released by mast cells and basophils, and can induce most of the characteristics of anaphylaxis when administered intravenously to humans and laboratory animals (see **Table 4**).[99] However, even the strongest inhibitors of histamines are not sufficient to block or reverse anaphylaxis, suggesting other mechanism may also be involved.[103,104] In the past few years, PAF has emerged as a major player in the propagation of anaphylaxis. PAF is a preformed mediator released by mast cells, monocytes, and tissue macrophages during anaphylaxis, and is capable of activating mast cells in the lung and peripheral blood but not in the skin.[105] Higher levels of PAF and lower levels of its metabolizing enzyme (PAF acetylhydrolase) have been found by Vadas and colleagues[106,107] to correlate with the severity of the anaphylactic attack. Recently, Arias and colleagues[108] showed that a molecule that blocks PAF prevents severe anaphylactic reactions and, when combined with antihistamines, abolishes nearly all signs of anaphylaxis. In a mouse model of peanut anaphylaxis it has been shown that peanut may contribute to induce anaphylactic shock by causing activation of the complement cascade and relative production of C3a, which stimulates macrophages, basophils, and mast cells to produce PAF and histamine.[109]

Patients with the lowest serum angiotensin-converting enzyme concentrations were also more likely to develop life-threatening pharyngeal edema in peanut-induced FIA, suggesting that this complication may be partly mediated by bradykinins.[50]

The intrinsic properties of the food allergens may contribute to whether the allergen favors allergic immune responses. Indeed, relatively few foods (egg, milk, peanut, tree nuts, fish, shellfish) account for most of the allergic reactions.[110] Characteristics common to major food allergens are that they are water-soluble glycoproteins, are 10 to 70 kDa in size, and are relatively stable to heat, acid, and proteases. To elicit a sustained immune response, the immunogenic molecule should ideally stimulate both T and B cells. The portion of the immunogenic molecule that binds specifically with membrane receptors on T or B cells is called an epitope, which can be sequential or conformational. Sequential epitopes are determined by contiguous amino acids, whereas conformational epitopes contain amino acids from different regions of the protein that are in close proximity because of the folding of the protein. Conformational epitopes can be destroyed with heating or partial hydrolysis, which alters the tertiary structure of the protein, hence they are less stable, heat/enzyme labile, and often cause less severe reactions especially when cooked.[83]

In addition, the presence of immunostimulatory factors in the food may also contribute to such sensitization. For example, the major glycoprotein allergen from peanut, Ara h 1, is not only very stable and resistant to heat-digestive enzyme degradation but also acts as a Th2 adjuvant, due to the expression of a glycan adduct.[111,112]

DIAGNOSIS
Clinical

Anaphylaxis remains first and foremost a clinical diagnosis. A good history remains the most powerful tool that physicians have to confirm both a history of FIA and the food trigger. Indeed anaphylaxis occurs soon after food ingestion (see **Box 1**), and patients themselves often notice the relationship with the eliciting food. However, the patient's own perceptions and knowledge may influence history, so the physician has to ensure correct compilation of the history. Thus a systematic review of all patient's symptoms, patient's diet, and the last meal before the reaction are a highly useful first step. As described in **Box 1**, anaphylaxis is characterized by a combination of cutaneous, respiratory, cardiovascular, and gastrointestinal factors. The presence of all of these symptoms need to be asked of patients and parents, because patients may only initially remember or mention the more severe or obvious ones. Reactions of skin and mucosal involvement such as urticaria, angioedema, itch, rhinorrhea, and conjunctivitis present in a high percentage (70%–98%) of patients, especially in young children.[35,48,56,113] However, anaphylaxis without skin or mucosal involvement have been described, and relying solely on skin manifestation may delay the diagnosis and could be fatal for the patient.[68] Perhaps because the gastrointestinal mucosa is the location of exposure in FIA, immediate gastrointestinal hypersensitivity is commonly seen as a manifestation of anaphylaxis.[27,90] Abdominal pain and vomiting is common especially in children, and can be the primary manifestation of anaphylaxis with only minimal involvement of other organs.[23,48,71] Cardiovascular symptoms can rapidly cause the death of the patient, and need to be recognized at an early stage. Close monitoring of blood pressure with the correct cuff size for age is essential in all patients with suspected or ongoing anaphylaxis. However, cardiovascular symptoms are much less common in FIA compared with other types of anaphylaxis, and are rarely found in isolation from respiratory arrest. In infant and preschool children, reactions tend to be less likely to involve the cardiovascular system.[23,48,71] Respiratory manifestation such edema of the glottis and asthma are the primary cause of death in patients with FIA and need to be treated aggressively, especially in asthmatic patients.[67–69]

The time from ingestion of food to the onset of FIA symptoms is usually on the order of minutes, and almost never occurs after 2 hours from ingestion of the triggering foods.[91] In small children timing can help to differentiate between anaphylaxis and food protein–induced enterocolitis (FPIES), a non-IgE–mediated food allergy that typically begins later than 1.5 hours after ingestion.

Additional elements of clinical history can be helpful. Knowing the quantity necessary to trigger a reaction is helpful in evaluating risk of anaphylaxis for trace amounts of foods and the severity of anaphylaxis.

One area of considerable controversy in the literature is the true frequency of biphasic reactions during anaphylaxis. In a biphasic reaction, symptoms of the initial reaction resolve but are followed by new symptoms without any further allergen exposure, and are never more severe than the first manifestation. The true incidence of biphasic reaction and prevention measures is not known. Published reports suggest that biphasic reactions occur in 5% to 28% of anaphylaxis cases, with the highest incidence in FIA. However, in children undergoing oral food challenge (OFC) reactions are extremely rare.[85,114] There is also conflicting evidence about whether administration of steroid or epinephrine can prevent a biphasic reaction.[114]

When history is not convincing, other diseases that may mimic FIA have to be considered (**Box 3**), and laboratory evaluation in the acute phase may be important. Especially important in the differential diagnosis of FIA are the restaurant syndromes and toxic reactions due to fish intake (see **Box 3** and **Table 5**).

Laboratory Studies

At present, there is no laboratory test that reliably confirms cases of FIA. Indeed histamine and tryptase serum levels are less helpful in FIA than in other types of anaphylaxis.

Box 3
Differential diagnosis of food-induced anaphylaxis

1. Vasovagal reactions
2. Non-IgE–mediated food allergy
   a. FPIES
3. "Flush" syndrome
   a. Carcinoid
   b. Postmenopausal
   c. Chlorpropamide alcohol
   d. Medullary and thyroid carcinoma
   e. Autonomic epilepsy
4. "Restaurant syndromes"
   a. Monosodium glutamate
   b. Sulfites
   c. Scombroid
5. Other shock
   a. Hemorrhagic
   b. Cardiac
   c. Endotoxic
   d. Monoclonal gammopathy (paroxysmal hyperpermeability)
6. Syndromes with excessive endogenous production of histamine
   a. Mastocytosis
   b. Urticaria pigmentosa
   c. Basophil leukemia
   d. Promyelocytic acute leukemia
   e. Hydatid cyst
7. Nonorganic syndromes
   a. Panic attack
   b. Munchausen
   c. Vocal cord dysfunction
   d. Hysteric bolus
8. Miscellaneous
   a. Hereditary angioedema
   b. Anaphylaxis due to progesterone
   c. Urticaria vasculitis
   d. Pheochromocytoma
   e. Hyper-IgE syndrome
   f. Neurologic diseases (seizures, stroke)
   g. Pseudoanaphylaxis
   h. Red man syndrome (vancomycin)

Table 5
Adverse reactions to seafood generated by different triggers

	Symptoms	Time of Reaction
Bacteria		
Aeromonas, Listeria, Salmonella, Vibrio, Klebsiella pneumoniae, Proteus morganii	Cutaneous, gastrointestinal, and neurologic (headache)	Minutes to several hours
Viruses		
Rotavirus, astrovirus, hepatitis A, small round viruses, etc	Gastrointestinal	Hours
Parasites		
Anisakis	Respiratory distress	Minutes to several hours
Toxins		
Algae toxins		

Serum histamine levels are elevated only for 30 to 60 minutes after the onset of reaction, so they are very rarely measured. The most commonly assessed mediator in clinical practice is tryptase, whose blood levels peak 1.5 hours after the onset of symptoms and are measurable for up to 5 hours. However, in FIA tryptase is less commonly elevated than in other types of anaphylaxis.[114] Other laboratory tests may be important in ruling out nonanaphylactic causes of symptoms, as shown in **Box 4**.

Box 4
Examinations in cases of nonconvincing anaphylaxis

Blood Tests

Serum histamine (within 1 hour)

Tryptase (within 5 hours)

CH_{50}, C1 esterase ⟶ Hereditary angioedema

IgA, IgM, IgG immunoelectrophoresis ⟶ monoclonal gammopathy

Cardiac enzymes ⟶ cardiac ischemia?

Serotonin ⟶ carcinoid syndrome?

Urine

Histamine

5-Indoleacetic acid, vanillylmandelic acid, catecholamines ⟶ carcinoid syndrome, pheochromocytoma

Other

Blood pressure monitoring

Electrocardiogram

Echocardiogram

Chest radiograph

Liver ultrasound examination

Parasites in feces

Diagnosis of the food allergen that caused anaphylaxis is the most important step in preventing future reaction; hence referral to an allergist is essential for the appropriate workup. Food allergy diagnosis is made primarily on the history and on a few tests done to confirm the history. An SPT examines for the presence of food protein–specific IgEs, having a positive predictive accuracy of about 50% that the patient will react to the tested food. The larger the size of wheal on SPT, the more accurate is such a predictive value; however, negative predictive values are in excess of 95%. Furthermore, the age of the patient, previous exposure reactions to the food, and the type of food change the predictive value for a wheal size. An alternative method to detect food protein–specific IgE is by in vitro methods (FEIA-CAP or "RAST test"). Some clinicians may prefer to use in vitro testing when there is persistent dermatographism (rare) in the few weeks following an anaphylactic shock (ie, mast cell refractory period), severe eczema, or when the patient is on antihistamines. Indeed in all these conditions skin tests may not be reliable. Similar to SPT, a cutoff value can be developed for predicting 50% to 95% of who will react to foods. SPT or levels of specific IgE give only an indication of the likelihood of clinical reactivity; however, individual results do not provide prognostic information or distinguish between likelihood of mild or severe reaction.[51,76,98,114,115] Recently, peptide microarrays have been developed for large-scale epitope mapping, with small quantities of serum allowing large-scale study to compare levels of IgE and their affinity toward specific epitopes of different allergens.[51,72,73,116–122] So far no single informative epitope that reliably distinguishes between the different phenotypes of milk, egg, or peanut allergy has been identified because of the heterogeneity of epitopes recognized by subjects within the different phenotypes. The number of epitopes recognized, rather than recognition of specific epitopes, might be more predictive of clinical features of food allergy.[15] However, the overlap in the number of epitopes recognized in different clinical group does not allow its clinical use.[51,72,73,116–122]

Oral Food Challenges

OFC are the key to establishing the identity of specific food triggers. The most rigorous method is double-blinded and placebo-controlled (DBPC), but single-blind (patient) and open challenges can be performed. The least time-intensive procedure is the open challenge. With a previous history of anaphylaxis they are not needed, and they can be very dangerous if history and allergy evaluation are concordant. OFC may be needed years after the anaphylactic reaction has occurred in order to establish the possible development of tolerance, especially in children. In such highly selected cases, they should be performed in the hospital setting with an intensive care unit readily available, and should be started from allergen doses of less than 100 mg of protein.[123]

TREATMENT
Epinephrine

Intramuscular injection of epinephrine into the vastus lateralis muscle (lateral thigh) is the life-saving treatment in cases of FIA as well as for all types of anaphylactic reactions. All other treatments such as antihistamines, glucocorticoids, and β-agonists, either alone or in combination, are to be considered ancillary in the treatment of anaphylaxis.

In animal models and in humans, injected epinephrine rapidly reverses anaphylaxis, because is an agonist for the adrenergic receptors (α-1, β-1, β-2).[3,67–69,101,103,114,124] In humans, prospective controlled studies on the use of epinephrine during an acute anaphylactic event have not been done, for obvious ethical reasons; however, retrospective studies have shown convincingly that lack of treatment with epinephrine within a few minutes of the beginning of the symptoms is one of the major risk factors for death from FIA.

There is wide agreement that the optimal method of administration of epinephrine is intramuscular, as subcutaneous injection can lead to local vasoconstriction with possible delayed absorption, and decreased peak levels, while the intravenous route lacks an established dosing regimen, is prone to dosing errors, is difficult to perform rapidly, and can induce lethal arrhythmias.

In cases of profound hypotension or failure to respond to intramuscular epinephrine, intraventricular epinephrine should be used while patients have continuous cardiac monitoring in place.[15,23,48,70,115,120,121,125]

The recommended dose for intramuscular epinephrine injection 1:1000 solution (1 mg/mL) is from 0.01 mg/kg to a maximum of 0.3 mg in children and 0.5 mg in adults. Commercially available prefilled syringes for autoinjection are available in strengths of 0.15 and 0.3 mg. The most recent guidelines from the NIH recommend switching to the 0.3-mg dose at approximately 25 kg (55 lbs) because of the risk of underdosing above this weight if the smaller dosage is used, even if the package instruction recommends the switch at 30 kg. For children who have asthma or other additional risk factors for fatality from anaphylaxis, switching to the higher dose at a lower weight might be considered. The same guidelines recommend the use of the 0.15-mg autoinjector for patients weighing down to 10 kg. In practice, self-injected epinephrine is prescribed even to smaller otherwise healthy infants, because the risks of overdose with autoinjector use is weighed against the demonstrated difficulty encountered by professionals and nonprofessionals with correctly and promptly drawing up a correct-for-age dose of epinephrine into the syringe. The dose may be repeated at intervals of at least 5 minutes if necessary. World Health Organization (WHO) and Anaphylaxis Canada recommend the availability of 1 dose for every 10 to 20 minutes of travel time to a medical emergency facility, and most guidelines recommend the prescription of 2 doses, as in some cases of anaphylaxis one dose may not be enough.[15,23,48,70,115,120,121,125]

Ideally epinephrine autoinjectors are prescribed on discharge from the emergency room after management of anaphylaxis, or following consultation with a pediatrician or pediatric allergist for suspected food allergy. Despite universal recommendations for the use of epinephrine in anaphylaxis, it is actually uncommonly used in home or emergency room treatment of FIA, and most patients with a history of anaphylaxis will discontinue its use within a few years of the anaphylactic episode, perhaps because patients perceive epinephrine as a dangerous medication or patients and practitioners do not think their symptoms are severe enough to merit epinephrine.[68,114,126] In general, it is recommended that epinephrine be given to food-allergic children at the first signs of a systemic reaction, before life-threatening symptoms such as respiratory distress and hypotension develop, as those symptoms may be harder to reverse and may cause permanent damage to the subjects (cerebral hypoxia). Patient with history of life-threatening reaction have to be instructed to recognize the early symptoms of anaphylaxis (**Box 5**).

H1 Antihistamines

H1 antihistamines are inverse agonists at the H1 histamine receptor in that that they bind the receptor in its inactive state, preventing signaling through the receptor. H1 antihistamines are the most commonly used medications in the treatment of anaphylactic episodes both in the hospital and outpatient setting. Although H1 antihistamines

---

Box 5
Early symptoms of anaphylaxis

Itch of scalp, palms of hands, or soles of feet extending to acoustic meatus, lips, genital area

Diffuse erythema

Oral or pharyngeal itch

Nasal congestion

Subjective sensation of throat tightness

Changes in the tone of voice: hoarseness

Swelling of lips and tongue

---

decrease skin symptoms (itch, flush, urticaria) and nasal symptoms (rhinorrhea, congestion), they do not prevent or treat life-threatening manifestations of anaphylaxis such as airway obstruction, wheeze, or hypotension. Hence they are considered secondary medications for the treatment of anaphylaxis, and their use in the outpatient setting is controversial. Indeed, even if the most recent practice parameter suggests that they may have utility for "control of cutaneous and cardiovascular manifestations" of anaphylaxis, others recommend against their use because of their potential for both delaying life-saving therapy and causing dangerous side effects such sedation (which could make assessment of the progression of anaphylaxis difficult), neurotoxicity such as seizure, and potentially fatal QT prolongation. If antihistamines are used for children, the dose should be 1 mg/kg up to 50 mg, whereas for adults the dose is 25 to 50 mg, whether given intramuscularly, intraventricularly, or by mouth.[3,68,114]

H2 Antihistamines

Like H1 antihistamines, H2 antihistamines are inverse agonists that preferentially bind to the inactive state of the receptor. The H2 receptor participates in the anaphylactic response, and even if theoretically blockade of this receptor may have an additive effect with the H1 antihistamines, their efficacy has been only suggested and not proved in cases of any kind of anaphylaxis including FIA. The most recent United States practice parameter for anaphylaxis states "an H2 antagonist added to the H1 antagonist may be helpful in the management of anaphylaxis." If used, ranitidine can be given intraventricularly or intramuscularly at 1 mg/kg in children and 12.5 to 50 mg in adults. Infusion of cimetidine should be done slowly to prevent hypotension.[3,68,114]

Glucocorticoids

Like antihistamines, the efficacy of glucocorticoids in the treatment of anaphylaxis has not been proved in a randomized, double-blind, placebo-controlled trial, but is widely used in the emergency room and outpatient settings. The onset of action of glucocorticoids is slow, occurring hours after administration, and it is well known that pretreatment for 48 hours with glucocorticoids prevents the late-phase response to allergen challenge; it does not affect the acute-phase response. Glucocorticoids can cause significant adverse events if used long term, but short-term use is generally much safer and mostly limited to mood changes, increase in peripheral blood concentration of glucose, and occasional high blood pressure. Their use may reduce the biphasic reaction but, given the rarity of such reactions, a double-blind placebo-controlled study to prove such an effect is difficult to realize.[3,68,114]

β-Agonists

β-Agonists may be used as an adjunct to epinephrine for the treatment of wheeze, but should not replace epinephrine because they lack the widespread effects of epinephrine and do not effectively treat angioedema.[3,68,114]

Others

β-Blockers are associated with anaphylaxis that is difficult to treat in adults. If the patient is taking β-blockers, glucagon can be useful.

Additional potentially life-saving supportive measures include placing the patient in a supine position to maximize cardiac return, administering oxygen if needed, and giving intraventricular fluids if hypotension develops.[3,68,114]

PREVENTION OF ANAPHYLAXIS AND FATAL ANAPHYLAXIS

Until recently the only proven prevention strategy for FIA has been food elimination in subjects with a history of food allergy to a specific food. To facilitate allergen avoidance in the United States the Food Allergen Labeling and Consumer Protection Act was enacted in 2005 to publish help on food labels to prevent accidental exposure to foods for the 8 most common food allergens (milk, egg, peanut, tree nuts, fish, shellfish, soy, and wheat). Similar legislation has been introduced in Japan, Europe, and Australia. All patients at risk for anaphylaxis must be trained to identify relevant food allergens on the labels, and written instruction should be given.[115,124]

Even if a correct diagnosis is made, accidental exposure and recurrence of anaphylaxis induced by the same or different foods are frequent in subjects with FIA. Indeed most patients who died of anaphylaxis knew they were allergic to the food that eventually killed them.[67–69,126] All patients with a history of anaphylaxis or at high risk of anaphylaxis should be taught to recognize early symptoms (see **Box 5**) and be taught the use of autoinjectable epinephrine with written and verbal instruction immediately after the diagnosis of anaphylaxis is made. All patients at risk of anaphylaxis should leave the clinician's office or the hospital with a written plan indicating clearly the food allergies, the dose of epinephrine to be used, and symptoms that should induce epinephrine use.[1,3]

In a recent report, Pumphrey and Gowland[68] noted that more than half FIA-related deaths occurred in patients whose previous reactions had been so mild that it was unlikely that a doctor would have recommended they should carry self-injectable epinephrine. Indeed recent NIH guidelines for food allergy management encourage clinicians to consider prescribing an epinephrine autoinjector for all patients with food allergy having IgE-mediated reactions, based on the fact that it is impossible to predict the severity of any subsequent reactions with accuracy (**Box 6**)[45] WHO and Anaphylaxis Canada recommend the availability of 1 dose for every 10 to 20 minutes of travel time to a medical emergency facility.

More recently oral immunotherapy has been proved to be effective in the short term in preventing anaphylaxis attributable to several foods such as milk, hazelnut, and eggs.[127] Moreover, a unique combination of Chinese herbs, Zhi Fu Zi (Radix Lateralis Aconiti Carmichaeli Praeparata) and Xi Xin (Herba Asari), could also help with the induction of tolerance.[127]

Box 6

Epinephrine autoinjector (or 2-dose prescription) NIH food allergy guidelines 2010

All patients experiencing anaphylaxis should be provided directly with an epinephrine autoinjector or, if this is not possible, with a prescription (recommended prescription is for 2 doses of epinephrine), and advised to fill it immediately.

Other patients who should be prescribed an epinephrine autoinjector include:

1. Patients with a history of a prior systemic allergic reaction

2. Patients with food allergy and asthma

3. Patients with a known food allergy to peanut, tree nuts, fish, and crustacean shellfish (ie, allergens known to be associated with more fatal and near-fatal allergic reactions)

4. In addition, consideration should be given to prescribing an epinephrine autoinjector for all patients with food allergy having IgE-mediated reactions because it is impossible to predict the severity of any subsequent reactions with accuracy

Data from Boyce JA, Assa'ad A, Burks AW, et al. Guidelines for the diagnosis and management of food allergy in the United States: report of the NIAID-sponsored expert panel. J Allergy Clin Immunol 2010;126(Suppl 6):S1–58.

FOOD-DEPENDENT EXERCISE-INDUCED ANAPHYLAXIS

Exercise-induced anaphylaxis (EIA) is a particular type of anaphylaxis that occurs while performing intense exercise. It is estimated that 5% to 15% of anaphylactic episodes are caused by or are associated with exercise. EIA may occur independently of food ingestion (pure EIA) or in close time relationship with food ingestion (30% to 50% of EIA).[128] Food-dependent exercise-induced anaphylaxis (FDEIA) is diagnosed when anaphylactic episodes occur only when exercise follows food ingestion (up to 6 hours, usually within 1–3 hours), and is otherwise well tolerated. The most common foods reported in adults with FDEIA include crustacean shellfish, celery, cheese, tomatoes, and alcohol. In adults with FDEIA about 75% are female. Fifty percent report seasonal allergic rhinitis and 19% report asthma.[129] In children, FDEIA may be more frequent in teenage males and in association with wheat allergy.[130] Water-insoluble omega-5-gliadin (Tri a 19) has been identified as a major allergen in Finnish subjects with FDEIA.[40,41] However, a long list of foods including many vegetables (ie, celery), cereals, milk, eggs, and meat has been reported as a cause of FDEIA.[14,131,132] Clinical presentations of FDEIA include pruritus, urticaria, angioedema, flushing, shortness of breath, dysphagia, chest tightness, syncope, profuse sweating, headache, nausea, diarrhea, colicky abdominal pain, throat closing, and hoarseness.[128]

FDEIA can manifest in teen years or adulthood in subjects without any prior history of food allergy. In patients with suspected FDEIA, SPT to foods ingested prior to the exercise can identify the offending food, although negative allergy test results do not rule out FDEIA. Suspected FDEIA is one of the few situations for which a large panel of food skin tests needs to be performed if the meal eaten before the exercise included many ingredients. A food challenge followed by exercise on a treadmill may be necessary to confirm the diagnosis in selected cases. Food challenges in FDEIA are a high-risk procedure, as the dose of food and intensity of exercise required to induce a reaction cannot be well controlled, and severe anaphylactic reactions have been reported.[133] A positive challenge provides definitive diagnosis. However, a negative challenge does not rule out FDEIA because the intensity of exercise might have not been well reproduced, or because of the potential necessary association of additional cofactors, such as pollen exposure or concomitant ingestions of drugs such as nonsteroidal anti-inflammatory drugs or, in women, the concomitant presence of menses.[133] Management of FDEIA includes prompt treatment with epinephrine during an acute episode.

To prevent FDEIA, the following strategies are recommended: (1) avoidance of exercise within 4 to 6 hours following the incriminated food ingestion; (2) avoidance of exercising alone or in hot or humid weather or during pollen allergy season; and (3) carrying emergency medications. Patients with FDEIA often have environmental allergies to pollens, and one of the major challenges is to distinguish between FDEIA and exercise-induced asthma especially in those subjects in whom FDEIA is associated with dyspnea or wheezing. Elevated serum tryptase levels have been reported in subjects with FDEIA following an acute episode, and can be helpful in determining the diagnosis.[128]

SUMMARY

FIA is a serious allergic reaction that may cause death rapidly in otherwise healthy individuals. There is no universal agreement on its definition or criteria for diagnosis.

Food is one of the most common causes of anaphylaxis, with most surveys indicating that food-induced reactions account for 30% to 50% of anaphylaxis cases in North America, Europe, Asia, and Australia, with up to 81% of anaphylaxis occurring in children.

Although a wide range of foods has been reported as a cause of FIA, the most commonly implicated foods worldwide are peanut, tree nuts, milk, egg, sesame seeds, fish, and shellfish, in both adults and children.

Allergens and patients' characteristics are probably important in determining an anaphylactic reaction. The major risk factor for FIA appears to be food allergy, in particular for those with asthma with allergy to peanut, tree nuts, and shellfish, adolescents, and young adults. The severity of previous allergic reaction is not predictive of the severity of any future allergic reaction. The only life-saving treatment for anaphylaxis is allergen avoidance and intramuscular epinephrine injection if an anaphylactic event occurs. All patients at risk for FIA should be provided with an anaphylaxis plan that indicates allergen and treatment modalities, as well as with self-injectable epinephrine.

REFERENCES

1. Sampson HA, Munoz-Furlong A, Campbell RL, et al. Second symposium on the definition and management of anaphylaxis: summary report—second National Institute of Allergy and Infectious Disease/Food Allergy and Anaphylaxis Network symposium. Ann Emerg Med 2006;47(4):373–80.
2. Neugut AI, Ghatak AT, Miller RL. Anaphylaxis in the United States: an investigation into its epidemiology. Arch Intern Med 2001;161(1):15–21.
3. Muraro A, Roberts G, Clark A, et al. The management of anaphylaxis in childhood: position paper of the European Academy of Allergology and Clinical Immunology. Allergy 2007;62(8):857–71.
4. Liew WK, Williamson E, Tang ML. Anaphylaxis fatalities and admissions in Australia. J Allergy Clin Immunol 2009;123(2):434–42.
5. Clark S, Camargo CA Jr. Epidemiology of anaphylaxis. Immunol Allergy Clin North Am 2007;27(2):145–63, v.
6. Decker WW, Campbell RL, Manivannan V, et al. The etiology and incidence of anaphylaxis in Rochester, Minnesota: a report from the Rochester Epidemiology Project. J Allergy Clin Immunol 2008;122(6):1161–5.

7. Bohlke K, Davis RL, DeStefano F, et al. Epidemiology of anaphylaxis among children and adolescents enrolled in a health maintenance organization. J Allergy Clin Immunol 2004;113(3):536–42.

8. Yocum MW, Butterfield JH, Klein JS, et al. Epidemiology of anaphylaxis in Olmsted County: A population-based study. J Allergy Clin Immunol 1999; 104(2 Pt 1):452–6.

9. Mullins RJ. Anaphylaxis: risk factors for recurrence. Clin Exp Allergy 2003;33(8): 1033–40.

10. Moneret-Vautrin DA, Romano MC, Kanny G, et al. The individual reception project (IRP) for anaphylactic emergencies. The situation in France and French overseas territories in 2002. Presse Med 2003;32(2):61–6 [in French].

11. Simons FE, Peterson S, Black CD. Epinephrine dispensing patterns for an out-of-hospital population: a novel approach to studying the epidemiology of anaphylaxis. J Allergy Clin Immunol 2002;110(4):647–51.

12. Patel DA, Holdford DA, Edwards E, et al. Estimating the economic burden of food-induced allergic reactions and anaphylaxis in the United States. J Allergy Clin Immunol 2011;128(1):110–5 e115.

13. Sicherer SH, Munoz-Furlong A, Sampson HA. Prevalence of peanut and tree nut allergy in the United States determined by means of a random digit dial telephone survey: a 5-year follow-up study. J Allergy Clin Immunol 2003;112(6): 1203–7.

14. Sicherer SH, Munoz-Furlong A, Burks AW, et al. Prevalence of peanut and tree nut allergy in the US determined by a random digit dial telephone survey. J Allergy Clin Immunol 1999;103(4):559–62.

15. Tariq SM, Stevens M, Matthews S, et al. Cohort study of peanut and tree nut sensitisation by age of 4 years. BMJ 1996;313(7056):514–7.

16. Nicolaou N, Poorafshar M, Murray C, et al. Allergy or tolerance in children sensitized to peanut: prevalence and differentiation using component-resolved diagnostics. J Allergy Clin Immunol 2010;125(1):191–7 e1–13.

17. Green TD, LaBelle VS, Steele PH, et al. Clinical characteristics of peanut-allergic children: recent changes. Pediatrics 2007;120(6):1304–10.

18. Rance F, Bidat E, Bourrier T, et al. Cashew allergy: observations of 42 children without associated peanut allergy. Allergy 2003;58(12):1311–4.

19. Sicherer SH, Munoz-Furlong A, Sampson HA. Prevalence of seafood allergy in the United States determined by a random telephone survey. J Allergy Clin Immunol 2004;114(1):159–65.

20. Turner P, Ng I, Kemp A, et al. Seafood allergy in children: a descriptive study. Ann Allergy Asthma Immunol 2011;106(6):494–501.

21. Lopata AL, O'Hehir RE, Lehrer SB. Shellfish allergy. Clin Exp Allergy 2010;40(6): 850–8.

22. Macdougall CF, Cant AJ, Colver AF. How dangerous is food allergy in childhood? The incidence of severe and fatal allergic reactions across the UK and Ireland. Arch Dis Child 2002;86(4):236–9.

23. Cianferoni A, Novembre E, Mugnaini L, et al. Clinical features of acute anaphylaxis in patients admitted to a university hospital: an 11-year retrospective review (1985-1996). Ann Allergy Asthma Immunol 2001;87(1):27–32.

24. Wang J, Sampson HA. Food anaphylaxis. Clin Exp Allergy 2007;37(5):651–60.

25. Sampson HA, Munoz-Furlong A, Campbell RL, et al. Second symposium on the definition and management of anaphylaxis: summary report–Second National Institute of Allergy and Infectious Disease/Food Allergy and Anaphylaxis Network symposium. J Allergy Clin Immunol 2006;117(2):391–7.

26. Sampson HA, Munoz-Furlong A, Bock SA, et al. Symposium on the definition and management of anaphylaxis: summary report. J Allergy Clin Immunol 2005;115(3):584–91.

27. Boyce JA, Assa'ad A, Burks AW, et al. Guidelines for the diagnosis and management of food allergy in the United States: report of the NIAID-sponsored expert panel. J Allergy Clin Immunol 2010;126(Suppl 6):S1–58.

28. Silva R, Gomes E, Cunha L, et al. Anaphylaxis in children: a nine years retrospective study (2001-2009). Allergol Immunopathol (Madr) 2011. [Epub ahead of print].

29. Asero R, Antonicelli L, Arena A, et al. Causes of food-induced anaphylaxis in Italian adults: a multi-centre study. Int Arch Allergy Immunol 2009;150(3):271–7.

30. Beyer K, Morrow E, Li XM, et al. Effects of cooking methods on peanut allergenicity. J Allergy Clin Immunol 2001;107(6):1077–81.

31. Sicherer SH, Burks AW, Sampson HA. Clinical features of acute allergic reactions to peanut and tree nuts in children. Pediatrics 1998;102(1):e6.

32. Lack G, Fox D, Northstone K, et al. Factors associated with the development of peanut allergy in childhood. N Engl J Med 2003;348(11):977–85.

33. Lifschitz CH, Hawkins HK, Guerra C, et al. Anaphylactic shock due to cow's milk protein hypersensitivity in a breast-fed infant. J Pediatr Gastroenterol Nutr 1988;7(1):141–4.

34. Monti G, Marinaro L, Libanore V, et al. Anaphylaxis due to fish hypersensitivity in an exclusively breastfed infant. Acta Paediatrica 2006;95(11):1514–5.

35. Romano A, Fernandez-Rivas M, Caringi M, et al. Allergy to peanut lipid transfer protein (LTP): frequency and cross-reactivity between peanut and peach LTP. Eur Ann Allergy Clin Immunol 2009;41(4):106–11.

36. Asero R, Mistrello G, Amato S, et al. Peach fuzz contains large amounts of lipid transfer protein: is this the cause of the high prevalence of sensitization to LTP in Mediterranean countries? Eur Ann Allergy Clin Immunol 2006;38(4):118–21.

37. Asero R, Mistrello G, Roncarolo D, et al. Relationship between peach lipid transfer protein specific IgE levels and hypersensitivity to non-Rosaceae vegetable foods in patients allergic to lipid transfer protein. Ann Allergy Asthma Immunol 2004;92(2):268–72.

38. Prieto A, Razzak E, Lindo DP, et al. Recurrent anaphylaxis due to lupin flour: primary sensitization through inhalation. J Investig Allergol Clin Immunol 2010;20(1):76–9.

39. Wassenberg J, Hofer M. Lupine-induced anaphylaxis in a child without known food allergy. Ann Allergy Asthma Immunol 2007;98(6):589–90.

40. Palosuo K, Alenius H, Varjonen E, et al. Rye gamma-70 and gamma-35 secalins and barley gamma-3 hordein cross-react with omega-5 gliadin, a major allergen in wheat-dependent, exercise-induced anaphylaxis. Clin Exp Allergy 2001;31(3):466–73.

41. Palosuo K, Alenius H, Varjonen E, et al. A novel wheat gliadin as a cause of exercise-induced anaphylaxis. J Allergy Clin Immunol 1999;103(5 Pt 1):912–7.

42. Commins SP, Satinover SM, Hosen J, et al. Delayed anaphylaxis, angioedema, or urticaria after consumption of red meat in patients with IgE antibodies specific for galactose-alpha-1,3-galactose. J Allergy Clin Immunol 2009;123(2):426–33.

43. Commins SP, James HR, Kelly LA, et al. The relevance of tick bites to the production of IgE antibodies to the mammalian oligosaccharide galactose-alpha-1,3-galactose. J Allergy Clin Immunol 2011;127(5):1286–93 e1286.

44. Van Nunen SA, O'Connor KS, Clarke LR, et al. An association between tick bite reactions and red meat allergy in humans. Med J Aust 2009;190(9):510–1.

45. Bock SA. The incidence of severe adverse reactions to food in Colorado. J Allergy Clin Immunol 1992;90(4 Pt 1):683–5.
46. Iribarren C, Tolstykh IV, Miller MK, et al. Asthma and the prospective risk of anaphylactic shock and other allergy diagnoses in a large integrated health care delivery system. Ann Allergy Asthma Immunol 2010;104(5):371–7.
47. Hompes S, Kohli A, Nemat K, et al. Provoking allergens and treatment of anaphylaxis in children and adolescents—data from the anaphylaxis registry of German-speaking countries. Pediatr Allergy Immunol 2011;22(6):568–74.
48. Rudders SA, Banerji A, Clark S, et al. Age-related differences in the clinical presentation of food-induced anaphylaxis. J Pediatr 2011;158(2):326–8.
49. Crespo JF, James JM, Fernandez-Rodriguez C, et al. Food allergy: nuts and tree nuts. Br J Nutr 2006;96(Suppl 2):S95–102.
50. Summers CW, Pumphrey RS, Woods CN, et al. Factors predicting anaphylaxis to peanuts and tree nuts in patients referred to a specialist center. J Allergy Clin Immunol 2008;121(3):632–8 e632.
51. Flinterman AE, Knol EF, Lencer DA, et al. Peanut epitopes for IgE and IgG4 in peanut-sensitized children in relation to severity of peanut allergy. J Allergy Clin Immunol 2008;121(3):737–43 e710.
52. Asarnoj A, Moverare R, Ostblom E, et al. IgE to peanut allergen components: relation to peanut symptoms and pollen sensitization in 8-year-olds. Allergy 2010;65(9):1189–95.
53. Pastorello EA, Vieths S, Pravettoni V, et al. Identification of hazelnut major allergens in sensitive patients with positive double-blind, placebo-controlled food challenge results. J Allergy Clin Immunol 2002;109(3):563–70.
54. Teuber SS, Comstock SS, Sathe SK, et al. Tree nut allergy. Curr Allergy Asthma Rep 2003;3(1):54–61.
55. Sicherer SH. Clinical implications of cross-reactive food allergens. J Allergy Clin Immunol 2001;108(6):881–90.
56. Monreal P, Botey J, Pena M, et al. Mustard allergy. Two anaphylactic reactions to ingestion of mustard sauce. Ann Allergy 1992;69(4):317–20.
57. Gloor M, Kagi M, Wuthrich B. Poppyseed anaphylaxis. Schweiz Med Wochenschr 1995;125(30):1434–7 [in German].
58. Dechamp C, Bessot JC, Pauli G, et al. First report of anaphylactic reaction after fig (Ficus carica) ingestion. Allergy 1995;50(6):514–6.
59. Subiza J, Subiza JL, Hinojosa M, et al. Anaphylactic reaction after the ingestion of chamomile tea: a study of cross-reactivity with other composite pollens. J Allergy Clin Immunol 1989;84(3):353–8.
60. Miell J, Papouchado M, Marshall AJ. Anaphylactic reaction after eating a mango. BMJ 1988;297(6664):1639–40.
61. Savonius B, Kanerva L. Anaphylaxis caused by banana. Allergy 1993;48(3):215–6.
62. Bock SA. Anaphylaxis to coriander: a sleuthing story. J Allergy Clin Immunol 1993;91(6):1232–3.
63. Blaiss MS, McCants ML, Lehrer SB. Anaphylaxis to cabbage: detection of allergens. Ann Allergy 1987;58(4):248–50.
64. Parker JL, Yunginger JW, Swedlund HA. Anaphylaxis after ingestion of millet seeds. J Allergy Clin Immunol 1981;67(1):78–80.
65. Wild LG, Lehrer SB. Fish and shellfish allergy. Curr Allergy Asthma Rep 2005;5(1):74–9.
66. Schabelman E, Witting M. The relationship of radiocontrast, iodine, and seafood allergies: a medical myth exposed. J Emerg Med 2010;39(5):701–7.

67. Bock SA, Munoz-Furlong A, Sampson HA. Further fatalities caused by anaphylactic reactions to food, 2001-2006. J Allergy Clin Immunol 2007;119(4): 1016–8.

68. Pumphrey RS, Gowland MH. Further fatal allergic reactions to food in the United Kingdom, 1999-2006. J Allergy Clin Immunol 2007;119(4):1018–9.

69. Bock SA, Munoz-Furlong A, Sampson HA. Fatalities due to anaphylactic reactions to foods. J Allergy Clin Immunol 2001;107(1):191–3.

70. Hoffer V, Scheuerman O, Marcus N, et al. Anaphylaxis in Israel: experience with 92 hospitalized children. Pediatr Allergy Immunol 2011;22(2):172–7.

71. Novembre E, Cianferoni A, Bernardini R, et al. Anaphylaxis in children: clinical and allergologic features. Pediatrics 1998;101(4):E8.

72. Fiocchi A, Bouygue GR, Albarini M, et al. Molecular diagnosis of cow's milk allergy. Curr Opin Allergy Clin Immunol 2011;11(3):216–21.

73. Restani P, Ballabio C, Di Lorenzo C, et al. Molecular aspects of milk allergens and their role in clinical events. Anal Bioanal Chem 2009;395(1):47–56.

74. Nowak-Wegrzyn A, Bloom KA, Sicherer SH, et al. Tolerance to extensively heated milk in children with cow's milk allergy. J Allergy Clin Immunol 2008; 122(2):342–7, 347.e1–2.

75. Jarvinen KM, Beyer K, Vila L, et al. B-cell epitopes as a screening instrument for persistent cow's milk allergy. J Allergy Clin Immunol 2002;110(2):293–7.

76. Jarvinen KM, Chatchatee P, Bardina L, et al. IgE and IgG binding epitopes on alpha-lactalbumin and beta-lactoglobulin in cow's milk allergy. Int Arch Allergy Immunol 2001;126(2):111–8.

77. Vila L, Beyer K, Jarvinen KM, et al. Role of conformational and linear epitopes in the achievement of tolerance in cow's milk allergy. Clin Exp Allergy 2001;31(10): 1599–606.

78. Chatchatee P, Jarvinen KM, Bardina L, et al. Identification of IgE and IgG binding epitopes on beta- and kappa-casein in cow's milk allergic patients. Clin Exp Allergy 2001;31(8):1256–62.

79. Chatchatee P, Jarvinen KM, Bardina L, et al. Identification of IgE- and IgG-binding epitopes on alpha(s1)-casein: differences in patients with persistent and transient cow's milk allergy. J Allergy Clin Immunol 2001;107(2):379–83.

80. Shreffler WG, Wanich N, Moloney M, et al. Association of allergen-specific regulatory T cells with the onset of clinical tolerance to milk protein. J Allergy Clin Immunol 2009;123(1):43–52 e47.

81. Kattan JD, Cocco RR, Jarvinen KM. Milk and soy allergy. Pediatr Clin North Am 2011;58(2):407–26, x.

82. Tewari A, Du Toit G, Lack G. The difficulties of diagnosing food-dependent exercise-induced anaphylaxis in childhood—a case study and review. Pediatr Allergy Immunol 2006;17(2):157–60.

83. Eigenmann PA. Anaphylactic reactions to raw eggs after negative challenges with cooked eggs. J Allergy Clin Immunol 2000;105(3):587–8.

84. Caubet JC, Wang J. Current understanding of egg allergy. Pediatr Clin North Am 2011;58(2):427–43, xi.

85. Jarvinen KM, Amalanayagam S, Shreffler WG, et al. Epinephrine treatment is infrequent and biphasic reactions are rare in food-induced reactions during oral food challenges in children. J Allergy Clin Immunol 2009;124(6): 1267–72.

86. Sicherer SH, Morrow EH, Sampson HA. Dose-response in double-blind, placebo-controlled oral food challenges in children with atopic dermatitis. J Allergy Clin Immunol 2000;105(3):582–6.

87. Holzhauser T, Wackermann O, Ballmer-Weber BK, et al. Soybean (Glycine max) allergy in Europe: Gly m 5 (beta-conglycinin) and Gly m 6 (glycinin) are potential diagnostic markers for severe allergic reactions to soy. J Allergy Clin Immunol 2009;123(2):452–8.

88. Bernhisel-Broadbent J, Taylor S, Sampson HA. Cross-allergenicity in the legume botanical family in children with food hypersensitivity. II. Laboratory correlates. J Allergy Clin Immunol 1989;84(5 Pt 1):701–9.

89. Bernhisel-Broadbent J, Sampson HA. Cross-allergenicity in the legume botanical family in children with food hypersensitivity. J Allergy Clin Immunol 1989; 83(2 Pt 1):435–40.

90. Sicherer SH. Clinical aspects of gastrointestinal food allergy in childhood. Pediatrics 2003;111(6 Pt 3):1609–16.

91. Spergel JM, Beausoleil JL, Fiedler JM, et al. Correlation of initial food reactions to observed reactions on challenges. Ann Allergy Asthma Immunol 2004;92(2): 217–24.

92. Gonzalez-Perez A, Aponte Z, Vidaurre CF, et al. Anaphylaxis epidemiology in patients with and patients without asthma: a United Kingdom database review. J Allergy Clin Immunol 2010;125(5):1098–104 e1091.

93. Imamura T, Kanagawa Y, Ebisawa M. A survey of patients with self-reported severe food allergies in Japan. Pediatr Allergy Immunol 2008;19(3):270–4.

94. Lemon-Mule H, Nowak-Wegrzyn A, Berin C, et al. Pathophysiology of food-induced anaphylaxis. Curr Allergy Asthma Rep 2008;8(3):201–8.

95. Mullins RJ, Clark S, Camargo CA Jr. Regional variation in epinephrine autoinjector prescriptions in Australia: more evidence for the vitamin D-anaphylaxis hypothesis. Ann Allergy Asthma Immunol 2009;103(6):488–95.

96. Camargo CA Jr, Clark S, Kaplan MS, et al. Regional differences in EpiPen prescriptions in the United States: the potential role of vitamin D. J Allergy Clin Immunol 2007;120(1):131–6.

97. Sampson HA. Food allergy. Part 2: diagnosis and management. J Allergy Clin Immunol 1999;103(6):981–9.

98. Sicherer SH, Sampson HA. Food allergy: recent advances in pathophysiology and treatment. Annu Rev Med 2009;60:261–77.

99. Lieberman P. Anaphylaxis. Med Clin North Am 2006;90(1):77–95, viii.

100. Stone SF, Cotterell C, Isbister GK, et al. Elevated serum cytokines during human anaphylaxis: identification of potential mediators of acute allergic reactions. J Allergy Clin Immunol 2009;124(4):786–92 e784.

101. Simons FE. Anaphylaxis. J Allergy Clin Immunol 2010;125(2 Suppl 2):S161–81.

102. Arias K, Chu DK, Flader K, et al. Distinct immune effector pathways contribute to the full expression of peanut-induced anaphylactic reactions in mice. J Allergy Clin Immunol 2011;127(6):1552–61 e1551.

103. Simons FE. Pharmacologic treatment of anaphylaxis: can the evidence base be strengthened? Curr Opin Allergy Clin Immunol 2010;10(4):384–93.

104. Sheikh A, Ten Broek V, Brown SG, et al. H1-antihistamines for the treatment of anaphylaxis: Cochrane systematic review. Allergy 2007;62(8):830–7.

105. Kajiwara N, Sasaki T, Bradding P, et al. Activation of human mast cells through the platelet-activating factor receptor. J Allergy Clin Immunol 2010;125(5): 1137–45 e1136.

106. Lee JK, Vadas P. Anaphylaxis: mechanisms and management. Clin Exp Allergy 2011;41(7):923–38.

107. Vadas P, Gold M, Perelman B, et al. Platelet-activating factor, PAF acetylhydrolase, and severe anaphylaxis. N Engl J Med 2008;358(1):28–35.

108. Arias K, Baig M, Colangelo M, et al. Concurrent blockade of platelet-activating factor and histamine prevents life-threatening peanut-induced anaphylactic reactions. J Allergy Clin Immunol 2009;124(2):307–14, 314.e1–2.

109. Khodoun M, Strait R, Orekov T, et al. Peanuts can contribute to anaphylactic shock by activating complement. J Allergy Clin Immunol 2009;123(2):342–51.

110. Radauer C, Breiteneder H. Evolutionary biology of plant food allergens. J Allergy Clin Immunol 2007;120(3):518–25.

111. Ditto AM, Neilsen CV, Neerukonda S, et al. Clinical reactivity to raw peanut correlates with IgE binding to conformational epitopes of Ara h 1: a case report. Allergy 2010;65(11):1485–6.

112. Shreffler WG, Castro RR, Kucuk ZY, et al. The major glycoprotein allergen from *Arachis hypogaea*, Ara h 1, is a ligand of dendritic cell-specific ICAM-grabbing nonintegrin and acts as a Th2 adjuvant in vitro. J Immunol 2006;177(6): 3677–85.

113. Lieberman P, Nicklas RA, Oppenheimer J, et al. The diagnosis and management of anaphylaxis practice parameter: 2010 update. J Allergy Clin Immunol 2010;126(3):477–80 e471–442.

114. Keet C. Recognition and management of food-induced anaphylaxis. Pediatr Clin North Am 2011;58(2):377–88, x.

115. Cianferoni A, Spergel JM. Food allergy: review, classification and diagnosis. Allergol Int 2009;58(4):457–66.

116. Fiocchi A, Terracciano L, Bouygue GR, et al. Incremental prognostic factors associated with cow's milk allergy outcomes in infant and child referrals: the Milan Cow's Milk Allergy Cohort study. Ann Allergy Asthma Immunol 2008;101(2): 166–73.

117. Restani P, Gaiaschi A, Plebani A, et al. Cross-reactivity between milk proteins from different animal species. Clin Exp Allergy 1999;29(7):997–1004.

118. Caubet JC, Kondo Y, Urisu A, et al. Molecular diagnosis of egg allergy. Curr Opin Allergy Clin Immunol 2011;11(3):210–5.

119. Yamada K, Urisu A, Kakami M, et al. IgE-binding activity to enzyme-digested ovomucoid distinguishes between patients with contact urticaria to egg with and without overt symptoms on ingestion. Allergy 2000;55(6):565–9.

120. Urisu A, Yamada K, Tokuda R, et al. Clinical significance of IgE-binding activity to enzymatic digests of ovomucoid in the diagnosis and the prediction of the outgrowing of egg white hypersensitivity. Int Arch Allergy Immunol 1999; 120(3):192–8.

121. van Nieuwaal NH, Lasfar W, Meijer Y, et al. Utility of peanut-specific IgE levels in predicting the outcome of double-blind, placebo-controlled food challenges. J Allergy Clin Immunol 2010;125(6):1391–2.

122. Wang J, Lin J, Bardina L, et al. Correlation of IgE/IgG4 milk epitopes and affinity of milk-specific IgE antibodies with different phenotypes of clinical milk allergy. J Allergy Clin Immunol 2010;125(3):695–702, 702 e691–702 e696.

123. Nowak-Wegrzyn A, Assa'ad AH, Bahna SL, et al. Work Group report: oral food challenge testing. J Allergy Clin Immunol 2009;123(Suppl 6):S365–83.

124. Nowak-Wegrzyn A, Sampson HA. Adverse reactions to foods. Med Clin North Am 2006;90(1):97–127.

125. Hourihane JO. Peanut allergy. Pediatr Clin North Am 2011;58(2):445–58, xi.

126. Cianferoni A, Novembre E, Pucci N, et al. Anaphylaxis: a 7-year follow-up survey of 46 children. Ann Allergy Asthma Immunol 2004;92(4):464–8.

127. Nowak-Wegrzyn A, Muraro A. Food allergy therapy: is a cure within reach? Pediatr Clin North Am 2011;58(2):511–30, xii.

128. Du Toit G. Food-dependent exercise-induced anaphylaxis in childhood. Pediatr Allergy Immunol 2007;18(5):455–63.
129. Shadick NA, Liang MH, Partridge AJ, et al. The natural history of exercise-induced anaphylaxis: survey results from a 10-year follow-up study. J Allergy Clin Immunol 1999;104(1):123–7.
130. Aihara Y, Kotoyori T, Takahashi Y, et al. The necessity for dual food intake to provoke food-dependent exercise-induced anaphylaxis (FEIAn): a case report of FEIAn with simultaneous intake of wheat and umeboshi. J Allergy Clin Immunol 2001;107(6):1100–5.
131. Baek CH, Bae YJ, Cho YS, et al. Food-dependent exercise-induced anaphylaxis in the celery-mugwort-birch-spice syndrome. Allergy 2010;65(6):792–3.
132. Silverstein SR, Frommer DA, Dobozin B, et al. Celery-dependent exercise-induced anaphylaxis. J Emerg Med 1986;4(3):195–9.
133. Fujita H, Osuna H, Kanbara T, et al. Wheat anaphylaxis enhanced by administration of acetylsalicylic acid or by exercise. Arerugi 2005;54(10):1203–7 [in Japanese].

Index

Note: Page numbers of article titles are in **boldface** type.

A

Acupuncture, 136, 138
Adjuvants
 in CAM, 144
 sensitization and, 3–4
Alpha-amylase, 16
Alternative treatment. *See* Complementary and alternative medicine.
Anaphylaxis, food-induced
 biphasic reactions in, 180
 clinical criteria for, 166
 definition of, 165
 diagnosis of, 179–183
 differential diagnosis of, 180–181
 epidemiology of, 38–40, 165–167
 exercise-induced, 187–188
 fatal, 165, 185–187
 impact on family, 88
 pathogenesis of, 177–179
 prevention of, 185–187
 risk factors for, 177
 treatment of, 183–186
 triggers of, 167–177
Animal allergens, 12–13, 17
Antihistamines, for anaphylaxis, 184–185
Anxiety, in food allergy, 86
Ara allergens, 18, 20, 170–173
Ayurvedic medicine, 139

B

Baked milk diet and baked egg diet, **151–164**
Basophil activation testing, 102–103
Beans, allergens in, 174
Ber allergens, 174
Bet v 1-related proteins, 16
Beta agonists, for anaphylaxis, 186
Beta blockers, for anaphylaxis, 186
Bos allergens, 172–173
Bovine serum albumin, clinical relevance of, 173
Breastfeeding, food allergy prevention practices in, 52–57
Budesonide, for eosinophilic esophagitis, 73–75
Bullying, with food allergy, 89–90

Immunol Allergy Clin N Am 32 (2012) 197–206
doi:10.1016/S0889-8561(12)00009-4
0889-8561/12/$ – see front matter © 2012 Elsevier Inc. All rights reserved.

immunology.theclinics.com

Moving?

Make sure your subscription moves with you!

To notify us of your new address, find your **Clinics Account Number** (located on your mailing label above your name), and contact customer service at:

Email: journalscustomerservice-usa@elsevier.com

800-654-2452 (subscribers in the U.S. & Canada)
314-447-8871 (subscribers outside of the U.S. & Canada)

Fax number: 314-447-8029

Elsevier Health Sciences Division
Subscription Customer Service
3251 Riverport Lane
Maryland Heights, MO 63043

*To ensure uninterrupted delivery of your subscription,
please notify us at least 4 weeks in advance of move.

Printed and bound by CPI Group (UK) Ltd, Croydon, CR0 4YY

03/10/2024

01040446-0004